1500 Questions in Psychiatry
for the MRCPsych

Edited by

Albert Michael MB BS DPM MD MRCPsych

Consultant in Adult Psychiatry, West Suffolk Hospital, Bury St Edmunds; Course Organizer, Cambridge MRCPsych Course, UK

Ben Underwood MA MB BS MRCPsych

Specialist Registrar in Psychiatry, Cambridge; Assistant Organizer, Cambridge MRCPsych Course, UK

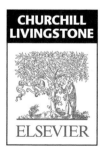

Edinburgh   London   New York   Oxford   Philadelphia   St Louis   Sydney   Toronto

2007

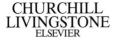

CHURCHILL LIVINGSTONE
ELSEVIER

An imprint of Elsevier Limited

First published 2007

ISBN-13: 978-0-443-10338-4
ISBN-10: 0-443-10338-0

British Library Cataloguing in Publication Data
A catalogue record for this book is available from the British Library

Library of Congress Cataloging in Publication Data
A catalog record for this book is available from the Library of Congress

Notice
Knowledge and best practice in this field are constantly changing. As new research and experience broaden our knowledge, changes in practice, treatment and drug therapy may become necessary or appropriate. Readers are advised to check the most current information provided (i) on procedures featured or (ii) by the manufacturer of each product to be administered, to verify the recommended dose or formula, the method and duration of administration, and contraindications. It is the responsibility of the practitioner, relying on their own experience and knowledge of the patient, to make diagnoses, to determine dosages and the best treatment for each individual patient, and to take all appropriate safety precautions. To the fullest extent of the law, neither the Publisher nor the Editors assume any liability for any injury and/or damage to persons or property arising out of or related to any use of the material contained in this book.

The Publisher

ELSEVIER your source for books, journals and multimedia in the health sciences

www.elsevierhealth.com

Working together to grow
libraries in developing countries

www.elsevier.com | www.bookaid.org | www.sabre.org

ELSEVIER   BOOK AID International   Sabre Foundation

The Publisher's policy is to use **paper manufactured from sustainable forests**

Printed in China

Contents

Contents

Preface

The advent of Modernising Medical Careers (MMC), the Postgraduate Medical Education and Training Board (PMETB) and possibly other bodies yet to come will keep the format of the MRCPsych examinations in a state of evolution for the foreseeable future. Preparing for changing exam formats poses an added challenge for candidates. Two things make this challenge less formidable than it may seem at first. Firstly, though the format of the exam may change, the core knowledge that it tests will not. Secondly, reformatting exams from scratch is an extremely time-consuming process and therefore future exams are likely to be based on previous exam questions. At the time of writing ISQs are still intended to be part of the exam format.

In this book we have picked over 1500 questions which are at the heart of each topic in the syllabus. We have selected the questions very carefully based on our many years of successful experience at the Cambridge course.

There is little time for study in the junior doctor's working life. For this reason we have organized the book into manageable chapters of 25 questions each which can be answered in 15 minutes. Each chapter covers one specialty only. This will enable readers to assess their knowledge (or ignorance) in each area separately and hence identify their weak and strong areas. This will prove exceptionally useful if the exams become modular.

Each question is answered True or False, followed by an explanation and references where more information can be found. The reader is advised to answer all questions in one chapter before looking up the answers. Simply knowing whether an answer is true or false is of limited value. Taking time to understand the explanations will help the reader to remember the true/false answer and also enable them to answer different questions in the exam which are on the same topic as the questions answered in this book.

Though we originally intended to provide 1500 questions and answers, you will find an extra 25. Whilst every effort has been made to ensure the accuracy of the answers it is hoped that these extra questions will compensate for any unintentional repetitions, deviations, errors or omissions.

This book provides a useful revision and teaching aid well beyond simple question answering. It is likely to stand the reader in good stead in future examinations whatever their format.

We wish you every success in the examination and look forward to you becoming a member of the Royal College of Psychiatrists.

A.M.

B.U.

Cambridge

2007

Contributors

Rudwan Abdul-Al MD MPH MRCPsych
Specialist Registrar in Psychiatry, Sheffield, UK

Regi T. Alexander MRCPsych
Consultant Psychiatrist, Norfolk, UK

Chittaranjan Andrade MD
Professor of Psychopharmacology, National Institute of Mental Health and
Neuroscience, Bangalore, India; Visiting Professor of Statistics and Research
Methodology, St John's Medical College, Bangalore, India

Alison Battersby MA MB BChir MRCPsych
Consultant in Substance Misuse, Plymouth, UK

K. Martin Beckmann Sataasexamen MRCPsych
Locum Consultant in Child and Adolescent Psychiatry, Isle of Man

Irma Beyers MB ChB MSt MRCPsych
Consultant Addiction Psychiatrist, Hertfordshire, UK

Judy Chan MB BS MRCPsych
Specialist Registrar in Child and Adolescent Psychiatry, Portsmouth, UK

Kit Wa Chan MB BS MRCPsych
Specialist Registrar in Psychiatry, Cambridge, UK

Ricci Chang MB ChB MRCPsych
Specialist Registrar in Psychiatry, Manchester, UK

Catherine Corby MB BCh BAO MSc MRCPsych
Consultant Psychiatrist, Limerick, Ireland

Claire Dibben BSc MB BS MRCPsych
Specialist Registrar in Psychiatry, Cambridge, UK

Fiona Hynes MMedSci MRCPsych
Specialist Registrar in Forensic Psychiatry, Birmingham, UK

Furhan Iqbal MA MSc MRCPsych
Specialist Registrar in Psychiatry, Cambridge, UK

Salbu Krishnan MB BS DFM
Senior House Officer in Psychiatry, Ipswich, UK

Rudi Kritzinger MBChB MMed Psych
Consultant in Liaison Psychiatry and Community Neurobehavioral Service,
Auckland, New Zealand

Fernando Lazaro-Perlado LMS MSc MRCPsych
Consultant Neuropsychiatrist, Brain Injury Service, Grafton Manor,
Northampton, UK

Louisa Mann MB ChB MRCPsych
Consultant Psychiatrist, Cambridge, UK

Deborah McCartney BA(Hons)
Research Psychologist, Cambridge, UK

Graham Murray BA MB MRCPsych
Clinical Lecturer in Psychiatry, Cambridge, UK

Alan Murtagh MRCPsych
Research Registrar in Psychiatry, Dublin, Ireland

Christopher O'Loughlin MRCP MRCPsych
Specialist Registrar in Psychiatry, Cambridge; Assistant Organizer, Cambridge
MRCPsych Course, UK

Nadir Omara MB BS MRCPsych
Consultant Psychiatrist in Substance Misuse, Suffolk, UK

Bipin Ravindran MB BS
Senior House Officer in Psychiatry, Ipswich, UK

Piyal Sen DPM Dip.Forensic Psych, MRCPsych
Consultant Forensic Psychiatrist, Milton Keynes, UK

Carla Sharp MA PhD
Menninger Department of Psychiatry and Behavioral Sciences, Baylor College of
Medicine, Houston, Texas, USA

Michael D. Spencer MA MB MRCPsych
Clinical Research Fellow and Honorary Clinical Lecturer in Child and Adolescent
Psychiatry, University of Edinburgh, UK

Konstantinos Stagias MSc MRCPsych
Research Registrar in Psychiatry, West Suffolk Hospital, Bury St Edmunds, UK

Paul Wilkinson MA MB BCh DCH MRCPsych
Clinical Lecturer in Child and Adolescent Psychiatry,
University of Cambridge, UK

Asif Zia MRCPsych
Consultant in Learning Disability Psychiatry, Peterborough, UK

Alcohol – 1

Irma Beyers

	T	F

1. Drug and alcohol problems are more prevalent among homosexuals. ☐ ☐

2. Moderate drinkers are a greater public health problem than very heavy drinkers. ☐ ☐

3. The prevalence of alcohol-related problems in a population depends on the average consumption per person. ☐ ☐

4. Alcohol misuse is more common in the elderly than in the middle-aged. ☐ ☐

5. The prevalence of alcohol misuse in patients admitted to general hospitals is 5–10%. ☐ ☐

6. Aldehyde dehydrogenase is the rate-limiting enzyme in the metabolism of alcohol. ☐ ☐

7. Women get drunk more easily than men because women have relatively more body water. ☐ ☐

8. Sons of male alcoholics have a 10 times increased risk of alcoholism. ☐ ☐

9. A raised GGT (gamma glutamyl transpeptidase) level indicates demonstrable liver damage. ☐ ☐

10. Salience of drink-seeking behaviour is an indicator of alcohol dependence. ☐ ☐

11. Alcohol withdrawal starts as early as 6 hours after the last drink. ☐ ☐

12. Delirium tremens starts 2–4 days after the last drink. ☐ ☐

13. Alcoholic blackouts refer to memory loss following intoxication to the point of losing consciousness. ☐ ☐

14. Alcohol abuse during pregnancy causes facial abnormalities in the fetus. ☐ ☐

15. Alcoholic hallucinosis resolves spontaneously in 6 months. ☐ ☐

16. Implicit memory is preserved in Korsakoff's syndrome. ☐ ☐

17. Korsakoff's psychosis is commonly associated with suggestibility. ☐ ☐

18. Methanol poisoning may cause acidosis. ☐ ☐

19. Pathological drunkenness is followed by amnesia for the episode. ☐ ☐

20. In Wernicke's encephalopathy, ophthalmoplegia starts to improve within hours of treatment with thiamine. ☐ ☐

T F

21. In the management of alcoholism, admission to specialist alcohol treatment units is more effective than admission to general psychiatric wards. ☐ ☐

22. Acamprosate inhibits alcohol dehydrogenase. ☐ ☐

23. Stimulus control is more useful in the precontemplation phase of stages of change than in the action phase. ☐ ☐

24. Disulfiram inhibits the conversion of dopamine to noradrenaline. ☐ ☐

25. Suicide in the elderly is associated with alcohol abuse. ☐ ☐

ANSWERS

1. Drug and alcohol problems are more prevalent among homosexuals.

True: Alcohol and other substance use and abuse may be 2–3 times higher among homosexuals than in the general population. However, homosexuals do not have higher rates of drug or alcohol dependence (Sadock & Sadock 2005, p. 1960).

2. Moderate drinkers are a greater public health problem than very heavy drinkers.

True: Heavy drinkers have more alcohol-related problems than moderate and light drinkers. However, their contribution to the total alcohol-related harm in the community is less compared to that of the far greater numbers of moderate and light drinkers. Hence, preventive measures should focus on the whole population, rather than only on the very high-risk group. This is called the 'prevention paradox' (Chick & Cantwell 1994, p. 85).

3. The prevalence of alcohol-related problems in a population depends on the average consumption per person.

True: The prevalence of alcohol-related problems in a population is linked to the alcohol consumption per person in that population. There is a close correlation between cirrhosis mortality and national average consumption (Gelder et al 2006, p. 435; Johnstone et al 2004, p. 359).

4. Alcohol misuse is more common in the elderly than in the middle-aged.

False: Alcohol consumption decreases with age. This may be because of decreased tolerance and increased financial pressures in old age and the premature mortality of heavy drinkers. Alcohol abuse in the elderly is often undiagnosed. This is partly because the commonly used screening questionnaires and blood indices are less sensitive tools in the elderly. In the elderly, alcohol abuse is 3 times more common in men than in women (Gelder et al 2000, p. 1637; Johnstone et al 2004, p. 649).

5. The prevalence of alcohol misuse in patients admitted to general hospitals is 5–10%.

False: 20–30% of male admissions and 5–10% of female admissions misuse alcohol (Gelder et al 2006, p. 434).

6. Aldehyde dehydrogenase is the rate-limiting enzyme in the metabolism of alcohol.

False: Alcohol dehydrogenase metabolizes 90–95% of the alcohol consumed in social drinkers. This is the rate-limiting enzyme (King 2004, p. 492; Sadock & Sadock 2005, p. 1171).

7. Women get drunk more easily than men because women have relatively more body water.

False: A given dose of ethanol per kg bodyweight produces a higher peak blood level in women than in men. This is because women have relatively more body fat than water and lower activity of alcohol dehydrogenase in the gastric mucosa compared to men (Johnstone et al 2004, p. 366).

8. Sons of male alcoholics have a 10 times increased risk of alcoholism.

False: Those with alcoholic parents and/or siblings are 3–4 times more likely to become alcoholics than those without such family history. The rate of alcohol problems increases with the number of alcoholic relatives, the severity of their problems and the closeness of their genetic relationship (Gelder et al 2000, p. 479; Sadock & Sadock 2005, p. 1174).

9. A raised GGT indicates demonstrable liver damage.

False: GGT may be raised even when there is no demonstrable liver damage (Gelder et al 2006, p. 445).

10. Salience of drink-seeking behaviour is an indicator of alcohol dependence.

True: Salience of drinking was proposed as a feature of alcohol dependence by Edwards & Gross in 1976. Preoccupation with substance use as manifest by neglect of alternative pleasures or interests is an ICD-10 criterion for alcohol dependence (Gelder et al 2000, p. 483).

11. Alcohol withdrawal starts as early as 6 hours after the last drink.

True: Alcohol withdrawal starts 4–12 hours after cessation of/reduction in alcohol use. This may last for up to 4–5 days (DSM-IV 1994, p. 198; Gelder et al 2000, p. 489).

12. Delirium tremens starts 2–4 days after the last drink.

True: Delirium tremens starts 48–72 hours following stopping or reducing alcohol intake. It usually lasts for 2–3 days (Chick & Cantwell 1994, p. 174).

13. Alcoholic blackouts refer to memory loss following intoxication to the point of losing consciousness.

False: Alcoholic blackouts are periods of intoxication during which the patient appeared alert and performed complex tasks, but which are followed by amnesia for this period. This can last for hours or even days. Brain damage increases the susceptibility to developing alcoholic blackouts (Gelder et al 2000, p. 489; Sadock & Sadock 2005, p. 1178).

14. Alcohol abuse during pregnancy causes facial abnormalities in the fetus.

True: The effects of maternal alcohol intake on organogenesis were first described by Lemoine and colleagues. The features of fetal alcohol syndrome include the triad of pre- and postnatal growth retardation, learning difficulties and craniofacial abnormalities. The craniofacial abnormalities include midfacial hypoplasia, microcephaly, thin upper lip, small palpebral fissure, flat maxillary area, poorly developed philtrum, etc. In addition, they have congenital dislocation of the hip and atrial septal defects, delayed language development, sleep disturbance and overactivity (Gelder et al 2006, p. 437; Ghodse 2002, p. 151; Johnstone et al 2004, p. 745).

15. Alcoholic hallucinosis resolves spontaneously in 6 months.

True: The prognosis of alcoholic hallucinosis is good. It usually resolves spontaneously within days or weeks in patients who are abstinent. Cases that persist beyond 6 months have a poor prognosis (Gelder et al 2000, p. 490).

16. Implicit memory is preserved in Korsakoff's syndrome.

True: Implicit memory is preserved in Korsakoff's syndrome.

Explicit or declarative memory is memory to which we have conscious access. The anatomical basis includes the limbic and temporal neocortical structures.

Implicit or procedural memory involves conditioned reflexes and motor tasks, e.g. the ability to ride a bicycle. The anatomical substrate is less clear and may involve the basal ganglia, cerebral cortex and possibly even the cerebellum.

Recall, retrieval or conscious recollection applies to explicit memory whereas recognition applies equally to both (Hodges 1994, p. 18).

17. Korsakoff's psychosis is commonly associated with suggestibility.

True: The patient with Korsakoff's syndrome is often highly suggestible (Lishman 1997, p. 31).

18. Methanol poisoning may cause acidosis.

True: Methanol has relatively low toxicity. Methanol is oxidized by alcohol dehydrogenase to formaldehyde. Formaldehyde is oxidized to formic acid by formaldehyde dehydrogenase. Formic acid is converted to carbon dioxide and water by 10-formyl tetrahydrofolate synthetase.

Methanol poisoning causes nausea, vomiting, abdominal pain and CNS (central nervous system) depression. After a latent phase of 12–24 hours, metabolic acidosis develops with blurring of vision, altered visual fields and blindness. It can cause necrosis of the putamen. Mortality is 20%.

Management includes general support, correction of metabolic acidosis using sodium bicarbonate, blocking further production of formic acid using fomepizole or ethanol as antidotes, enhancing metabolism of formic acid using folinic acid and haemodialysis to eliminate methanol and formate (Barcelous et al 2002).

19. Pathological drunkenness is followed by amnesia for the episode.

True: There is amnesia for the entire episode (Lishman 1997, p. 595).

20. In Wernicke's encephalopathy, ophthalmoplegia starts to improve within hours of treatment with thiamine.

True: Sixth nerve palsies and other ocular abnormalities recover with thiamine treatment. The improvement often starts within hours of starting treatment. Sometimes it takes several days or weeks to disappear completely. The only exception is horizontal nystagmus which persists in two-thirds of patients (Lishman 1997, p. 579).

21. In the management of alcoholism, admission to specialist alcohol treatment units is more effective than admission to general psychiatric wards.

False: There is no evidence to support this claim (Gelder et al 2006, p. 449; Johnstone et al 2004, p. 377).

22. Acamprosate inhibits alcohol dehydrogenase.

False: The excitatory (glutamate) and inhibitory (GABA) neurotransmitters are important in alcohol dependence. Acamprosate, a GABA analogue, has an effect on both. It is a dose-dependent antagonist to NMDA receptors in the neocortex and hippocampus. Acamprosate has no effect on the metabolism of alcohol or acetaldehyde (Gelder et al 2006, p. 448; Ghodse 2002, p. 158; Johnstone et al 2004, p. 375; King 2004, p. 495; Sadock & Sadock 2005, p. 1187).

23. Stimulus control is more useful in the precontemplation phase of stages of change than in the action phase.

False: CBT for addictions identifies five phases:

1. Precontemplation: Individuals are relatively content with their behaviour and they are unlikely to consider any need for change.
2. Contemplation: Beginning to feel two ways about their behaviour. Costs and benefits are identified.
3. Preparation for change: Planning for behaviour change and making firm resolution to change.
4. Action stage: Initial attempt at modifying the behaviour. Stimulus control is useful.
5. Maintenance stage: Sustaining change (Chick & Cantwell 1994, p. 132).

24. Disulfiram inhibits the conversion of dopamine to noradrenaline.

True: Disulfiram inhibits the conversion of dopamine to noradrenaline by inhibiting dopamine-beta-hydroxylase due to depletion of its cofactor copper. The depletion of noradrenaline in the heart and blood vessels allows acetaldehyde to act directly on these tissues to cause flushing, tachycardia and hypertension (ABPI 2005, p. 125; Anderson & Reid 2002, p. 160).

25. Suicide in the elderly is associated with alcohol abuse.

True: The main predictors of suicide in the elderly include age above 75 years, male gender, physical illness (35–85%), social isolation, widowed or separated status, recent bereavement, alcohol or other substance abuse, depression (70–80%) and past history of depression. The estimates of prevalence of alcohol abuse in the elderly vary widely. The prevalence of alcohol and substance misuse and dependence in the elderly may be 1–2% in the community and 40–65% in those admitted to medical wards, those admitted with mood disorders and in suicide victims. Older people with alcohol dependence are at higher risk for suicide, possibly due to depression, social isolation and alcohol-induced impulsive behaviour (Gelder et al 2006, p. 410; Johnstone et al 2004, p. 648; Sadock & Sadock 2005, pp. 3713, 3715, 3805; Wright et al 2005, p. 488).

Alcohol – 2

Ben Underwood

	T	F
1. Heavy alcohol consumption increases the risk of pharyngeal carcinoma.	☐	☐
2. Convictions for driving with blood level over 80 mg/L are strongly suggestive of alcohol dependence.	☐	☐
3. Binge drinking is more harmful than regular drinking.	☐	☐
4. Alcoholic liver disease is more common in bus conductors than in the general population.	☐	☐
5. Chronic alcohol intake enhances GABA (gamma-aminobutyric acid)-benzodiazepine receptor function.	☐	☐
6. The microsomal ethanol oxidizing system metabolizes only 5–10% of the alcohol consumed.	☐	☐
7. Cloninger's type 1 alcoholism is predominantly genetically determined.	☐	☐
8. Acute alcohol intoxication elevates gamma glutamyl transpeptidase (GGT) levels.	☐	☐
9. In the EEG (electroencephalogram), there is a pattern associated with alcohol use.	☐	☐
10. Withdrawal delirium is an essential feature of alcohol dependence syndrome.	☐	☐
11. Auditory hallucinations occur in alcohol withdrawal.	☐	☐
12. In delirium tremens, cogwheel rigidity may suggest nicotinic acid deficiency.	☐	☐
13. Approximately 10% of chronic heavy drinkers develop seizures.	☐	☐
14. Alcoholic hallucinosis characteristically occurs when alcohol intake is reduced.	☐	☐
15. Confabulation is a feature of Korsakoff's psychosis.	☐	☐
16. In Korsakoff's psychosis, semantic memory is impaired.	☐	☐
17. Increased fast activity in the EEG is a characteristic feature of hepatic encephalopathy.	☐	☐
18. 80% of survivors of Wernicke's encephalopathy suffer from Korsakoff's syndrome.	☐	☐
19. In chronic alcoholism suicide risk is increased only in the depressed.	☐	☐

T F

20. The Minnesota model of treatment for alcoholism recommends strict daily limits on alcohol consumption rather than abstinence. ☐ ☐

21. Acamprosate is an NMDA (N-methyl-D-aspartic acid) antagonist. ☐ ☐

22. Alcohol detoxification cannot usually be done at home in a 65-year-old man. ☐ ☐

23. Disulfiram can cause peripheral neuritis. ☐ ☐

24. In the management of alcoholism, group therapy is more effective than individual therapy. ☐ ☐

25. Marchiafava–Bignami syndrome is associated with demyelination of the corpus callosum. ☐ ☐

ANSWERS

1. Heavy alcohol consumption increases the risk of pharyngeal carcinoma.

   True: The gastrointestinal effects of heavy alcohol consumption include gastritis, vomiting, Mallory–Weiss tear, stomach and duodenal ulcers, cirrhosis of the liver, pancreatitis and an increased risk of cancer of the mouth, pharynx, oesophagus, stomach and liver. Garro and Lieber concluded that excess drinking increases the risk of cancer of the oropharynx by threefold, cancer of the oesophagus by twofold and cancer of the larynx by fourfold. Those who smoke or abuse other drugs are at even higher risk (DSM-IV 1994, p. 200; Chick & Cantwell 1994, p. 81; Johnstone et al 2004, p. 370).

2. Convictions for driving with blood level over 80 mg/L are strongly suggestive of alcohol dependence.

   True: The majority of people charged by the police with drunkenness offences are alcohol dependent. Drink-driving offences are common among dependent drinkers. Though one instance of high alcohol concentration does not differentiate between an isolated episode of heavy drinking and chronic misuse, if the person has high blood levels and is not intoxicated, it would suggest tolerance and, hence, habitual heavy drinking.

   Offenders with exceptionally high blood levels of alcohol, i.e. over 150 mg/L, or who have previous drink-driving convictions are particularly likely to be alcohol dependent. Drink-driving offences are also common in patients with other alcohol-related problems. This question is about convictions being strongly suggestive, not about one single conviction being diagnostic (Ghodse 2002, p. 159; Johnstone et al 2004, p. 372).

3. Binge drinking is more harmful than regular drinking.

   True: Binge drinking is defined as consumption of at least half of the recommended weekly limits per occasion, i.e. ≥10 units/occasion for men and ≥7 units/occasion for women.

Binge drinkers can be identified by dividing number of units of alcohol consumed in the last week by usual drinking frequency. Binge drinking, and particularly frequent binge drinking, is more likely than regular moderate drinking to be associated with alcohol-related problems. Many of the binge drinkers have low average consumption. This has resulted in the 'second order prevention paradox'.

4. Alcoholic liver disease is more common in bus conductors than in the general population.

True: Bus conductors and bus drivers' mates have a higher risk than the general population of developing alcoholic liver disease. Bus drivers are not considered a high-risk group (Chick & Cantwell 1994, p. 115).

5. Chronic alcohol intake enhances GABA-benzodiazepine receptor function.

False: The indirect effect of alcohol on the GABA-$_A$ receptor is responsible for sedating, sleep-inducing, anticonvulsant and muscle-relaxant effects of alcohol. Chronic alcohol intake decreases GABA-benzodiazepine receptor function. This may be causally related to dependence (King 2004, p. 494; Sadock & Sadock 2005, p. 1171).

6. The microsomal ethanol oxidizing system metabolizes 5–10% of the alcohol consumed.

True: The microsomal ethanol oxidizing system (MEOS) metabolizes 5–10% of the alcohol consumed. Its activity increases with tolerance (Ghodse 2002, p. 149; King 2004, p. 492; Sadock & Sadock 2005, p. 1171).

7. Cloninger's type 1 alcoholism is predominantly genetically determined.

False: Type 1 is environmentally caused, milieu limited, affects both men and women, starts after age 20 years, the severity is mild and there is minimal criminality.

Type 2 is genetically determined, starts before age 20, affects mostly males and is associated with severe alcoholism, criminality and other substance misuse (Gelder et al 2006, p. 441).

8. Acute alcohol intoxication elevates gamma glutamyl transpeptidase (GGT) levels.

False: Acute alcohol intoxication does not raise GGT levels. Regular moderate drinking in the preceding weeks raises the levels slightly. The heavier the drinking, the higher the levels (Ghodse 2002, p. 149).

9. In the EEG, there is a pattern associated with alcohol use.

False: There is no particular pattern associated with alcohol use. There is increased fast activity, decreased alpha activity and decreased EEG coherence in alcoholics and even their alcohol-naïve offspring. This may reflect higher arousal levels and may be a possible marker of susceptibility to alcoholism. Acute ingestion of alcohol increases alpha activity and slows alpha frequency. Higher blood levels increase theta activity. Chronic alcohol use may be associated with a lower voltage and slightly faster resting EEG. Withdrawal is associated with increased higher frequency beta activity. Delirium tremens is associated with dominant fast activity. A state of subacute encephalopathy with seizures has been described in chronic alcohol users who are not withdrawing, associated with prominent slowing and periodic lateralized paroxysmal discharges (Chick & Cantwell 1994, p. 97; Sadock & Sadock 2005, p. 185).

10. Withdrawal delirium is an essential feature of alcohol dependence syndrome.

False: Withdrawal delirium is not a criterion for ICD-10 diagnosis of dependence syndrome, although withdrawal symptoms are (ICD-10 1992, p. 79).

11. Auditory hallucinations occur in alcohol withdrawal.

True: Transient visual, tactile or auditory hallucinations or illusions occur in alcohol withdrawal (DSM-IV, p. 198; Gelder et al 2000, p. 489).

12. In delirium tremens, cogwheel rigidity may suggest nicotinic acid deficiency.

True: Nicotinic acid deficiency can manifest in 3 ways:

1. Inborn error of metabolism, e.g. Hartnup disease – may be asymptomatic or may have photosensitive rash, episodic confusion, etc.
2. Chronic deficiency – dermatitis, diarrhoea and dementia.
3. Acute deficiency – following physical illness or surgery, especially in patients with alcoholism. There is often catastrophic development of delirium and stupor. There may be lethargy, weakness, anxiety and agitation, glossitis and stomatitis. They often have extrapyramidal symptoms with cogwheel rigidity, grasp reflexes and sucking reflexes. This responds extremely well to nicotinic acid replacement (Lishman 1997, p. 574).

13. Approximately 10% of chronic heavy drinkers develop seizures.

True: Approximately 10% of hospitalized alcoholics develop seizures – 'rum fits'. Causes include direct toxic effect of alcohol, alcohol withdrawal, hypoglycaemia and head injury. An epileptic fit for the first time in an adult should alert to the possibility of alcohol dependence. Withdrawal fits can occur without other gross features (Ghodse 2002, p. 153; Johnstone et al 2004, p. 373).

14. Alcoholic hallucinosis characteristically occurs when alcohol intake is reduced.

False: Alcoholic hallucinosis is a rare condition. In people who have been drinking heavily for many years, auditory hallucinations are present in clear consciousness and without autonomic overactivity. The hallucinations are fragmentary to start with, but soon become second or third person auditory hallucinations. It is classified as a substance-induced psychotic disorder in both ICD-10 1992 and DSM-IV 1994.

In contrast, in alcohol withdrawal and delirium tremens the hallucinations are transient and disorganized. They are mainly visual, but also auditory and tactile. Delirium tremens is also associated with altered consciousness (Gelder et al 2000, p. 490; Johnstone et al 2004, p. 368).

15. Confabulation is a feature of Korsakoff's psychosis.

True: Confabulation is the unconscious filling of gaps in memory by imagined or untrue but often plausible experiences, occurring in clear sensorium. It is associated with organic pathology, e.g. neurodegenerative conditions, dementias, amnesic disorders and psychotic disorders. It is not synonymous with lying or factitious disorders where symptoms are deliberately distorted or feigned. It is more common in damage to diencephalic structures than in bilateral hippocampal damage. In Korsakoff's syndrome it is most often seen in the acute stages but is not universal. The provoked or momentary type is more common and usually has reference to the recent past, sometimes a memory that is displaced. The spontaneous or fantastic type does not have a stimulus and has been linked to frontal lobe damage. Suggestibility may facilitate confabulation (Lishman 1997, p. 30).

16. In Korsakoff's psychosis, semantic memory is impaired.

False: Semantic memory deals with organized knowledge about the world, i.e. knowledge of objects, labels, vocabulary, principles and concepts.

Korsakoff's syndrome is characterized by severe impairment of episodic memory. Other deficits, although they may exist, are comparatively modest (Hodges 1994, pp. 5, 19; Lishman 1997, p. 30).

17. Increased fast activity in the EEG is a characteristic feature of hepatic encephalopathy.

False: The EEG is useful in the diagnosis, prognosis and monitoring of severity of hepatic encephalopathy. EEG changes appear even before psychological abnormalities. First there is alpha slowing and appearance of 5–7-Hz theta waves, most prominently in the frontal and temporal regions. As consciousness deteriorates, alpha waves are increasingly replaced by theta. Then the characteristic triphasic waves appear. This is followed by a decrease in amplitude, blunting of triphasic waves and periods of flattening. Similar changes occur also in uraemia, hypokalaemia, anoxia, vitamin B12 deficiency and raised intracranial pressure (Lishman 1997, p. 564).

18. 80% of survivors of Wernicke's encephalopathy suffer from Korsakoff's syndrome.

True: In Victor et al's (1971) series of 245 patients 84% developed a typical amnesic syndrome (Gelder et al 2000, p. 491; Gelder et al 2006, p. 328).

19. In chronic alcoholism suicide risk is increased only in the depressed.

False: The risk of suicide in alcoholism is 15%. Alcoholics form 15–25% of all completed suicides. Their risk is 6–20%, i.e. 100 times that of the general population.

20. The Minnesota model of treatment for alcoholism recommends strict daily limits on alcohol consumption rather than abstinence.

False: The Minnesota model, 28-day programme or 12-step programme is a refined and expanded version of the 12-step principles of Alchoholics

Anonymous. It is usually used in private residential treatment programmes. Like the AA, the focus is on abstinence (Gelder et al 2000, p. 507; Sadock & Sadock 2005, p. 1151).

21. Acamprosate is an NMDA antagonist.

True: Acamprosate antagonizes the excitatory neurotransmitter glutamate by antagonizing NMDA receptors.

Acamprosate is an analogue of taurine and structurally resembles GABA. Some believe that acamprosate stimulates GABAergic inhibitory neuro-transmission (Gelder et al 2006, p. 448; Johnstone et al 2004, p. 375; King 2004, p. 495; Sadock & Sadock 2005, p. 1187).

22. Alcohol detoxification cannot usually be done at home in a 65-year-old man.

False: Indications for inpatient detoxification include severe symptoms, medical/psychiatric complications, a history of withdrawal seizures or DT, comorbid severe mental illness, frail and elderly patients, intercurrent acute physical illness, failure of previous outpatient detoxification and lack of social support (Chick & Cantwell 1994, p. 132; Wright et al 2005, p. 431).

23. Disulfiram can cause peripheral neuritis.

True: (See ABPI 2005, p. 125).

24. In the management of alcoholism, group therapy is more effective than individual therapy.

False: There is no evidence that the results of group psychotherapy differ in general from those of individual therapy of similar form and duration and used for the same problem. Moreover, different styles of group therapy produce almost similar results (Gelder et al 2006, p. 449; Johnstone et al 2004, p. 377).

25. Marchiafava–Bignami syndrome is associated with demyelination of the corpus callosum.

True: Marchiafava–Bignami syndrome involves extensive demyelination of the corpus callosum and adjacent subcortical white matter, optic tracts and cerebellar peduncles. The clinical features include dysarthria, ataxia, epilepsy and impaired consciousness. Dementia and limb paralysis are seen in the more slowly progressive forms. Mortality is high and recovery is rare. The cause may be nutritional and/or alcohol-related (Gelder et al 2006, p. 437; Lishman 1997, p. 586).

Antidepressants

Louisa Mann and Ricci Chang

T F

1. Antidepressants relieve pain mainly by their antidepressant effect.

2. Amitriptyline decreases REM sleep in the elderly.

3. Clomipramine is used for studies of noradrenaline neurotransmission.

4. Duloxetine is an SNRI (serotonin-noradrenaline reuptake inhibitor).

5. Bifrontal ECT (electroconvulsive therapy) is effective in depression.

6. ECT is contraindicated in patients with cognitive impairment.

7. Retrograde amnesia is a side-effect of ECT.

8. EEG (electroencephalogram) change is still apparent 2 months after ECT.

9. ECT and amitriptyline have synergistic action.

10. Bilateral ECT is more rapidly effective than unilateral ECT in severe depression.

11. Memory problems improve towards the end of a course of ECT.

12. Imipramine and CBT (cognitive behavioural therapy) are equally effective in treating moderate depression.

13. Erectile dysfunction is more common than ejaculatory failure with clomipramine.

14. mCPP is a 5-HT$_{2A}$ antagonist.

15. Mirtazapine is an antagonist at H$_1$ receptors.

16. Mirtazapine causes indirect 5-HT$_{1A}$ stimulation.

17. Moclobemide does not cause a tyramine reaction.

18. Pindolol blocks postsynaptic 5-HT$_{1A}$ receptors.

19. Reboxetine blocks 5-HT$_2$ receptors.

20. SSRIs cause insomnia due to their action on the 5-HT$_{2A}$ receptor.

21. Tricyclic antidepressants (TCAs) can cause peripheral neuropathy.

22. TCAs increase REM latency.

23. Gastric lavage is of no use 6 hours after severe TCA overdose.

24. Venlafaxine has a half-life of 12 hours.

25. Venlafaxine at a dose of 75 mg enhances noradrenergic effects.

ANSWERS

1. Antidepressants relieve pain mainly by their antidepressant effect.

False: Whilst the majority believe that the improvement in pain in patients with psychogenic pain and somatoform pain disorder is not related to changes in mood (Sadock & Sadock 2005, p. 1822), some believe that the pain relief is partly related to the alleviation of the accompanying depression (King 2004, p. 206).

2. Amitriptyline decreases REM sleep in the elderly.

True: Depression is associated with decreased REM latency and increased total REM sleep. Tricyclic antidepressants increase REM latency and reduce total REM sleep (Johnstone et al 2004, p. 788; King 2004, p. 203; Wright et al 2005, p. 306).

3. Clomipramine is used for studies of noradrenaline neurotransmission.

False: Clomipramine is a potent serotonin reuptake inhibitor and an anticholinergic, and its metabolite N-desmethylclomipramine is a potent noradrenaline reuptake inhibitor. Hence, it would be unsuitable for studies of noradrenaline neurotransmission (King 2004, p. 197).

4. Duloxetine is an SNRI.

True: Duloxetine is an SNRI, i.e. a serotonin and noradrenaline reuptake inhibitor. It works as an antidepressant at a dose of 60 mg/day. It is used in moderate to severe stress incontinence in women at a dose of 20–40 mg twice daily (BNF 2005, 4.3.4).

5. Bifrontal ECT is effective in depression.

True: However, some types of bifrontal electrode placement may not be as efficacious as bifrontotemporal placement. Moreover, the advantage in terms of less cognitive impairment is yet to be confirmed (King 2004, p. 282; Sadock & Sadock 2005, p. 2976).

6. ECT is contraindicated in patients with cognitive impairment.

False: Cognitive impairment including dementia is not a contraindication to ECT for the treatment of coexistent depression. However, pre-existing cognitive impairment would increase the risk of adverse cognitive effects such as post-treatment delirium and prolonged confusion (Johnstone et al 2004, p. 647; Sadock & Sadock 2005, p. 2981).

7. Retrograde amnesia is a side-effect of ECT.

True: Short- and long-term retrograde amnesia and long-term anterograde amnesia for personal and impersonal events are side-effects of ECT. However, short-term retrograde amnesia could partly be caused by the depression itself. The long-term retrograde amnesia is difficult to evaluate (Gelder et al 2006, p. 568; Scott 2005).

8. EEG change is still apparent 2 months after ECT.

True: The post-ECT EEG shows greater slowing with bilateral ECT than with unilateral ECT. It may be detectable for several weeks after a course of ECT.

9. ECT and amitriptyline have synergistic action.

False: There is no evidence that the concurrent administration of antidepressant drugs increases either the response rate or the speed of response (Sadock & Sadock 2005, p. 2980).

10. Bilateral ECT is more rapidly effective than unilateral ECT in severe depression.

False: The speed of response to ECT depends on the extent to which the administered stimulus is suprathreshold, and not on the electrode placement.

Hence, bilateral ECT is no more rapidly effective than unilateral ECT. However, patients who do not improve with unilateral ECT may improve with bilateral ECT (Scott 2005).

11. Memory problems improve towards the end of a course of ECT.

False: Memory problems are usually worst towards the end of a course of ECT. Memory begins to improve after ECT is stopped and usually recovers fully within 6 months (Scott 2005).

12. Imipramine and CBT are equally effective in treating moderate depression.

True: CBT has been shown to be equivalent to pharmacotherapy and superior to waiting list for unipolar depressive disorders of moderate severity (Gelder et al 2006, p. 258; Johnstone et al 2004, p. 323).

13. Erectile dysfunction is more common than ejaculatory failure with clomipramine.

False: The prevalence of sexual side-effects in male patients on clomipramine are: decreased libido = 21%, erectile dysfunction = 20%, ejaculatory failure = 42% (Crenshaw & Goldberg 1996, p. 276).

14. mCPP is a 5-HT$_{2A}$ antagonist.

True: Meta-chlorophenyl piperazine (mCPP) is a metabolite of nefazodone. It is an agonist at 5-HT$_{2C}$ and 5-HT$_{1A}$ receptors and an antagonist at 5-HT$_{2A}$ and 5-HT$_3$ receptors (King 2004, p. 230).

15. Mirtazapine is an antagonist at H$_1$ receptors.

True: Mirtazapine is a histamine 1, a_2, 5-HT$_2$ and 5-HT$_3$ receptor antagonist. Antagonism of presynaptic a_2 receptors enhances the release of noradrenaline and serotonin.

Blockade of 5-HT$_2$, 5-HT$_3$ and H$_1$ receptors enhances sedation and appetite (Anderson & Reid 2002, p. 71; King 2004, p. 227; Sadock & Sadock 2005, p. 2852).

16. Mirtazapine causes indirect 5-HT$_{1A}$ stimulation.

True: Mirtazapine blocks a_2 adrenergic, 5-HT$_2$, 5-HT$_3$ and histamine 1 receptors. Inhibition of alpha 2 adrenergic receptors enhances the release of noradrenaline and serotonin. Antagonism of 5-HT$_2$ and 5-HT$_3$ receptors enhances the availability of serotonin to act on 5-HT$_1$ receptors. Thus mirtazapine acts as an indirect 5-HT$_{1A}$ receptor agonist. Blockade of 5-HT$_2$ and 5-HT$_3$ receptors and the indirect stimulation of 5-HT$_{1A}$ receptors minimize sexual dysfunction (Anderson & Reid 2002, p. 71; King 2004, p. 227; Sadock & Sadock 2005, p. 2852).

17. Moclobemide does not cause a tyramine reaction.

False: Moclobemide is a reversible MAO-A inhibitor. It is much less likely to provoke tyramine reaction than conventional MAOIs. However, tyramine reaction is possible with high doses (600 mg/day) or if a large quantity of tyramine is ingested (Anderson & Reid 2002, p. 69; King 2004, p. 194).

18. Pindolol blocks postsynaptic 5-HT$_{1A}$ receptors.

True: SSRIs increase extracellular fluid concentration of 5-HT. This causes negative feedback and activation of 5-HT$_{1A}$ autoreceptors that inhibit cell firing, resulting in decreased release of 5-HT from the synaptic terminal.

Pindolol is a non-selective β-adrenoceptor antagonist. It blocks β_1 and β_2 as well as 5-HT$_{1A}$ autoreceptors.

Therefore, pindolol can potentiate the ability of SSRIs to facilitate 5-HT neurotransmission. For this reason, pindolol has been used with SSRIs in treatment-resistant depression. Pindolol may accelerate, though may not augment, antidepressant effect of SSRIs (Sadock & Sadock 2005, p. 2726; Stahl 2000, p. 278).

19. Reboxetine blocks 5-HT$_2$ receptors.

False: Reboxetine is a potent and selective noradrenaline reuptake inhibitor. Other than a mild sympathomimetic activity it has no other actions of significance. It has no actions on neuroreceptors (Anderson & Reid 2002, p. 70; King 2004, p. 215).

20. SSRIs cause insomnia due to their action on the 5-HT$_{2A}$ receptor.

True: Stimulation of 5-HT$_{2A}$ receptors in brainstem sleep centres may disrupt slow-wave sleep and cause nocturnal awakening. It can cause or worsen anxiety, restlessness, akathisia, agitation and insomnia. It may also cause myoclonus during the night (King 2004, p. 461; Stahl 2000, p. 230).

21. Tricyclic antidepressants (TCAs) can cause peripheral neuropathy.

False: The catch here is that TCAs may be used to treat peripheral neuropathy.

22. TCAs increase REM latency.

True: TCAs increase REM latency, decrease total REM sleep, cause distressing dreams, decrease the number of awakenings, increase stage IV sleep, cause daytime sedation and prolong reaction times. This may be due to the blockade of H$_1$, a_1 adrenergic and muscarinic cholinergic receptors (Johnstone et al 2004, p. 273; King 2004, p. 203).

23. Gastric lavage is of no use 6 hours after severe TCA overdose.

False: In TCA overdose, the anticholinergic activity reduces gastric motility and absorption. Therefore, gastric lavage may be useful for several hours after TCA overdose (Gelder et al 2006, p. 543; Johnstone et al 2004, p. 283).

24. Venlafaxine has a half-life of 12 hours.

False: Venlafaxine has a half-life of 5 hours. The active metabolite of venlafaxine, o-methylvenlafaxine, has a half-life of 10 hours (Johnstone et al 2004, p. 280).

25. Venlafaxine at a dose of 75 mg enhances noradrenergic effects.

False: The actions of venlafaxine are dose-dependent. At doses below 150 mg, venlafaxine blocks reuptake of serotonin. At 150–300 mg, venlafaxine blocks reuptake of 5-HT and noradrenaline. At doses above 300 mg, venlafaxine blocks reuptake of 5-HT, noradrenaline and dopamine (Johnstone et al 2004, p. 281; King 2004, p. 211).

4 Antipsychotics

Ben Underwood

	T	F
1. Atypical antipsychotics have a longer D_2 receptor occupancy than typical antipsychotics.	☐	☐
2. Clozapine is a potent D_2 antagonist.	☐	☐
3. Clozapine dissociates from D_2 receptors slowly.	☐	☐
4. Clozapine antagonizes D_3 and D_4 receptors.	☐	☐
5. Clozapine causes less postural hypotension than typical antipsychotics.	☐	☐
6. Clozapine produces less sedation than typical antipsychotic drugs.	☐	☐
7. Clozapine is contraindicated in the elderly.	☐	☐
8. The risk of clozapine-induced seizures is dose-related.	☐	☐
9. Aripiprazole is a D_2 partial agonist.	☐	☐
10. Olanzapine causes diabetes mellitus only at doses above 20 mg.	☐	☐
11. Quetiapine causes clinically significant hyperprolactinaemia.	☐	☐
12. Quetiapine has antihistaminic properties.	☐	☐
13. Quetiapine has a half-life of 6 hours.	☐	☐
14. Risperidone induces less akathisia than clozapine.	☐	☐
15. Akathisia usually starts within a week of initiating treatment with antipsychotics.	☐	☐
16. Neuroleptic malignant syndrome is characterized by gradual onset.	☐	☐
17. Neuroleptic malignant syndrome is associated with clear consciousness.	☐	☐
18. Neuroleptic malignant syndrome can be treated with a combination of a dopamine agonist and a calcium channel blocker.	☐	☐
19. Tardive dyskinesia can occur in antipsychotic naïve patients.	☐	☐
20. The prevalence of tardive dyskinesia in people on long-term antipsychotic treatment is more than 50%.	☐	☐
21. Tardive dyskinesia disappears during sleep.	☐	☐
22. Procyclidine can cause visual hallucinations.	☐	☐
23. Physical dependence can occur in long-term procyclidine use.	☐	☐
24. Antimuscarinic drugs are useful in the treatment of acute dystonia.	☐	☐

T F

25. Bradykinesia responds better to antimuscarinic drugs than rigidity. ☐ ☐

ANSWERS

---

1. Atypical antipsychotics have a longer D_2 receptor occupancy than typical antipsychotics.

False: Clozapine, quetiapine, amisulpride and other atypical antipsychotics bind less strongly to the D_2 receptor and dissociate more rapidly from the D_2 receptor than the typical antipsychotics or dopamine. This may facilitate more 'normal' dopamine transmission by allowing endogenously released brief pulses of dopamine to compete with these drugs for occupancy of the receptor. This may explain why atypical antipsychotics cause fewer extrapyramidal symptoms than the typical antipsychotics (King 2004, p. 325; Sadock & Sadock 2005, p. 2918).

2. Clozapine is a potent D_2 antagonist.

False: Clozapine binds more loosely to and has only modest affinity for the D_2 receptor compared to the older typical antipsychotic drugs (King 2004, p. 323; Sadock & Sadock 2005, p. 2918).

3. Clozapine dissociates from D_2 receptors slowly.

False: Clozapine is the archetypal atypical antipsychotic drug. One explanation for its low propensity to cause extrapyramidal side-effects is that it binds less strongly to the D_2 receptor than dopamine which may allow more 'normal' dopamine transmission (King 2004, p. 325; Sadock & Sadock 2005, p. 2918).

4. Clozapine antagonizes D_3 and D_4 receptors.

True: Clozapine antagonizes D_2-like (D_2, D_3, D_4) and D_1-like (D_1, D_5) receptors. Clozapine has the lowest affinity for D_2 receptor and a 10-fold higher affinity for D_4 receptor compared to other antipsychotics (Cookson et al 2002, p. 312; Sadock & Sadock 2005, p. 2918).

5. Clozapine causes less postural hypotension than typical antipsychotics.

False: Clozapine and most typical and atypical antipsychotics cause postural hypotension due to a_1 adrenergic receptor blockade. Postural hypotension is less marked with amisulpride, sulpiride, haloperidol, trifluoperazine and aripiprazole. Even though, 'typical antipsychotics' are a large group that includes drugs with widely differing hypotensive effects, postural hypotension is particularly problematic with clozapine (Gelder et al 2006, p. 536; King 2004, p. 351; Taylor et al 2005, p. 27).

6. Clozapine produces less sedation than typical antipsychotic drugs.

False: Clozapine is more sedative than the most sedative typical antipsychotics, e.g. thioridazine, chlorpromazine, mesoridazine, trifluoperazine, etc. Clozapine is the most sedative atypical antipsychotic. Sedation is the most common side-effect of clozapine. Sedation occurs early in treatment and tends to subside over time (BNF 2005 4.2.1; Sadock & Sadock 2005, p. 2923).

7. Clozapine is contraindicated in the elderly.

False: Clozapine is not commonly used in the elderly due to its sedative, hypotensive, anticholinergic and haematological side-effects. It may be cautiously considered for treatment-resistant schizophrenia. The usual dose range is 12.5–100 mg (Sadock & Sadock 2005, p. 3729).

8. The risk of clozapine-induced seizures is dose-related.

True: Clozapine reduces seizure threshold in a dose-dependent fashion. The risk starts increasing at doses above 300 mg and increases sharply at doses above 600 mg.

EEG changes occur in 75% and paroxysmal discharges in 40% of patients on clozapine. Rapid increase in dose, pre-existing seizure disorder and history of head injury increase the risk. Monitoring blood clozapine levels and doing an EEG before increasing the dose above 600 mg may help reduce the risk. Sodium valproate is often used concomitantly as an anticonvulsant (Gelder et al 2000, p.1322; Johnstone et al 2004, p. 267; King 2004, p. 350).

9. Aripiprazole is a D_2 partial agonist.

True: Aripiprazole is a partial agonist at both 5-HT_{1A} and D_2 receptors and an antagonist at 5-HT_{2A} receptors. Partial agonists bind to receptor sites to give a partial response which is less than that of a full agonist but greater than an antagonist. Partial agonists compete with endogenous ligand and therefore give an attenuated response if the ligand is in excess, whilst increasing response where there is a deficit (Sadock & Sadock 2005, p. 2933).

10. Olanzapine causes diabetes mellitus only at doses above 20 mg.

False: Various degrees of glucose intolerance including hyperglycaemia, type II diabetes mellitus and even diabetic keto-acidosis can occur with atypical antipsychotics, especially clozapine and olanzapine. Most cases of hyperglycaemia occur within 6 months of initiating treatment. The exact mechanism is unknown but does not seem to be dose-related (King 2004, p. 533; Sadock & Sadock 2005, p. 2927; Taylor et al 2005, p. 10).

11. Quetiapine causes clinically significant hyperprolactinaemia.

False: Quetiapine, ziprasidone, sertindole, aripiprazole, olanzapine and clozapine do not cause clinically meaningful elevation of prolactin (Taylor et al 2005, p. 92).

12. Quetiapine has antihistaminic properties.

True: Quetiapine has its highest affinity for H_1 receptors. H_1 antagonism is considered responsible for its sedative effects (King 2004, pp. 328, 349).

13. Quetiapine has a half-life of 6 hours.

True: The steady state half-life is 6.9 hours (Sadock & Sadock 2005, p. 2929).

14. Risperidone induces less akathisia than clozapine.

False: Clozapine, risperidone and other atypical antipsychotics have low propensity to cause extrapyramidal side-effects. However, risperidone is more likely to cause extrapyramidal side-effects than clozapine. This may be related to clozapine's lower affinity for the D_2 receptors. Risperidone-induced extrapyramidal side-effects tend to be dose-related (Sadock & Sadock 2005, p. 2914).

15. Akathisia usually starts within a week of initiating treatment with antipsychotics.

True: Akathisia usually quickly follows initiating or increasing the dose of antipsychotic drugs, often within hours of oral administration and within 30 minutes of parenteral administration (Johnstone et al 2004, p. 268; Sadock & Sadock 2005, p. 2716).

16. Neuroleptic malignant syndrome is characterized by gradual onset.

False: Neuroleptic malignant syndrome is generally considered to be an acute, severe syndrome that develops rapidly over 1–3 days and lasts 5–10 days. However, the onset may appear more gradual if one monitors creatinine phosphokinase (CPK), blood pressure and white cell counts (King 2004, p. 579; David Taylor, personal communication).

17. Neuroleptic malignant syndrome is associated with clear consciousness.

False: The diagnostic features include:

1. Hyperthermia and muscle rigidity associated with neuroleptic medication.
2. Two or more of the following: diaphoresis, dysphagia, tremor, incontinence, altered sensorium, mutism, tachycardia, elevated or labile blood pressure, leucocytosis and evidence of muscle injury, i.e. elevated creatinine phosphokinase (CPK). Changes in the level of consciousness may range from confusion to coma (DSM-IV 1994, p. 739; Gelder et al 2006, p. 536; Sadock & Sadock 2005, p. 2714; Stein & Wilkinson 1998, p. 426).

18. Neuroleptic malignant syndrome can be treated with a combination of a dopamine agonist and a calcium channel blocker.

False: The definitive treatments include stopping the offending drug, excluding other possible causes for the presentation and general supportive measures. No drug treatment is of proven value. Treatments that have been used include amantidine, bromocriptine, L-dopa (dopamine agonists), dantrolene (muscle relaxant), benzodiazepines (sedative, muscle relaxant) and antimuscarinic drugs. There have only been anecdotal reports of using calcium channel blockers. Some centres use nifedipine as a prophylactic agent when restarting antipsychotics in patients who had neuroleptic malignant syndrome (King 2004, p. 579; Robert Kerwin, personal communication).

19. Tardive dyskinesia can occur in antipsychotic naïve patients.

False: Spontaneous dyskinesias indistinguishable from neuroleptic-induced tardive dyskinesia have been recorded in 5% of patients with schizophrenia prior to the introduction of antipsychotic drugs and occur in 2% of the normal elderly. However, strictly speaking, the term tardive dyskinesia is used only for dyskinesias developing secondary to exposure to antipsychotic drugs (Taylor et al 2005, p. 8).

20. The prevalence of tardive dyskinesia in people on long-term antipsychotic treatment is more than 50%.

False: Although some studies report rates as high as 56%, most studies report rates of 15–20% prevalence of tardive dyskinesia in chronic institutionalized patients. Rates are higher (up to 40%) in the over 65s on long-term treatment (Gelder et al 2006, p. 535; King 2004, p. 347; Sadock & Sadock 2005, p. 2716).

21. Tardive dyskinesia disappears during sleep.

True: Tardive dyskinesia disappears during sleep. It can be temporarily suppressed voluntarily or by purposeful action or distraction. Some other movement disorders (e.g. the chorea associated with Huntington's disease) also decrease during sleep (Sadock & Sadock 2005, p. 997).

22. Procyclidine can cause visual hallucinations.

True: Antimuscarinic agents can cause acute organic reactions in the elderly. In adults they can cause delirium in high doses. Symptoms include confusion, excitement, agitation, paranoid delusions and hallucinations (Gelder et al 2000, p. 1323; Gelder et al 2006, p. 539; Lishman 1997, p. 657).

23. Physical dependence can occur in long-term procyclidine use.

True: Tolerance, withdrawal symptoms and psychological and physical dependence can occur. Abrupt discontinuation may cause akinesia, rigidity and cholinergic rebound, i.e. nausea, diarrhoea, restlessness and agitation (Cookson et al 2002, p. 305; Gelder et al 2006, p. 540).

24. Antimuscarinic drugs are useful in the treatment of acute dystonia.

True: The acute dystonias, e.g. oculogyric crisis and torticollis, respond rapidly to antimuscarinic drugs such as procyclidine. Acute dystonia is caused by relative excess cholinergic activity compared to dopaminergic activity in the nigrostriatal pathway following blockade of dopamine receptors. Acute dystonias are more common in men and in younger patients, with high potency drugs, higher doses and rapid increase in dose. 90% of cases occur within 5 days of exposure or dose increment (Johnstone et al 2004, p. 267; King 2004, p. 345).

25. Bradykinesia responds better to antimuscarinic drugs than rigidity.

False: On treatment with typical antipsychotic drugs 15–40% of patients develop Parkinsonian symptoms such as bradykinesia, tremor and rigidity. The risk increases with age, drug potency and the rate of dose increments. In drug-induced Parkinsonism, bradykinesia is more prominent and more disabling than rigidity and tremor. Unfortunately, antimuscarinic drugs have least effect on bradykinesia (Johnstone et al 2004, p. 269; Neal 1992, p. 57).

Child and adolescent psychiatry – 1

5

Paul Wilkinson

T F

1. Using ICD-10 results in diagnosing more cases of hyperkinetic disorder than using DSM-IV.

2. A child with ADHD is likely to experience peer rejection.

3. Clonidine and methylphenidate combination is more effective than either alone in treatment of ADHD with associated tics.

4. Autistic children do not show attachment to mother.

5. Autism is associated with epilepsy in adolescence.

6. One in six people with autism manage to live independently as adults.

7. Children who are aggressive are likely to develop antisocial traits in adulthood.

8. Conduct disorder children have normal executive function if there is no ADHD.

9. Maternal smoking in pregnancy is associated with conduct disorders.

10. Shoplifting is a feature of social anxiety in children.

11. Being the first child in the family increases the risk of violence.

12. Adolescent girls have more depressive cognitions than boys.

13. Mutation of the methyltetrahydrofolate reductase (MTHFR) allele is associated with adolescent onset depression.

14. Dyslexic children have decreased temporal lobe activity during attempts to read.

15. Encopresis is associated with school refusal.

16. In children with both faecal and urinary soiling the urinary problem needs to be treated first.

17. In divorce, adjustment difficulties are seen in children before the event even if there is a lack of parental conflict.

18. Gender identity disorder in childhood is associated with decreased contact with the father.

19. The prevalence of specific reading disorder is higher in China compared to the US.

T   F

20. Severe specific reading disorder is associated with impaired non-verbal task performance in an IQ test.

21. In children with specific reading disorders there is an increased risk of schizophrenia in adulthood.

22. In a 14-year-old boy with school refusal, depression is a likely diagnosis if there is no history of missing school.

23. If a 12-year-old girl discloses repeated sexual abuse by her father, an interview using 'anatomically correct' dolls is indicated.

24. Night terrors are associated with depression.

25. Death of a parent is associated with truancy.

ANSWERS

1. Using ICD-10 results in diagnosing more cases of hyperkinetic disorder than using DSM-IV.

False: DSM-IV criteria for ADHD are looser, and there can be the predominantly inattentive subtype or the predominantly hyperactive–impulsive subtype. The combined type better matches the stricter ICD-10 criteria for hyperkinetic disorder. Hence, using DSM-IV results in more cases being diagnosed than using ICD-10. This must be considered when interpreting research findings in ADHD.

2. A child with ADHD is likely to experience peer rejection.

False: Children with ADHD are at increased risk of peer relationship problems, as they are often overactive, intrusive and have difficulty following rules of games. However, the majority do not suffer from these problems so much that they 'experience peer rejection'.

3. Clonidine and methylphenidate combination is more effective than either alone in treatment of ADHD with associated tics.

False: A recent RCT compared clonidine, methylphenidate, clonidine and methylphenidate combination and placebo in patients with ADHD and tic disorder. All three active groups led to significant clinical improvement compared to placebo. While the greatest difference was between combined treatment and placebo, the study was not adequately powered to demonstrate significant differences between combined and single treatments. Tics reduced in all active treatments compared with placebo (Tourette's Syndrome Study Group 2002).

4. Autistic children do not show attachment to mother.

False: Attachment is the infant's predisposition to seek proximity to certain people and to be more secure in their presence. Attachment is variable in autistic children: often attachment is very poor. They have little interest in the human face. They rarely seek others for comfort or attention. They are aloof and indifferent to people. However, sometimes an autistic child is very affectionate and shows strong attachment behaviours. While attachment is possible, autistic children still normally show poor social reciprocity with their attachment figures, for example, giving hugs only on their terms, whether or not their mother is able to give a hug in that situation (Johnstone et al 2004, p. 583).

5. Autism is associated with epilepsy in adolescence.

True: About 20–25% of those with autism develop epilepsy, particularly in adolescence (Gelder et al 2000, p. 1726; Johnstone et al 2004, p. 590).

6. One in six people with autism manage to live independently as adults.

False: One in 10 lives independently (Gelder et al 2000, p. 1726).

7. Children who are aggressive are likely to develop antisocial traits in adulthood.

False: Aggressive children are more likely to be antisocial in adulthood, but as a group, they are still more likely to be non-antisocial. 40% of children with conduct disorder go on to be delinquent as young adults (Goodman & Scott 1997, p. 66).

8. Conduct disorder children have normal executive function if there is no ADHD.

False: Conduct disordered children have impairments of executive control functions such as planning, initiation of actions, inhibition of responses and self-monitoring behaviour. These are present even if there is no ADHD (Rutter & Taylor 2002, p. 424).

9. Maternal smoking in pregnancy is associated with conduct disorders.

True: This association is stronger for males, stronger for persistent conduct disorders and stronger for violent than non-violent criminality.

10. Shoplifting is a feature of social anxiety in children.

False: Shoplifting is not a common feature of childhood emotional disorders.

11. Being the first child in the family increases the risk of violence.

False: There is no evidence of this. However, behavioural problems are associated with large family size.

12. Adolescent girls have more depressive cognitions than boys.

True: Community studies of adolescent girls show higher levels of depressive symptoms and cognitions than boys.

13. Mutation of the methyltetrahydrofolate reductase (MTHFR) allele is associated with adolescent onset depression.

False: MTHFR is a regulatory enzyme in homocysteine metabolism. A mutation in the gene results in decreased enzyme activity, contributing to increased homocysteine levels and decreased folate levels. This is implicated in coronary artery disease and possibly Alzheimer's disease, but there is no evidence linking it with depression.

14. Dyslexic children have decreased temporal lobe activity during attempts to read.

True: PET and fMRI studies have shown that when attempting phonologic tasks, e.g. rhythm detection, dyslexic children show reduced activation in parts of the left hemisphere, including the superior temporal, parieto-temporal, middle temporal, middle occipital and inferior frontal gyri; parts of the right hemisphere, including the inferior frontal gyrus; and two posterior sites – the parieto-temporal region and the occipito-temporal region. There is also an unusual degree of symmetry of planum temporale (Lishman 1997, p. 49).

15. Encopresis is associated with school refusal.

False: There is no evidence that children with encopresis are more likely to refuse to go to school.

16. In children with both faecal and urinary soiling the urinary problem needs to be treated first.

False: Faecal soiling is often as a result of overflow from constipation. Constipation can make enuresis worse due to pressure on the bladder. Therefore, constipation needs to be addressed first.

17. In divorce, adjustment difficulties are seen in children before the event even if there is a lack of parental conflict.

False: Conflict before divorce and the actual divorce are the major risk factors for adjustment problems. If there is no pre-divorce conflict, there is no increased risk for adjustment difficulties before the divorce (Gelder et al 2000, p. 1693).

18. Gender identity disorder in childhood is associated with decreased contact with the father.

True: Cross-gender behaving boys have been shown to spend less time with their fathers in their early years than conventionally masculine boys. There was no difference between times spent with mothers in the two groups. It is possible that, rather than the reduced contact with fathers causing feminine behaviour, boys with feminine identification were less interesting to their fathers (Gelder et al 2000, p. 1821).

19. The prevalence of specific reading disorder is higher in China compared to the US.

False: Despite great differences in the nature of printed words, there is no difference in the prevalence of specific reading disorder in USA, China and Japan.

20. Severe specific reading disorder is associated with impaired non-verbal task performance in an IQ test.

False: By definition, specific reading disorder tells us nothing about IQ other than that the level of reading is less than that expected from IQ. Specific reading disorder is associated with some neuropsychological and neurodevelopmental difficulties, e.g. left–right confusion, difficulty in construction and coordination, motor persistence and abnormalities of language. However, these would be unlikely to affect performance IQ tests significantly (Goodman & Scott 1997, p. 193).

21. In children with specific reading disorders there is an increased risk of schizophrenia in adulthood.

False: There is no association between specific reading disorder and schizophrenia (Goodman & Scott 1997, p. 197).

22. In a 14-year-old boy with school refusal, depression is a likely diagnosis if there is no history of missing school.

False: Depression is possible, but much less likely than anxiety or no formal psychiatric disorder (Goodman & Scott 1997, p. 76).

23. If a 12-year-old girl discloses repeated sexual abuse by her father, an interview using 'anatomically correct' dolls is indicated.

False: The use of anatomically correct dolls is controversial. Some practitioners find them useful but others feel that they should not be used, due to concerns that they may lead answers or bring up traumatic memories (Gelder et al 2006, p. 701).

24. Night terrors are associated with depression.

False: Night terror is a parasomnia occurring in non-REM deep sleep. The asleep child screams, appearing terrified with autonomic arousal. There is no relationship between night terrors and social or psychological problems.

25. Death of a parent is associated with truancy.

False: However, death of a parent is associated with the onset of school refusal.

6 Child and adolescent psychiatry – 2

Paul Wilkinson

T F

1. Very low birthweight is a risk factor for ADHD.

2. ADHD is associated with alcohol dependence in later life.

3. In ADHD, combined drugs and behaviour treatment is better than drug treatment alone.

4. Autistic children have poor imaginative play.

5. In autism, IQ is usually less than 70.

6. Half of autistic children never develop language.

7. Heritability of conduct disorder is about 0.1–0.2.

8. Conduct disordered boys usually get approval from their non-deviant peers.

9. Conduct disorder is associated with mood disorders in adulthood.

10. In a 14-year-old boy caught shoplifting, depression is a likely diagnosis.

11. Perinatal insult increases chances of violence in later life.

12. After adolescence, girls get more depressive symptoms than boys.

13. Fluoxetine is more effective than cognitive behavioural therapy in the short-term treatment of depression in adolescents.

14. Encopresis is related to parenting style.

15. Several studies have linked the MMR vaccine to autism.

16. Primary enuresis in an 8-year-old boy is an indication for an intravenous urogram.

17. Genetic influences are as important as family factors in children's adjustment.

18. More than 50% of mothers with Munchausen's syndrome by proxy have psychiatric illness.

19. Specific reading disorder is more common in boys.

20. Specific reading disorder is associated with low IQ.

21. School refusal is more common in girls than in boys.

22. Antidepressants are likely to be useful in the treatment of school refusal if depressive symptoms are present.

T F

23. If a 12-year-old girl is complaining of repeated sexual abuse by her father, this is an indication for immediately securing a Child Protection Order for her. ☐ ☐

24. Night terrors are likely to be related to relationship difficulties. ☐ ☐

25. Truancy is associated with somatization in children. ☐ ☐

ANSWERS

1. Very low birthweight is a risk factor for ADHD.

True: Aetiological factors include fetal exposure to the mother's use of alcohol, drugs, or cigarettes; perinatal obstetric complications and prematurity (Gelder et al 2000, p. 1739).

2. ADHD is associated with alcohol dependence in later life.

True: People with ADHD are at increased risk for substance use disorders, e.g. alcohol, tobacco, illicit drugs (Gelder et al 2000, p. 1739).

3. In ADHD, combined drugs and behaviour treatment is better than drug treatment alone.

False: The Multimodal Treatment study of children with ADHD (MTA) in 1999 randomized children with ADHD to 4 groups – drug treatment, behavioural treatment, combined drug and behavioural treatments or treatment as usual. Both drug and combined treatments were better than treatment as usual, but there was no significant difference between drug and combined groups. The behavioural management was not significantly more effective than treatment as usual, except for improving social skills and self-esteem (Gelder et al 2000, p. 1743; Johnstone et al 2004, p. 595).

4. Autistic children have poor imaginative play.

True: The symptom triad of autism includes restricted and repetitive activities and interests, social impairment and communication impairment. Poor imaginative play is a symptom in the area of restricted and repetitive activities. Delays or abnormalities in symbolic or imaginative play are a DSM-IV criterion for autism. Autistic children fail to develop the usual patterns of symbolic-imaginative play.

Poor imaginative play is also seen in non-autistic children with language delay because the capacity for abstract and imaginative play is linked with the ability to use words as representations of objects. Therefore, when trying to assess whether a child has autism, compare imaginative play with what would be normal for a child with that level of language (Sadock & Sadock 2005, p. 3169).

5. In autism, IQ is usually less than 70.

True: 50% of those with autism have IQ<50, 70% have IQ<70 and 95% have IQ<100. Verbal IQ is almost always lower than performance IQ (Goodman & Scott 1997, p. 43).

6. Half of autistic children never develop language.

True: Around 50% of people with autism never develop useful speech. In those who develop language, the abnormalities include delayed and deviant language acquisition, echolalia, poor comprehension, poor use of gesture, pronominal reversal, non-reciprocal communication and abnormalities in intonation, rhythm and tone (Goodman & Scott 1997, p. 42).

7. Heritability of conduct disorder is about 0.1–0.2.

False: Heritability of conduct disorder is 0.4. Heritability is greater for early onset and persistent conduct disorder. Latent class analysis suggests that there is a strong genetic influence for ADHD/conduct disorder symptoms rather than 'pure' conduct disorder symptoms.

8. Conduct disordered boys usually get approval from their non-deviant peers.

False: Peer relationships of conduct disordered boys are consistently poor. Non-deviant peers are more likely to reject them.

9. Conduct disorder is associated with mood disorders in adulthood.

True: Conduct disorder is associated with increased antisocial personality traits, substance abuse, anxiety, depression, somatic complaints, self-harm, suicide and time spent in psychiatric hospitals (Gelder et al 2000, p. 1758).

10. In a 14-year-old boy caught shoplifting, depression is a likely diagnosis.

False: Most shoplifting has no association with any mental disorder. However, children with conduct disorder are more likely to develop depression than children without conduct disorder (Johnstone et al 2004, p. 715).

11. Perinatal insult increases chances of violence in later life.

True: Perinatal insults including fetal exposure to alcohol and cocaine can impair brain development, resulting in minimal brain dysfunction, low IQ and impulsivity, increasing the risk of later violence. Obstetric complications also have been implicated (Gelder et al 2000, p. 1756; Stone et al 2000, p. 265).

12. After adolescence, girls get more depressive symptoms than boys.

True: Before puberty, boys are more vulnerable than girls to depression. Over the course of adolescence, the girls have a precipitous rise in depression rates compared to the boys. By age 15 years, girls are twice as likely as boys to have experienced an episode of major depression. This gender difference persists for the next 35–40 years (Sadock & Sadock 2005, p. 2295).

13. Fluoxetine is more effective than cognitive behavioural therapy in the short-term treatment of depression in adolescents.

True: The TADS study showed fluoxetine to be more effective than CBT in the short-term treatment of depressed adolescents. CBT was no more effective than placebo. Fluoxetine plus CBT was better than fluoxetine alone (March et al 2004).

14. Encopresis is related to parenting style.

True: In particular, primary encopresis (not having yet developed bowel control) may be caused by insensitive, inconsistent or neglectful toilet training, which is likely to be within a context of generally suboptimal parenting.

15. Several studies have linked the MMR vaccine to autism.

False: A hypothesis that MMR vaccines cause autism arose after reports that some children underwent developmental regression soon after MMR vaccination. However, developmental regression in autism can be seen around the age of the MMR vaccine (12–15 months) in non-vaccinated children. Epidemiological studies have shown that the incidence of autism is no different in children given or not given MMR.

16. Primary enuresis in an 8-year-old boy is an indication for an intravenous urogram.

False: Around 5% of 8-year-old boys have primary enuresis. This is usually a specific developmental disorder, often hereditary. 70% will have an affected first-degree relative. Behavioural treatment, initially with star charts and rewards, later with pad and bell if necessary, is the best treatment approach, with high success rates.

17. Genetic influences are as important as family factors in children's adjustment.

False: Familial factors, particularly how the parents treat the child, are more important than genes.

18. More than 50% of mothers with Munchausen's syndrome by proxy have psychiatric illness.

True: In Munchausen's syndrome by proxy, also termed factitious illness by proxy, a parent/carer produces a state of ill health or falsely describes ill health in a child they are responsible for. The majority of children are under 5 years of age, with boys and girls equally represented. Most fabricators are female. 79% have a somatization disorder themselves and half have a personality disorder (Gelder et al 2000, p. 1832).

19. Specific reading disorder is more common in boys.

True: Specific reading disorder affects 3–10% of children. It is two to three times more common in boys than girls (Goodman & Scott 1997, p. 189; Rutter & Taylor 2002, p. 682).

20. Specific reading disorder is associated with low IQ.

False: By definition, specific reading disorder tells us nothing about IQ; just that the level of reading is less than that expected from IQ.

21. School refusal is more common in girls than in boys.

False: No sex difference.

22. Antidepressants are likely to be useful in the treatment of school refusal if depressive symptoms are present.

True: If school refusal is associated with major depression and anxiety, treatment with CBT and imipramine is more effective than treatment with CBT and placebo, both in improving school attendance and reducing depressive symptoms (Bernstein et al 2000).

23. If a 12-year-old girl is complaining of repeated sexual abuse by her father, this is an indication for immediately securing a Child Protection Order for her.

False: All cases need decisions based on their own merits. If child sexual abuse is disclosed, the immediate safety of the child (and other children living in the family) is paramount. The case should be referred to Social Services who, among other things, should investigate the safety at home. If an alleged abuser is living at the same home, options would include the alleged abuser living away from the family home or the child being removed to another home. Social Services would make the decision about whether to ask a court to secure a Child Protection Order.

24. Night terrors are likely to be related to relationship difficulties.

False: Night terror is a parasomnia occurring in the non-REM deep sleep. The sleeping child screams, appearing terrified with autonomic arousal. There is no relationship between night terrors and social/psychological problems.

25. Truancy is associated with somatization in children.

False: However, school refusal is associated with somatization.

Child and adolescent psychiatry – 3

Paul Wilkinson

	T	F
1. Perinatal insult increases the risk of ADHD.	☐	☐
2. Atomoxetine has a half-life of 24 hours.	☐	☐
3. In children who are adopted, genetic factors explain emotional problems more than environmental factors.	☐	☐
4. Most children with autism have a learning disability.	☐	☐
5. Autism is associated with an increased risk of schizophrenia.	☐	☐
6. Autistic children become less isolated as they grow older.	☐	☐
7. Temperament in the first 6 months of life can accurately predict conduct disorder in adolescence.	☐	☐
8. Children with unsocialized conduct disorder have low self-esteem.	☐	☐
9. About 10% of British urban teenagers are delinquent.	☐	☐
10. Truancy is often a group activity.	☐	☐
11. Children who are rejected by peers are likely to have a mother who is unsociable.	☐	☐
12. 80% of depressed children have a positive dexamethasone suppression test.	☐	☐
13. Tricyclic antidepressants (TCAs) have been clearly shown to have better efficacy than placebo in children with depression.	☐	☐
14. Encopresis is associated with primary enuresis.	☐	☐
15. Encopretic children are more difficult to treat if there is associated nocturnal enuresis.	☐	☐
16. Fluid restriction is indicated in 7-year-olds with primary enuresis.	☐	☐
17. Children of parents with personality disorder are more likely to have mental disorder than children of parents with schizophrenia.	☐	☐
18. The management of pica is mainly pharmacological.	☐	☐
19. The prevalence of specific reading disorder in Japanese school children is 1%.	☐	☐
20. Specific reading disorder is associated with other psychiatric problems.	☐	☐
21. In large families, the oldest child is most likely to show school refusal.	☐	☐
22. School refusal is usually treated with gradual reintegration and support.	☐	☐

T   F

23. Memories of childhood sexual abuse are relived through flashbacks. ☐ ☐

24. Coprophagia is a feature of Gilles de la Tourette's syndrome. ☐ ☐

25. Children with chronic fatigue syndrome have more emotional problems than those with chronic juvenile arthritis. ☐ ☐

ANSWERS

1. Perinatal insult increases the risk of ADHD.

True: Aetiological factors in ADHD include fetal exposure to the mother's use of alcohol, drugs, or cigarettes; perinatal obstetrical complications and prematurity (Gelder et al 2000, p. 1739).

2. Atomoxetine has a half-life of 24 hours.

False: Atomoxetine is a noradrenaline reuptake inhibitor used in the treatment of ADHD. It has a half-life of approximately 5 hours. It is extensively metabolized principally by CYP 2D6. In poor metabolizers, i.e. 7% of whites and 2% of blacks, the half-life is 21 hours. It is administered once daily (King 2004, p. 427; Sadock & Sadock 2005, p. 2942).

3. In children who are adopted, genetic factors explain emotional problems more than environmental factors.

False: Adoption studies have not been able to tease out whether environmental factors within the adoptive family or genetic factors are more important contributors to emotional problems. There are also likely to be interactions between genetic and environmental factors (for example, in girls, genetic family history of alcohol dependence interacts with adoptive parental psychiatric illness to increase risk of mood disorder). Early environmental adversities are more common in children who are later adopted, increasing their risk of later emotional problems. Adopted children are likely to have better outcomes than their non-adopted peers who are not removed from adverse environments (Gelder et al 2000, pp. 697, 1843).

4. Most children with autism have a learning disability.

True: 70% of autistic children have learning disabilities. Only 5% have an IQ above 100. On the Wechsler scales, they perform poorly on Similarities and Comprehension, but do relatively well on Block design and Digit recall subtests. Up to 10% may have islets of special abilities called splinter skills or savant skills, i.e. high or prodigious performance on a specific skill in presence of learning disability (Johnstone et al 2004, p. 590; Sadock & Sadock 2005, p. 3170).

5. Autism is associated with an increased risk of schizophrenia.

False: There is no evidence of increased risk for schizophrenia. Depressive and anxiety symptoms may occur in high-functioning adolescents who become painfully aware of their inability to form friendships (Johnstone et al 2004, p. 590).

6. Autistic children become less isolated as they grow older.

True: 'Autistic aloofness' tends to improve in over half of cases. This is often replaced by being interested in social interactions, but behaving abnormally in social situations – 'active but odd' (Goodman & Scott 1997, p. 48).

7. Temperament in the first 6 months of life can accurately predict conduct disorder in adolescence.

False: The New York Longitudinal Study showed that children with certain temperamental characteristics were more likely to develop problems. However, correlations are low and the prediction is not 'accurate'.

8. Children with unsocialized conduct disorder have low self-esteem.

True: Unsocialized conduct disorder is conduct disorder with pervasively abnormal peer relationships. There is isolation, unpopularity and peer rejection. Relationships with adults are often marked by discord and hostility. All these increase the risk for low self-esteem.

9. About 10% of British urban teenagers are delinquent.

False: Juvenile delinquency is a legal term. It refers to an act committed by a young person, for which they are convicted, and which would have been regarded as criminal if they were adults. 3–6% of males are 'persistent' young offenders, while 20% of boys are convicted at some point in adolescence. 10% is therefore likely to be wrong (Gelder et al 2006, p. 680).

10. Truancy is often a group activity.

True: Truancy is staying away from school to engage in more appealing activities. It is often carried out with peers, and there is an association with other aspects of conduct disorder.

11. Children who are rejected by peers are likely to have a mother who is unsociable.

False: There are many possible reasons for peer rejection of children. Having an unsociable mother increases the risk. However, the majority of children who are rejected by peers do not have a mother who is unsociable.

12. 80% of depressed children have a positive dexamethasone suppression test (DST).

False: 50–70% of depressed children and 40–60% of depressed adolescents are DST non-suppressors (Kaufman et al 2001).

13. Tricyclic antidepressants (TCAs) have been clearly shown to have better efficacy than placebo in children with depression.

False: The Cochrane review of TCAs in young people has shown no difference in remission rates between TCAs and placebo in children and adolescents, and a small benefit of TCAs in reducing depressive symptoms in adolescents but not children (Hazell et al 2002).

14. Encopresis is associated with primary enuresis.

True: Specific developmental delays in bladder and bowel control are due to delays in maturation of similar mechanisms and so are associated. In addition, constipation can cause overflow encopresis and also makes bladder control harder, due to pressure from the overloaded bowel.

15. Encopretic children are more difficult to treat if there is associated nocturnal enuresis.

False: The opposite, however, is true. Encopresis may be due to constipation, and constipation makes nocturnal enuresis harder to treat, due to pressure effects from the overloaded bowel on the bladder.

16. Fluid restriction is indicated in 7-year-olds with primary enuresis.

False: Fluid restriction may reduce the number of episodes of wetting and is often used by parents of younger children in the early stages of nighttime toilet training to make the process easier. However, it does not actually cure the enuresis in 7-year-olds. The aim of treatment is for the child to associate a full bladder with the need to wake up and go to the toilet. Behavioural treatment (initially with 'star charts and rewards' and later with 'pad and bell' if necessary) is the best treatment approach and has high success rates. Overlearning, giving the child larger quantities of bedtime fluids, is sometimes used, and this reduces relapse rates (Gelder et al 2000, p. 1793).

17. Children of parents with personality disorder are more likely to have mental disorder than children of parents with schizophrenia.

False: No studies have directly compared these. There is more research for schizophrenia. Parental schizophrenia leads to increased risk of schizophrenia and also sub-syndromal schizophrenic symptoms. It also increases the risk of suboptimal parenting and family disruption. There is also evidence for increased risk of problems in children of parents with personality disorders, e.g. conduct disorders in children of those with antisocial personality disorders.

18. The management of pica is mainly pharmacological.

False: Pica, the eating of items normally regarded as inedible, is often associated with other behaviour problems and is more likely in children with learning disabilities. It is sometimes associated with emotional distress. Management is the identification and treatment of the underlying factors, which almost never involves medication.

19. The prevalence of specific reading disorder in Japanese school children is 1%.

False: Despite an earlier report that reading disorder was rare in Japan, more recent studies found that among Japanese children aged 8 to 13 years, 16% had a 1-year delay and 15% had a 2-year delay in reading. The definition of specific reading disorder is reading ability more than two standard deviations below that predicted by age and overall IQ, which corresponds to a 2½-year delay in a 10-year-old. Hence, the prevalence is the same as in the West.

20. Specific reading disorder is associated with other psychiatric problems.

True: Particularly hyperactivity. There is also a link between specific reading disorder and conduct disorder, but this may mainly be mediated by ADHD (Goodman & Scott 1997, p. 197).

21. In large families, the oldest child is most likely to show school refusal.

False: The youngest child may be at the greatest risk.

22. School refusal is usually treated with gradual reintegration and support.

False: A behavioural 'back to school' approach is particularly likely to be successful when refusal to attend school began recently and relatively suddenly. A rapid return to full-time school is often possible once the parents are persuaded that consistent firmness is in the child's best interests. In the majority of cases, the child goes straight back to school and mental health services are not involved. In cases with severe anxiety, gradual reintegration may be needed (Goodman & Scott 1997, p. 77).

23. Memories of childhood sexual abuse are relived through flashbacks.

True: Post-traumatic stress disorder with associated flashbacks occurs in victims of childhood sexual abuse (44% in one study).

24. Coprophagia is a feature of Gilles de la Tourette's syndrome.

False: Coprophagia is the eating of faeces. Coprolalia is uttering swear words, which can be a vocal tic in Tourette's syndrome.

25. Children with chronic fatigue syndrome have more emotional problems than those with chronic juvenile arthritis.

True: Both increase the risk for emotional problems, but a direct comparative study showed this to be greater for chronic fatigue syndrome (Rutter & Taylor 2002, p. 815).

8 Child and adolescent psychiatry – 4

Paul Wilkinson

T F

1. ADHD is common in people with profound learning disability.

2. Atomoxetine is a noradrenaline uptake inhibitor.

3. Autistic disorders affect girls three times more often than boys.

4. When a child is diagnosed with autism, many parents look back and remember that something was wrong during infancy.

5. Autism has a 90% monozygotic twin concordance.

6. Difficulties with theory of mind are the same in patients with autistic spectrum disorders as in the general population.

7. Boys from large families are at higher risk of conduct disorder.

8. Unsocialized conduct disorder is associated with peer rejection.

9. Juvenile delinquency is more likely to be associated with future mental health problems in girls than in boys.

10. Truancy is often seen in children with somatization disorders.

11. Children rejected by peers tend to be aggressive.

12. The ratio of cortisol to DHEA is increased in adolescents with depression.

13. Tricyclic antidepressants are more effective than placebo in adolescent depression.

14. Encopresis is associated with a passive personality.

15. Primary enuresis in an 8-year-old boy with no urinary or psychiatric problems is an indication for IQ assessment.

16. Childhood complex partial seizures are commonly associated with emotional problems in childhood.

17. When a mother remarries, girls are more likely to be distressed than boys.

18. Adolescents have more symptoms related to body perception in psychosis.

19. Specific reading disorder is associated with spelling difficulties.

20. Specific reading disorder is associated with hard neurological signs.

21. School refusal may be secondary to a death in the family.

22. Child abuse is associated with an insecure attachment.

23. Children's reporting of sexual abuse is consistently accurate.

T F

24. There is increased cortical activity in children with tic disorders. ☐ ☐

25. Central abdominal pain is a common presentation in children with emotional problems. ☐ ☐

ANSWERS

1. ADHD is common in people with profound learning disability.

False: Learning disability increases the risk of ADHD. However, the majority of learning disabled children do not have ADHD. In addition, to diagnose ADHD, attentional abilities need to be impaired relative to the overall developmental stage of the child. People with profound learning disability (IQ<25) may never reach the developmental stage at which ADHD can be diagnosed (7 years). The statement is therefore false.

2. Atomoxetine is a noradrenaline uptake inhibitor.

True: Atomoxetine is a presynaptic noradrenaline reuptake inhibitor. This may be the basis of its therapeutic effect (Sadock & Sadock 2005, p. 2942).

3. Autistic disorders affect girls three times more often than boys.

False: Boys are 3.5–4 times more likely to have autism than girls. However, this varies with IQ levels. Among those within the normal IQ range the male:female ratio may be as high as 50:1 (Gelder et al 2000, p. 1726).

4. When a child is diagnosed with autism, many parents look back and remember that something was wrong during infancy.

True: Most parents would have been concerned by 12–24 months and all by 3 years about the child being slow to smile, being unresponsive and passive, disliking social contact or attention, poor language development and not responding to human voices.

However, 'infancy' is usually defined as the first year of life. Autism is rarely detected or suspected in the first year of life. Abnormalities must be evident by 36 months for the diagnosis to be made. When this happens, parents often retrospectively realize that development was never entirely normal (Goodman & Scott 1997, p. 43; Johnstone et al 2004, p. 589; Sadock & Sadock 2005, p. 3169).

5. Autism has a 90% monozygotic twin concordance.

False: Monozygotic twin concordance is in the range 36–91%, while dizygotic twin concordance is around 5%. Heritability is greater than 90% (Rutter & Taylor 2002, p. 643).

6. Difficulties with theory of mind are the same in patients with autistic spectrum disorders as in the general population.

False: Impairments in theory of mind tasks are more common in patients with autistic spectrum disorders than in the general population.

7. Boys from large families are at higher risk of conduct disorder.

True: Conduct disorder is associated with larger family size. This may be due to confounding variables associated with large family size rather than the direct effects of a large family (Gelder et al 2000, p. 1756).

8. Unsocialized conduct disorder is associated with peer rejection.

True: Poor integration with peers is the key differentiating factor for unsocialized conduct disorder.

9. Juvenile delinquency is more likely to be associated with future mental health problems in girls than in boys.

True: Juvenile delinquency is more common in boys than girls. Juvenile delinquency is more likely to be part of a group activity, without underlying mental illness, in boys. In girls, a higher proportion of delinquency is associated with mental health problems, especially substance misuse and personality disorders.

10. Truancy is often seen in children with somatization disorders.

False: However, children with somatization disorder are at increased risk of school refusal, i.e. not wanting to go to school due to anxiety around being at school.

11. Children rejected by peers tend to be aggressive.

False: Peer rejection may lead to aggression, but only in a minority.

12. The ratio of cortisol to DHEA is increased in adolescents with depression.

False: Some, but not all, studies have shown increased cortisol in adolescent depression. Raised cortisol:DHEA (dehydroepiandrosterone) ratio in depressed adolescents vs. controls has not been found. However, raised cortisol:DHEA ratio has been shown to predict persistent as opposed to remitting depression in currently depressed adolescents and adolescents at risk for future depressive episodes.

It has been postulated that DHEA levels vary at different stages of depression – in the early stages, there is an increase, to counteract the harmful effects of the cortisol; the body is eventually exhausted in persistent depression and so DHEA levels fall to below those of controls. Therefore an undifferentiated depressed sample will contain a mixture of raised, normal and lowered cortisol:DHEA ratios (Goodyer et al 1998, p. 2003; Kaufman et al 2001).

13. Tricyclic antidepressants (TCAs) are more effective than placebo in adolescent depression.

True: This is a difficult question to answer. The Cochrane meta-analysis of TCAs in adolescents showed that there is no statistically significant increase in numbers of participants meeting improvement criteria in the adolescent TCA group than control group. However, using differences in continuous rating scales, TCAs cause slightly more reduction in symptoms than placebo in adolescents (effect size = −0.47, 95% confidence interval −0.92 to −0.02) but not in children. There were significant side-effects in the TCA group. In view of the little efficacy and significant side-effects, NICE has recommended that TCAs should not be used in adolescents (Hazell et al 2002).

14. Encopresis is associated with a passive personality.

False: There is no evidence for this.

15. Primary enuresis in an 8-year-old boy with no urinary or psychiatric problems is an indication for IQ assessment.

False: Around 5% of 8-year-old boys will have primary enuresis. It is usually a specific, rather than global, developmental disorder. It is often hereditary, with 70% having an affected first-degree relative. Behavioural treatment, initially with star charts and rewards and later with pad and bell if necessary, is the best treatment approach and has high success rates.

16. Childhood complex partial seizures are commonly associated with emotional problems in childhood.

True: 29% of a sample of epileptic children showed some psychiatric disorder compared to only 6.8% of controls. Complex partial seizures are associated with higher rates of psychiatric disorder than other types of epilepsy (Gelder et al 2000, p. 1155; Lishman 1997, p. 260).

17. When a mother remarries, girls are more likely to be distressed than boys.

False: Boys are more likely to have problems than girls (Black & Cottrell 1993, p. 46).

18. Adolescents have more symptoms related to body perception in psychosis.

False: There is no evidence for this. Adolescents with psychosis have lower rates of formal thought disorder than adults.

19. Specific reading disorder is associated with spelling difficulties.

True. Specific reading disorder is associated with spelling difficulties. In fact, spelling difficulties may persist after reading has improved significantly (Goodman & Scott 1997, p. 189).

20. Specific reading disorder is associated with hard neurological signs.

False: Normally there are no focal neurological deficits.

21. School refusal may be secondary to a death in the family.

True: School refusal may be precipitated by problems in the family, such as illness, bereavement, or moving house (Gelder et al 2006, p. 689).

22. Child abuse is associated with an insecure attachment.

True: Child abuse is associated with inconsistent responses to the infant. This is a major risk factor for insecure attachment.

23. Children's reporting of sexual abuse is consistently accurate.

True: Children's reporting of childhood sexual abuse is usually accurate. The main reducer of accuracy is suggestion by poor interviewing, such as the use of closed questions. Deliberately false allegations are rare (1.5% in one study).

24. There is increased cortical activity in children with tic disorders.

True: PET and fMRI studies have shown decreased metabolism in frontal, cingulate and insular cortices (Gelder et al 2000, p. 1776).

25. Central abdominal pain is a common presentation in children with emotional problems.

True: Younger children may show their distress through abdominal pain, rather than by cognitive symptoms.

Child and adolescent psychiatry – 5

Paul Wilkinson

	T	F
1. ADHD is associated with hypofrontality.	☐	☐
2. Clonidine can be used to treat ADHD.	☐	☐
3. Autistic children are unable to make eye contact.	☐	☐
4. Autistic patients have greater difficulty than non-autistic controls in identifying someone's gender from their eyes.	☐	☐
5. Siblings of patients with autism have an 8% risk of developing autism.	☐	☐
6. Aggression is more common in urban teenagers than rural teenagers.	☐	☐
7. More than 50% of children with conduct disorder have EEG abnormalities.	☐	☐
8. Irrespective of the child's aggression, peer rejection on its own increases later antisocial behaviour.	☐	☐
9. Delinquency is associated with low IQ.	☐	☐
10. Truancy is commonly associated with antisocial behaviour.	☐	☐
11. 20% of adolescent males have a criminal record.	☐	☐
12. The effect of cortisol is more than that of DHEA in adolescent depression.	☐	☐
13. In dyslexia, automatic lexical recognition is normal.	☐	☐
14. Encopresis is associated with nocturnal enuresis.	☐	☐
15. Primary enuresis has genetic heterogeneity.	☐	☐
16. In high parental discord, child psychiatric illness is high.	☐	☐
17. Siblings of child and adolescent patients are more reliable historians than parents.	☐	☐
18. The prevalence of specific reading disorder in schoolchildren in England is 20%.	☐	☐
19. Severe specific reading disorder is associated with normal digit span.	☐	☐
20. Reading difficulties are associated with otitis media.	☐	☐
21. School refusal is associated with reading difficulties.	☐	☐
22. Girls are more likely than boys to tell someone about childhood sexual abuse.	☐	☐
23. Nightmares are frequently associated with nocturnal enuresis.	☐	☐
24. Body rocking is seen in 40% of normal children at 18 months.	☐	☐

T F

25. Non-accidental injury to the child is very rare if the mother has obsessive compulsive disorder.

ANSWERS

---

1. ADHD is associated with hypofrontality.

True: Neuroimaging studies show smaller and asymmetrical prefrontal and basal ganglia structures, particularly on the right side (Gelder et al 2000, p. 1739).

2. Clonidine can be used to treat ADHD.

True: Clonidine can be particularly useful if there is a co-morbid tic disorder, as clonidine may also improve tics. It was believed that stimulants worsened tics, although recent evidence does not support this (Tourette's Syndrome Study Group 2002).

3. Autistic children are unable to make eye contact.

False: Autistic children can make eye contact but it is usually markedly impaired. Children with autism fail to use eye-to-eye gaze and facial expression for social interaction. They usually focus exclusively on the mouth of the person speaking, avoiding the upper part of the face and not noticing the emotional responses of the listener (DSM-IV 1994; Johnstone et al 2004, p. 589; Sadock & Sadock 2005, p. 3171).

4. Autistic patients have greater difficulty than non-autistic controls in identifying someone's gender from their eyes.

False: Adults with high-functioning autism/Asperger syndrome have been shown to be impaired in inferring the mental state of a person just from the photographs of their eyes. However, they were not impaired on the control tasks of recognizing gender from the eye region or recognizing emotions from the whole face (Baron-Cohen et al 1997).

5. Siblings of patients with autism have an 8% risk of developing autism.

False: The rate of narrowly-defined autism in siblings is 3%. For milder variants of the autistic spectrum the sibling rate is 10–20% (Goodman & Scott 1997, p. 46).

6. Aggression is more common in urban teenagers than rural teenagers.

False: Early studies of conduct disorder in a rural area (the Isle of Wight) and an urban area (London) suggested a higher rate of conduct disorder in the urban area. More recent studies (Ontario and North Carolina) showed minimal urban–rural differences. The Ontario study suggested higher conduct disorder in urban compared with rural children, but also higher rates in rural adolescents than urban adolescents. Poverty was an important confounding factor, and it diminished the effect of geography. Aggression itself has not been compared between rural and urban areas (Rutter & Taylor 2002, p. 421).

7. More than 50% of children with conduct disorder have EEG abnormalities.

False: There is no evidence of EEG abnormalities. Consistent biological findings include lower levels of electrodermal conductivity, lower mean resting heart rate, lower heart rate reactivity and variability and reduced serotonergic activity.

8. Irrespective of the child's aggression, peer rejection on its own increases later antisocial behaviour.

False: Several studies have shown peer rejection to be predictive for later antisocial behaviour. However, Dodge et al (2003) also measured aggression at baseline and showed that peer rejection increases the risk for later antisocial development only in children initially disposed towards aggression.

9. Delinquency is associated with low IQ.

True: Low intelligence and attention problems, rather than educational performance, are associated with delinquency (Gelder et al 2000, p. 1862).

10. Truancy is commonly associated with antisocial behaviour.

True: Truancy is associated with antisocial behaviour rather than emotional symptoms (Gelder et al 2000, p. 1764).

11. 20% of adolescent males have a criminal record.

True: 20% of males are convicted at least once during adolescence (Gelder et al 2006, p. 680).

12. The effect of cortisol is more than that of DHEA in adolescent depression.

True: Some, though not all, studies have shown increased cortisol in adolescent depression. Raised cortisol:DHEA ratio in depressed adolescents vs. controls has not been found. However, raised cortisol:DHEA ratio has been shown to predict persistent as opposed to remitting depression in currently depressed adolescents and children. Goodyer et al showed that just the evening cortisol and not the cortisol:DHEA ratio differentiates depressed adolescents who will remain depressed over a longer time period (72 weeks) from those who will recover. It is thought that DHEA may be produced by the body to counteract the harmful effects of cortisol, possibly on neurogenesis in the hippocampus (Goodyer et al 1998, 2003).

13. In dyslexia, automatic lexical recognition is normal.

True: The majority of cases of specific reading disorder are 'phonological dyslexia', where people have difficulty decoding words by their letters. Automatic lexical recognition is recognizing whole words, and is usually normal in cases of phonological dyslexia.

14. Encopresis is associated with nocturnal enuresis.

True: Specific developmental delays in bladder and bowel control are due to delays in maturation of similar mechanisms and so are associated. In addition, constipation can cause overflow encopresis and also makes bladder control harder, due to pressure from the overloaded bowel.

15. Primary enuresis has genetic heterogeneity.

True: There is thought to be autosomal dominant inheritance, with high (>90%) penetrance. However, linkage with several different gene areas has been demonstrated, indicating genetic heterogeneity (Gelder et al 2006, p. 690).

16. In high parental discord, child psychiatric illness is high.

False: Parental discord is one significant risk factor for child psychiatric illness. However, without other risk factors, the majority of children with high parental discord will not have a psychiatric illness.

17. Siblings of child and adolescent patients are more reliable historians than parents.

False: History from patients and their parents is very important. History from siblings can be helpful, but normally the parents know a lot more relevant information.

18. The prevalence of specific reading disorder in schoolchildren in England is 20%.

False: The prevalence in England is 3–10% (Goodman & Scott 1997, p. 193).

19. Severe specific reading disorder is associated with normal digit span.

True: The severity of specific reading disorder refers to the disparity between reading ability and IQ. There is no evidence that working memory difficulties are associated with specific reading disorder.

20. Reading difficulties are associated with otitis media.

False: Reading difficulties are usually due to a specific developmental disorder of reading, globally impaired intelligence or an environment not conducive to learning. They are not associated with otitis media, which is associated with impaired hearing and resultant language problems.

21. School refusal is associated with reading difficulties.

False: Children with school refusal are of average intelligence and academic performance.

22. Girls are more likely than boys to tell someone about childhood sexual abuse.

True: 12–17% of girls and 5–8% of boys are sexually abused. More than half of the children who are abused do not disclose it, especially boys (Gelder et al 2000, p. 1827; Johnstone et al 2004, p. 589).

23. Nightmares are frequently associated with nocturnal enuresis.

False: Nightmares are frightening dreams that usually awaken the sleeper from REM sleep, with clear consciousness and detailed dream recall. Children experience nightmares with a peak frequency around ages 5–6 years. Approximately half of adults report occasional nightmares. Nightmares may be caused by frightening experiences during the day. Frequent nightmares occur during periods of anxiety. Other causes include PTSD, fever, psychotropic drugs and alcohol detoxification. While emotional disorders may increase the risk for both nightmares and nocturnal enuresis there is no direct association between the two (Gelder et al 2006, p. 689; Johnstone et al 2004, p. 786).

24. Body rocking is seen in 40% of normal children at 18 months.

False: Body rocking is uncommon at 18 months and is a symptom of disturbance. It can be for self-stimulation if the child is not given enough stimulation. It can be a motor stereotypy as in fragile X or Rubenstein–Taybi syndrome. It can be a sign of emotional disturbance in a (usually older) child unable to express themselves verbally.

25. Non-accidental injury to the child is very rare if the mother has obsessive compulsive disorder.

False: Mothers rarely act on obsessive thoughts to harm their children. However, non-accidental injury for other reasons is still possible.

10 Classification

Classification

Claire Dibben and Rudwan Abdul-Al

	T	F
1. Jaspers is associated with the hierarchical classification of disease.	☐	☐
2. Schneider's first rank symptoms are operational criteria.	☐	☐
3. Eysenck's classification is categorical.	☐	☐
4. Kraepelin's mixed affective states include depression with flight of ideas.	☐	☐
5. The principle of co-morbidity implies a hierarchical use of diagnoses.	☐	☐
6. The ICD-10 is an example of dimensional classification.	☐	☐
7. An adequate classification should include mutually exclusive categories.	☐	☐
8. An adequate classification should use a dimensional approach.	☐	☐
9. Multiaxial classification helps avoid combining clinical picture and aetiology in a single category.	☐	☐
10. Syndromal classification is based on aetiology.	☐	☐
11. Reliability of diagnosis is improved by operational definitions.	☐	☐
12. ICD-10 acknowledges that 'disorder' is not an exact term.	☐	☐
13. Impairment is an essential part of the WHO definition of disability.	☐	☐
14. The ICD-10 classification has a multiaxial version.	☐	☐
15. In epidemiology, 'caseness' can be correctly identified with disease.	☐	☐
16. In ICD-10, the cut-off between mild and moderate learning disability is 49/50.	☐	☐
17. Neurasthenia is retained as a diagnosis in ICD-10.	☐	☐
18. Explosive personality is included in ICD-10 as a subtype of emotionally unstable personality.	☐	☐
19. ICD-10 classifies only psychiatric disorders.	☐	☐
20. The ICD-10 uses operational definitions.	☐	☐
21. The ICD-10 classification includes the diagnosis 'hysteria'.	☐	☐
22. For an ICD-10 diagnosis of dependence, at least three criteria should be met.	☐	☐
23. Possession disorders are included under dissociative (conversion) disorders in the ICD-10.	☐	☐
24. The DSM-IV has fewer specific categories for childhood disorders than ICD-10.	☐	☐

T F

25. The letters TR in DSM-IV-TR stand for 'Test Revision'.

☐ ☐

ANSWERS

1. Jaspers is associated with the hierarchical classification of disease.

False: Karl Jaspers (1883–1969) is associated with descriptive psychopathology. He took a systemized approach to phenomenology and psychopathology. He described his approach to nosology as empirical, descriptive and free from theoretical explanations (Sadock & Sadock 2002, p. 275).

2. Schneider's first rank symptoms are operational criteria.

False: They are not operationally defined. They are a list of symptoms with no specific rules of application to make a diagnosis (Gelder et al 2006, p. 273; Johnstone et al 2004, p. 247).

3. Eysenck's classification is categorical.

False: Eysenck & Eysenck proposed a dimensional classification of personality. The dimensions are introversion–extroversion, neuroticism and psychoticism. Dimensional classification does not use discrete entities and instead assigns a position along one or more axes. It is a more flexible approach. It is often used in psychology (Gelder et al 2006, p. 28; Johnstone et al 2004, pp. 111, 254).

4. Kraepelin's mixed affective states include depression with flight of ideas.

True: Kraepelin described six mixed affective states based on the level of mood, psychic activity and motor activity:

1. Depressive or anxious mania
2. Excited depression
3. Mania with poverty of thought
4. Manic stupor
5. Depression with flight of ideas
6. Inhibited mania (Sato et al 2002; Sims 2004, p. 322).

5. The principle of co-morbidity implies a hierarchical use of diagnoses.

False: Categorical classification often implies a hierarchical use of diagnoses. The principle of co-morbidity avoids hierarchy by lending equal weight to the diagnoses (Gelder et al 2000, p. 111).

6. The ICD-10 is an example of dimensional classification.

False: Categorical (Gelder et al 2006, p. 28).

7. An adequate classification should include mutually exclusive categories.

True: An adequate classification should include separate and mutually exclusive categories and be wholly exhaustive. However, many psychiatric disorders do not neatly fall within the boundaries of one category and there is some overlap (Gelder et al 2006, p. 21; Johnstone et al 2004, p. 254).

8. An adequate classification should use a dimensional approach.

False: An adequate classification should be valid, reliable, mutually exclusive and wholly exhaustive. It can be dimensional (rejects use of separate categories) or categorical (uses discrete groups). Each approach has advantages and disadvantages (Gelder et al 2006, p. 21; Johnstone et al 2004, p. 254).

9. Multiaxial classification helps avoid combining clinical picture and aetiology in a single category.

True: Removing aetiology from definitions of psychiatric disorders improves diagnostic reliability, but impoverishes the diagnoses by removing information which would have explained why the patient fell ill at that particular time with that particular symptom. Multiaxial systems allow assessments on several axes, each of which refers to a different domain of information. They promote consideration of all relevant aspects of clinical situations and help plan treatment and predict outcome (DSM-IV 1994, p. 25; Gelder et al 2000, p. 112; Gelder et al 2006, p. 28; Stein & Wilkinson 1998, p. 1246).

10. Syndromal classification is based on aetiology.

False: Syndromal classification is based predominantly on groups of symptoms and signs that together make up a recognizable condition, e.g. schizophrenia and myxoedema. Classification may also be based on alternatives such as aetiology, e.g. delirium tremens and hypothyroidism, or pathophysiology, e.g. cancer, response to treatment or prognosis (Johnstone et al 2004, p. 244; Sadock & Sadock 2002, p. 275).

11. Reliability of diagnosis is improved by operational definitions.

True: There are three ways to improve reliability:
1. Using structured interviews
2. Providing definitions for all items of psychopathology
3. Using operational definitions (Gelder et al 2006, p. 29; Johnstone et al 2004, p. 252).

12. ICD-10 acknowledges that 'disorder' is not an exact term.

True: The term 'disorder' in ICD-10 refers to 'the existence of a clinically recognizable set of symptoms or behaviour associated in most cases with distress and with interference with personal functions'. ICD-10 acknowledges that disorder is not an exact term but is used throughout as defined above (ICD-10 1992, p. 5).

13. Impairment is an essential part of the WHO definition of disability.

True: Disability is any restriction or lack (resulting from an impairment) of ability to perform an activity in a manner or within the range considered normal for a human being. It is now also called activity limitation (World Health Organisation 2001).

14. The ICD-10 classification has a multiaxial version.

True: There are different versions of ICD-10 for different purposes. These include clinical descriptions and diagnostic guidelines, diagnostic criteria for research, a primary care version, and a multiaspect (axial) version. In the multiaxial version, Axis I covers psychiatric disorders (F1-5), personality disorders (F6) and mental retardation (F7). Axis II is for disability. Axis III covers psychosocial and other problems (Gelder et al 2000, p. 112; Gelder et al 2006, pp. 28, 32).

15. In epidemiology, 'caseness' can be correctly identified with disease.

True: Caseness refers to the way in which the presence of disease is operationalized for the purpose of definition and identification in epidemiological research. However, the extent to which caseness is synonymous with disease will depend on the validity of the instrument used. With instruments with high presumptive validity (e.g. the DSM and the NINCDS-ADRDA), caseness and disease are truly synonymous because there is little further clarification possible from a clinical perspective. With instruments used for screening (e.g. the GHQ or the MDQ), sensitivity is usually high and positive predictive value is usually low; in consequence, caseness is not synonymous with disease, and cases screened positive require to be further interviewed or tested for disease. In contemporary epidemiological research, quality standards demand that instruments of high validity are used; as a result, caseness tends to be correctly identified with disease (Gelder et al 2000, p. 1527; Wright et al 2005, p. 117).

16. In ICD-10 the cut-off between mild and moderate learning disability is 49/50.

True: According to ICD-10, the IQ ranges are 50–69 for mild learning disability, 35–49 for moderate learning disability, 20–34 for severe learning disability and below 20 for profound learning disability. Thus, 49/50 is the cut-off between mild (F70) and moderate learning disability (F71) (ICD-10 1992).

17. Neurasthenia is retained as a diagnosis in ICD-10.

True: Neurasthenia (F48.0) is classified under 'Other neurotic disorders' (F48) and includes fatigue syndrome.

18. Explosive personality is included in ICD-10 as a subtype of emotionally unstable personality.

True: Emotionally unstable personality disorder Impulsive subtype (ICD-10 1992, F60.30) includes the categories of explosive and aggressive personality types. Explosive personality disorder was originally described in ICD-9.

19. ICD-10 classifies only psychiatric disorders.

False: The ICD-10 classification of mental and behavioural disorders is just Chapter V (F) of the tenth revision of the International Classification of Diseases and Related Health Problems (Gelder et al 2000, p. 111; Johnstone et al 2004, p. 250).

20. The ICD-10 uses operational definitions.

True: Operational definitions are rules of application, i.e. specific criteria that must be met before a diagnosis can be made. They act as diagnostic aids specifying the appropriate diagnosis for every possible combination of symptoms. Operationalized diagnoses are reached by considering characteristic and discriminatory symptoms, their hierarchy and inclusion and exclusion statements. Most categories in ICD-10 have flexible diagnostic guidelines for everyday use and strict diagnostic criteria for research, which uses specific operational criteria in a very similar style to DSM-IV (Gelder et al 2000, p. 111; Gelder et al 2006, p. 31; Johnstone et al 2004, p. 247).

21. The ICD-10 classification includes the diagnosis 'hysteria'.

False: The term 'hysteria' is not used in the title for any mental disorder in ICD-10. The ICD-10 recommends avoiding the term 'hysteria' as far as possible in view of its many and varied meanings. However, hysteria, conversion hysteria and hysterical psychosis are inclusion terms for F44, Dissociative (conversion) disorders and anxiety hysteria are included under F41.8, Other specified anxiety disorders.

22. For an ICD-10 diagnosis of dependence, at least three criteria should be met.

True: For a diagnosis of dependence according to ICD-10, 3 or more out of 6 features should have been present together in the previous year. According to DSM-IV, 3 or more of 7 features should have been present in the same 12-month period.

23. Possession disorders are included under dissociative (conversion) disorders in the ICD-10.

True: Trance and possession disorders (F44.3) are included under Dissociative (conversion) disorders (F44).

24. The DSM-IV has fewer specific categories for childhood disorders than ICD-10.

False: In DSM-IV 'Disorders usually diagnosed in infancy, childhood or adolescence' include more separate categories (52-76) than ICD-10 'Disorders of childhood and adolescence' (F90-98). Mental retardation and disorders of psychological development are listed separately in ICD-10, whereas in DSM-IV they form part of this chapter.

25. The letters TR in DSM-IV-TR stand for 'Test Revision'.

False: Text Revision. DSM-IV was revised to correspond more closely to ICD-10. It lists 365 disorders in 17 sections. In addition, some diagnostic criteria proposed for further study are included in the appendix (DSM-IV-TR 2000; Sadock & Sadock 2002, p. 288; Sadock & Sadock, 2005, p. 1013).

Drug abuse – 1

Irma Beyers

	T	F

1. Up to 50% of intravenous drug users die within 10 years of their first intravenous injection. ☐ ☐

2. Amphetamine can cause physical dependence. ☐ ☐

3. Caffeine intake can reliably be calculated from the number of cups of tea and coffee drunk. ☐ ☐

4. Visual hallucinations are a recognized feature of cannabis use. ☐ ☐

5. Cocaine causes psychosis lasting up to 4 weeks. ☐ ☐

6. MDMA causes physical dependence. ☐ ☐

7. Ecstasy has been used in explorative psychotherapy. ☐ ☐

8. Ecstasy causes more physical dependence than cocaine. ☐ ☐

9. Lysergic acid diethylamide has a distinct odour. ☐ ☐

10. LSD intoxication is associated with formication. ☐ ☐

11. LSD causes physical dependence. ☐ ☐

12. Approximately 28% of people in the UK smoke. ☐ ☐

13. Only doctors licensed by the Secretary of State can prescribe methadone to a heroin addict. ☐ ☐

14. 31% of IV heroin addicts die in 10 years. ☐ ☐

15. Dipipanone can cause dependence. ☐ ☐

16. Opiate dependence is characterized by a relapsing course. ☐ ☐

17. Convulsions are a sign of opiate withdrawal. ☐ ☐

18. Methadone given before delivery in opiate addicts will prevent withdrawal symptoms in the neonate. ☐ ☐

19. Heroin withdrawal can be precipitated with naloxone. ☐ ☐

20. Lofexidine is an opiate antagonist. ☐ ☐

21. Naltrexone is an opiate antagonist. ☐ ☐

22. PCP antagonizes glutamate. ☐ ☐

23. 10% of 14-year-old boys in England will use volatile substances in the next 4 months. ☐ ☐

T F

24. Butane inhalation can cause mania-like symptoms. ☐ ☐

25. 'Roid rage' is the syndrome of anger and irritability caused by anabolic steroid abuse. ☐ ☐

ANSWERS

1. Up to 50% of intravenous drug users die within 10 years of their first intravenous injection.

False: The mortality rate for injecting drug users, including intravenous and subcutaneous, from all causes, is estimated to be 3–4% per year (Baciewicz 2005).

2. Amphetamine can cause physical dependence.

True: Many recreational amphetamine users do not progress to misuse and dependence but dependence can develop quickly in susceptible individuals. Tolerance is more likely in the more persistent users and in those taking high doses. A withdrawal syndrome called 'crash' may follow a binge of a few days or cessation following long-term use. The features vary from low mood, fatigue, increased sleep and increased appetite to severe depression with high risk of suicide (Ghodse 2002, p. 115; Gelder et al 2006, p. 464).

3. Caffeine intake can reliably be calculated from the number of cups of tea and coffee drunk.

False: In order to calculate caffeine intake one should know the caffeine content of the various sources of caffeine, how the drink is prepared, e.g. brewed vs. instant and if the drink is strong or diluted. The caffeine content of 6 oz or 177 mL of selected drinks is: brewed coffee = 100 mg, instant coffee = 70 mg, decaffeinated coffee = 4 mg, leaf or bag tea = 40 mg and instant tea = 25 mg (Sadock & Sadock 2005, p. 1202).

4. Visual hallucinations are a recognized feature of cannabis use.

True: Cannabis intoxication can cause visual hallucinations in the form of flashes of light, human faces, pictures of great complexity or flashbacks. This may be part of an acute toxic psychosis with confusion, persecutory delusions, auditory and visual hallucinations, anxiety, agitation and amnesia (Lishman 1997, p. 613; Solowij 1998, p. 30).

5. Cocaine causes psychosis lasting up to 4 weeks.

False: Amphetamine and cocaine can both cause drug-induced psychosis with persecutory delusions and hallucinations that may occur in clear consciousness. The condition will recover spontaneously over the course of a few days or 1 or 2 weeks at the most (Sadock & Sadock 2005, p. 1226; Wright et al 2005, p. 444).

6. MDMA causes physical dependence.

False: Tolerance to successive doses of MDMA develops quickly. Weekend users describe a midweek 'crash' in mood that may represent withdrawal symptoms. In Australia, 2% of a sample of ecstasy users reported feeling dependent, i.e. 'needing to use the drug every day to cope'. Dependence has also been reported in the UK. Overall, however, physical dependence has not convincingly been demonstrated (Gelder et al 2006, p. 465; Sadock & Sadock 2005, p. 1199; Wright et al 2005, p. 446).

7. Ecstasy has been used in explorative psychotherapy.

True: Ecstasy was initially patented as an appetite suppressant. It has been used as an adjunct to psychotherapy termed psycholytic therapy (Sadock & Sadock 2005, p. 1198; Wright et al 2005, p. 445).

8. Ecstasy causes more physical dependence than cocaine.

False: Cocaine is more likely than ecstasy to be associated with tolerance, withdrawal symptoms and dependence (Sadock & Sadock 2005, pp. 1198, 1226; Wright et al 2005, p. 446).

9. Lysergic acid diethylamide has a distinct odour.

False: LSD, commonly referred to as 'acid', is sold on the street in tablets, capsules, and, occasionally, liquid form. It is odourless, colourless, and has a mild bitter taste. Often LSD is added to absorbent paper, such as blotting paper, and divided into small decorated squares, each square representing one dose, usually 75 micrograms. The exact dose contained in such a square or 'tab' can vary widely. It is usually taken by mouth (NIDA).

10. LSD intoxication is associated with formication.

False: Formication is the tactile hallucination involving the sensation that tiny insects are crawling over the skin. It is seen in cocaine abuse and delirium tremens.

11. LSD causes physical dependence.

False: LSD is not considered an addictive drug because it does not produce compulsive drug-seeking behaviour, as do cocaine, amphetamine, heroin, alcohol, nicotine, etc. However, like other addictive drugs, LSD produces tolerance, and hence, those who take the drug repeatedly need progressively higher doses to achieve a state of intoxication. This is a dangerous practice, given the unpredictability of its effects. LSD does not cause physical dependence, but psychological dependence may occur (Gelder et al 2006, p. 466; http://www.drugabuse.gov).

12. Approximately 28% of people in the UK smoke.

True: According to the Office of National Statistics the prevalence of cigarette smoking in the UK during 2000–2001 was 27% in those aged 16 or over (http://www.statistics.gov.uk).

13. Only doctors licensed by the Secretary of State can prescribe methadone to a heroin addict.

False: In the UK, any medical practitioner can prescribe methadone for the treatment of dependence. There are no legal constraints on the dose, the dosage form or the frequency with which methadone may be dispensed (Wright et al 2005, p. 441).

14. 31% of IV heroin addicts die in 10 years.

False: The reported mortality figures range from 12% in 22 years in London to 18% in 12 years in Sweden. The Home Office figures show an annual crude death rate 7.7/1000 person/year (Ghodse 2002, p. 356).

15. Dipipanone can cause dependence.

True: Dipipanone is an opioid analgesic. The only preparation available in the UK (Diconal) contains an antiemetic – cyclizine. Like any other opiate, dipipanone can cause tolerance, and psychological and physical dependence (ABPI 2005, p. 674; BNF 2005 4.7.2).

16. Opiate dependence is characterized by a relapsing course.

True: In the early stages of opioid use, the typical course is one of periods of abstinence lasting weeks or months, followed by relapse and reinstatement of dependence. Following abstinence oriented treatments, most relapses occur within the first 3 months and two-thirds relapse within 6 months. Depression and psychosocial stresses contribute to these relapses (Sadock & Sadock 2005, p. 1276).

17. Convulsions are a sign of opiate withdrawal.

False: Convulsions are more associated with alcohol and benzodiazepine withdrawal, and cocaine and amphetamine intoxication (Gelder et al 2000, p. 524; Ghodse 2002, p. 97; Wright et al 2005, p. 438).

18. Methadone given before delivery in opiate addicts will prevent withdrawal symptoms in the neonate.

False: If the mother is dependent on heroin, withdrawal symptoms in the newborn start within 24 hours. They include hyperactivity, irritability, restlessness, tremors, GI disturbances, vomiting, etc. Giving methadone before delivery delays the onset of withdrawal symptoms in the newborn until 48–72 hours after birth (Ghodse 2002, p. 318).

19. Heroin withdrawal can be precipitated with naloxone.

True: Naloxone is an opiate antagonist that displaces opiates by competitive antagonism. In accelerated detoxification, naloxone is used to precipitate immediate opiate withdrawal that can be treated with neuroleptics, propranolol and atropine. This procedure requires close supervision and monitoring, and is done very infrequently (Ghodse 2002, pp. 248, 266).

20. Lofexidine is an opiate antagonist.

False: Lofexidine is not an opioid. It is a α_2 adrenergic agonist, similar to clonidine. They both act on the locus coeruleus and hence attenuate the release of noradrenaline. This reduces the autonomic symptoms of opiate withdrawal which are associated with noradrenergic overactivity (Sadock & Sadock 2005, p. 1280; Wright et al 2005, p. 441).

21. Naltrexone is an opiate antagonist.

True: Naltrexone is a long-acting (up to 72 hours) opiate antagonist. It is used to prevent relapse. As it can also precipitate withdrawal, it is recommended that patients should remain opiate free for 7–10 days before commencing treatment with naltrexone. It can be given 2–3 times per week (Ghodse 2002, p. 266).

22. PCP antagonizes glutamate.

True: There are several types of glutamate receptors: NMDA, AMPA and kainate. The NMDA glutamate-calcium channel has multiple receptors surrounding the ion channel. One of the inhibitory modulatory sites is called the PCP site because phencyclidine binds to it. By allosteric modulation it blocks the NMDA glutamate receptor and decreases the influx of calcium (Stahl 2000, p. 387).

23. 10% of 14-year-old boys in England will use volatile substances in the next 4 months.

False: A 2004 survey carried out by Mori on behalf of the Youth Justice Board revealed that 15% of 11 to 16-year-olds had taken cannabis and 5% had used solvents (Gelder et al 2006, p. 468; http://www.drugscope.org.uk).

24. Butane inhalation can cause mania-like symptoms.

True: Inhalant intoxication can present with elated mood, illusions, visual, tactile and auditory hallucinations, delusions of omnipotence and body image disturbances (Lishman 1997, p. 629; Sadock & Sadock 2005, p. 1253; Wright et al 2005, p. 452).

25. 'Roid rage' is the syndrome of anger and irritability caused by anabolic steroid abuse.

True: Athletes using anabolic steroids have long recognized the symptoms of anger and irritability which they call 'roid rage'. They may also experience hypomanic and even manic episodes (Sadock & Sadock 2005, p. 1325).

12 Drug abuse – 2

Nadir Omara

	T	F

1. Under the Misuse of Drugs Regulations (1985) amphetamines are Schedule 1 drugs. ☐ ☐

2. Amphetamine withdrawal is a recognized phenomenon. ☐ ☐

3. The heritability of cannabis abuse is 60–80%. ☐ ☐

4. Intravenous injection of a mixture of heroin and cocaine is called a 'speedball'. ☐ ☐

5. Ecstasy increases the release of both dopamine and serotonin. ☐ ☐

6. Ecstasy can cause a withdrawal state. ☐ ☐

7. MDMA is neurotoxic in humans. ☐ ☐

8. Hallucinogens have a significant effect on memory. ☐ ☐

9. A minimum of 25 mg of LSD is needed to induce psychedelic effects. ☐ ☐

10. Ataxia is a feature of LSD intoxication. ☐ ☐

11. LSD is a 5-HT$_{2A}$ receptor antagonist. ☐ ☐

12. 2% of smokers quit on brief advice from clinicians. ☐ ☐

13. Diamorphine can be prescribed by any doctor for the treatment of addiction. ☐ ☐

14. 4% of opiate addicts will die in 2 years. ☐ ☐

15. Intravenous administration of unadulterated heroin can cause seizures. ☐ ☐

16. Cramps are a feature of opiate withdrawal. ☐ ☐

17. Heroin is more potent than methadone. ☐ ☐

18. It is important to prescribe methadone to patients presenting to A&E with a history of heroin addiction and methadone maintenance treatment, in order to avoid withdrawal symptoms. ☐ ☐

19. In heroin addiction, inspection of the arms could reliably exclude intravenous use. ☐ ☐

20. Lofexidine is an opioid with agonist and antagonist properties. ☐ ☐

21. Buprenorphine is a GABA antagonist. ☐ ☐

22. PCP causes a more prolonged psychotic reaction than LSD. ☐ ☐

T   F

23. Solvent abuse has a peak incidence in boys aged 17–21 years. ☐ ☐

24. Solvent abuse commonly leads to physical dependence. ☐ ☐

25. Anabolic steroids increase the level of low-density lipoproteins. ☐ ☐

ANSWERS

1. Under the Misuse of Drugs Regulations (1985) amphetamines are Schedule 1 drugs.

False: Amphetamines are Schedule 2 drugs.

The Misuse of Drugs Regulations (1985) divides drugs into five schedules with specific rules for storing, prescribing and record keeping for each schedule.

Schedule 1 includes drugs for which there are no therapeutic indications, e.g. LSD and cannabis.

Schedule 2 includes drugs which are used in clinical medicine but are highly likely to cause dependence, e.g. heroin, methadone, morphine, pethidine, cocaine and amphetamine.

Schedule 3 includes barbiturates, buprenorphine and temazepam.

The term 'controlled drugs' is used as a collective description of the drugs in Schedules 2 and 3.

Schedule 4 includes mainly benzodiazepine drugs.

Schedule 5 drugs are preparations which contain drugs listed in Schedules 2 and 3 but in small quantities (Ghodse 2002, p. 394).

2. Amphetamine withdrawal is a recognized phenomenon.

True: The features include dysphoric mood, fatigue, vivid and unpleasant dreams, insomnia or hypersomnia, increased appetite, psychomotor retardation or agitation, anhedonia and impaired attention. It is not always recognized by the abuser (Gelder et al 2006, p. 464; Sadock & Sadock 2005, p. 1192; Wright et al 2005, p. 443).

3. The heritability of cannabis abuse is 60–80%.

True: In a large female twin study, Kendler & Prescott (1998) calculated the heritability for cannabis use at about 35%. However, heavy cannabis use, abuse and dependence had heritability ranging from 62–79%. The COGA (Collaborative Study on the Genetics of Alcoholism) concluded that cocaine, alcohol and cannabis abuse are all familial, with evidence of specific and common addictive factors. The relative risk for a sibling of a cannabis dependent proband to develop dependence was 1.78 (Bierut et al 1998; Kendler & Prescott 1998).

4. Intravenous injection of a mixture of heroin and cocaine is called a 'speedball'.

True: The mixture of cocaine and heroin taken intravenously – 'speedball' – is particularly euphorigenic (Sadock & Sadock 2005, p. 1226).

5. Ecstasy increases the release of both dopamine and serotonin.

True: Ecstasy has two optical isomers. The R (−) isomer has LSD-like effects and releases serotonin. The S (+) isomer has amphetamine-like effects and releases dopamine (Sadock & Sadock 2005, p. 1199; Wright et al 2005, p. 445).

6. Ecstasy can cause a withdrawal state.

True: The reported MDMA withdrawal symptoms include tiredness, feeling sleepy and weak, changes in appetite, low mood and trouble concentrating. Weekend users describe a midweek 'crash' in mood which may represent withdrawal symptoms. However, many do not consider them as true withdrawal symptoms (http://www.drugabuse.gov; Wright et al 2005, p. 446).

7. MDMA is neurotoxic in humans.

False: MDMA (ecstasy) is a substituted amphetamine. MDMA is metabolized to MDA. In animals, MDA causes selective, long-lasting damage to serotonergic nerve terminals. It is unclear if the usual dose of MDMA produces enough MDA to cause neurotoxicity in humans (Sadock & Sadock 2005, p. 1199; Wright et al 2005, p. 445).

8. Hallucinogens have a significant effect on memory.

False: Hallucinogenic drugs primarily affect perception, mood and cognition. At the usual doses they have relatively minimal effects on memory and orientation. Hallucinogens include ergot alkaloid derivatives, e.g. LSD; indolealkylamines, e.g. psilocybin and dimethyltryptamine (DMT); and phenethylamines, e.g. mescaline and ecstasy (MDMA) (Sadock & Sadock 2005, p. 1238; Wright et al 2005, p. 447).

9. A minimum of 25 mg of LSD is needed to induce psychedelic effects.

False: LSD is the most potent mood- and perception-altering drug known. The effects can be felt at doses as low as 25 micrograms. An oral dose of 30 micrograms can produce effects lasting 6 to 12 hours. The usual dose is 75–100 µg. (Sadock & Sadock 2005, p. 1242; Wright et al 2005, p. 447).

10. Ataxia is a feature of LSD intoxication.

True: The neurological symptoms of LSD intoxication are usually mild. Dilated pupils, increased deep tendon reflexes, muscle tension, mild incoordination and ataxia frequently occur (Sadock & Sadock 2005, p. 1242; Wright et al 2005, p. 447).

11. LSD is a 5-HT_{2A} receptor antagonist.

False: LSD is a postsynaptic 5-HT_{2A} receptor partial agonist. 5-HT_{2A} receptors are concerned with perception and also hallucinations (Anderson & Reid 2002, p. 18; Wright et al 2005, p. 447).

12. 2% of smokers quit on brief advice from clinicians.

True: Even brief simple advice provided by doctors about quitting smoking increases the likelihood that a smoker will successfully quit and remain a non-smoker 12 months later. Although the success rate of brief advice is modest, achieving cessation in about 1 in 40 smokers, brief advice is one of the most cost effective interventions in medicine (Coleman 2004).

A Cochrane review suggested that the increment in those giving up with brief advice is 2%. As this is an increment, the total numbers giving up would be higher still and, hence, the NNT of 40 must be viewed with caution (Lancaster & Stead 2004).

13. Diamorphine can be prescribed by any doctor for the treatment of addiction.

False: Only doctors who hold a special licence, issued by the Home Secretary, are permitted to prescribe heroin, dipipanone or cocaine for addiction. However, any doctor may prescribe them to any patient (including addicts) for the treatment of organic disease (Ghodse 2002, p. 396).

14. 4% of opiate addicts will die in 2 years.

True: The annual mortality rate is 1–2%. Approximately 5% die in the first 2 years (Ghodse 2002, p. 354; Wright et al 2005, p. 442).

15. Intravenous administration of unadulterated heroin can cause seizures.

False: However, some opioids, such as meperidine, have toxic metabolites that can cause delirium and occasionally seizures. Pethidine in high doses can cause seizures (Lishman 1997, p. 612; Sadock & Sadock 2005, p. 1274).

16. Cramps are a feature of opiate withdrawal.

True: Muscle twitching, aching muscles and joints and abdominal cramps are features of opiate withdrawal (Gelder et al 2000, p. 524; Ghodse 2002, p. 97; Wright et al 2005, p. 438).

17. Heroin is more potent than methadone.

True: Heroin (diacetylmorphine) is a μ receptor agonist. It is more potent than morphine as it is more lipid-soluble and crosses the blood–brain barrier more quickly.

Methadone is as potent, weight for weight, as morphine. The withdrawal symptoms are similar in nature and severity to heroin and morphine. However, the slower onset of action causes less euphoriant effect and the long half-life leads to withdrawal symptoms only after 36 hours. Hence, patients consider methadone less potent (Sadock & Sadock 2005, pp. 1268, 1283).

18. It is important to prescribe methadone to patients presenting to A&E with a history of heroin addiction and methadone maintenance treatment, in order to avoid withdrawal symptoms.

False: Accurate assessment of the patient requesting treatment is very important. This should include a full drug history, a life history, physical examination and drug screening by testing either urine sample or oral swab to confirm dependent pattern of use. Prescribing methadone without a comprehensive assessment could convert the occasional user to an opiate dependent patient or worse still kill him (Ghodse 2002, p. 164).

19. In heroin addiction, inspection of the arms could reliably exclude intravenous use.

False: Physical examination of the patient and in particular the skin is essential for diagnosis of injecting drug use. The skin bears stigmata of subcutaneous use, 'skin popping', with shallow sterile abscesses leaving shallow punched out marks. For intravenous use, the forearms are the most accessible and are often used first. Other sites would include the hands, legs, feet, neck and the groin. Evidence can range from needle puncture marks to infected and thrombosed veins, often with associated pigmentation 'tracking' (Ghodse 2002, p. 174).

20. Lofexidine is an opioid with agonist and antagonist properties.

False: Lofexidine is not an opioid. It is an α_2 adrenergic agonist, similar to clonidine, but causes less hypotension. It acts on the locus coeruleus and blocks the release of noradrenaline which is responsible for the autonomic symptoms of opiate withdrawal. Lofexidine is used in the symptomatic treatment of opiate withdrawal in patients who use small amounts of heroin and do not require methadone treatment; at the patient's request, i.e. not wanting opiate substitution; or where substitutions are not available, e.g. in prisons (Gelder et al 2006, p. 459; Sadock & Sadock 2005, p. 1280; Wright et al 2005, p. 441).

21. Buprenorphine is a GABA antagonist.

False: Buprenorphine is a partial μ receptor agonist with tight receptor binding resulting in a long duration of action. The partial opiate agonist action means less positive reinforcement and effective antagonism at low doses. It is administered sublingually, or, very rarely, by injection because oral administration results in rapid metabolism by the liver (Ghodse 2002, p. 105).

22. PCP causes a more prolonged psychotic reaction than LSD.

True: The effects of LSD are short lasting, typically 6–12 hours. Primary intoxication with PCP lasts 4–6 hours. However, the following dose dependent effects may last for several weeks: initially, overactivity, irritability and elevated mood or sedation and impaired attention. With levels above 30 ng/mL, mood lability, psychosis and ataxia may occur. Paranoia and aggressive behaviour are most likely to occur between 30 and 100 ng/mL. PCP is highly lipophilic. Storage in fatty tissue may be a reason for its longer lasting effect.

23. Solvent abuse has a peak incidence in boys aged 17–21 years.

False: Solvent abuse begins around 9–12 years, peaks between ages 13 and 15 years and is less common after 35 years. It is the commonest cause of death in 15-year-olds in the UK (DSM-IV 1994, p. 241; Johnstone et al 2004, p. 607; Wright et al 2005, p. 452).

24. Solvent abuse commonly leads to physical dependence.

False: There is no evidence for physical dependence. However, psychological dependence can occur. Tolerance can occur with sustained use over 6–12 months. Withdrawal symptoms including sleep disturbance, irritability, nausea, tachycardia, and, rarely, hallucinations and delusions have been reported (Gelder et al 2006, p. 468; Sadock & Sadock 2005, p. 1252).

25. Anabolic steroids increase the level of low-density lipoproteins.

True: Anabolic steroids affect the cholesterol profile negatively by increasing the level of low-density lipoproteins and decreasing the levels of high-density lipoproteins (Sadock & Sadock 2005, p. 1321).

13

Drug abuse – 3

Irma Beyers and Alison Battersby

	T	F
1. Akathisia is a recognized feature of amphetamine use.	☐	☐
2. Acute amphetamine withdrawal after chronic heavy use can cause seizures.	☐	☐
3. Chronic use of cannabis impairs concentration and motivation but improves conversational ability.	☐	☐
4. Cocaine has been used in Coca-Cola®.	☐	☐
5. Ecstasy has weaker reinforcement effects than cocaine.	☐	☐
6. NMDA antagonists are neurotoxic in humans.	☐	☐
7. Khat can cause hypomania-like symptoms.	☐	☐
8. LSD is the main hallucinogen in magic mushrooms.	☐	☐
9. Lysergic acid diethylamide can cause a psychosis.	☐	☐
10. LSD is associated with withdrawal delirium.	☐	☐
11. Bupropion is an antidepressant.	☐	☐
12. Heroin produces dependence in 10% of users.	☐	☐
13. Heroin has 3 times the strength of morphine, which has 10 times the strength of opium.	☐	☐
14. Opiate dependence is characterized by a tendency to reduce the dose.	☐	☐
15. Heroin withdrawal is associated with psychotic symptoms.	☐	☐
16. Oral methadone reduces opiate withdrawal symptoms.	☐	☐
17. HIV testing is mandatory in heroin addiction.	☐	☐
18. Clonidine may be used to treat opiate withdrawal.	☐	☐
19. Naloxone reduces the severity of opiate withdrawal.	☐	☐
20. Phencyclidine is an NMDA receptor blocker.	☐	☐
21. Most prisoners have substance misuse problems.	☐	☐
22. Butane abuse can cause visual hallucinations.	☐	☐
23. Solvent abuse can impair cerebellar function.	☐	☐
24. Anabolic steroids can cause mania.	☐	☐

T   F

25. Confrontation of a person in the pre-contemplation phase about their substance misuse most readily brings about a change to action phase.

□ □

ANSWERS

1. Akathisia is a recognized feature of amphetamine use.

False: Amphetamines, especially dexamphetamine and methamphetamine, predominantly release dopamine. The clinical effects of agitation, restlessness and paranoid psychosis can be treated with antipsychotics. Blockade of the postsynaptic D_2 receptors in the mesolimbic pathway is hypothesized to mediate the action of antipsychotic drugs. Blockade of the D_2 receptors in the nigrostriatal pathway causes movement disorders including akathisia (Stahl 2000, pp. 509, 404).

2. Acute amphetamine withdrawal after chronic heavy use can cause seizures.

False: Amphetamine is a stimulant. Acute intoxication may cause seizures, but not withdrawal (Lishman 1997, p. 245).

3. Chronic use of cannabis impairs concentration and motivation but improves conversational ability.

False: Chronic use of cannabis can cause poor social judgement, poor attention span, poor concentration, confusion, anxiety, depression, apathy, passivity, indifference and often slowed and slurred speech. In addition, the patients can be incapable of completing thoughts during verbal communication (Solowij 1998, p. 30).

4. Cocaine has been used in Coca-Cola®.

True: Cocaine was an ingredient of Coca-Cola® until 1902 (Sadock & Sadock 2005, p. 1221).

5. Ecstasy has weaker reinforcement effects than cocaine.

True: Cocaine is a powerful positive reinforcer in animals. It causes strong dependence in humans. This results from cocaine's ability to block the reuptake of dopamine into presynaptic terminals, leading to high extracellular dopamine levels in the nucleus accumbens and consequent activation of the 'reward system'. Even though MDMA acts as a reinforcer in animals, this effect is weaker than that of cocaine (Gelder et al 2006, p. 464).

6. NMDA antagonists are neurotoxic in humans.

False: Phencyclidine, ketamine and other NMDA antagonists can cause neuronal vacuolization and necrosis at doses significantly greater than those required for their behavioural effects. Direct evidence for neurotoxicity in humans is lacking, despite the widespread use of ketamine as an anaesthetic.

Neurotoxicity may explain the cognitive deficits seen in heavy or repeated intoxication (Sadock & Sadock 2005, p. 1293).

7. Khat can cause hypomania-like symptoms.

True: Khat is used as a recreational drug. Its mild stimulant effects appear to promote social interaction. Users report loquacity, disinhibition and improved concentration. It reduces appetite and the need for sleep. It can cause a toxic psychosis or a schizophreniform psychosis (Gelder et al 2000, p. 545; Ghodse 2002, p. 122).

8. LSD is the main hallucinogen in magic mushrooms.

False: Psilocybin and related homologues are found in up to a hundred species of mushrooms, mainly the *Psilocybe* genus. These mushrooms are used for religious activities, e.g. in Mexico, and by Westerners who prefer 'naturally occurring' drugs. LSD is a synthetic ergot alkaloid derivative (Sadock & Sadock 2005, p. 1242).

9. Lysergic acid diethylamide can cause a psychosis.

True: The hallucinogen persisting perception disorder may be caused by toxic stimulation and destruction of 5-HT_{2A} receptor bearing inhibitory neurons, resulting in chronic disinhibition of visual information processing. Post-LSD psychosis resembles schizoaffective disorder with chronic visual disturbances, mystic preoccupations, delusions and auditory hallucinations. However, whether LSD can cause longstanding psychosis is still controversial (Gelder et al 2000, p. 537).

10. LSD is associated with withdrawal delirium.

False: Tolerance to the psychological effects of LSD occurs. It is controversial if psychological or physical dependence occurs. Withdrawal symptoms are not observed in humans (Gelder et al 2006, p. 467; Ghodse 2002, p. 125; http://www.drugabuse.gov).

11. Bupropion is an antidepressant.

True: Bupropion is a dopamine and noradrenaline reuptake inhibitor. It may have similar antidepressant effects to tricyclics and may produce improvement in 70% of patients with depression. It is marketed with the trade name Zyban as an aid to smoking cessation and with the trade name Wellbutrin as an antidepressant (Sadock & Sadock 2005, p. 2791).

12. Heroin produces dependence in 10% of users.

False: Approximately one-third of those who ever use heroin become dependent. Approximately 7.5% of those who use opioid analgesics (other than heroin) outside of a medical context develop dependence (Sadock & Sadock 2005, p. 1267).

13. Heroin has 3 times the strength of morphine, which has 10 times the strength of opium.

True: Heroin is 3–6 times as potent as morphine, although the pharmacology of the drugs is identical. Opium is the air-dried latex from the unripe capsules of *Papaver somniferum*. It contains 10–17% morphine, 2–4% codeine and a variable mixture of other alkaloids including noscapine and papaverine (King 2004, p. 498).

14. Opiate dependence is characterized by a tendency to reduce the dose.

False: Like dependence on most other drugs, opiate dependence is characterized by tolerance, withdrawal symptoms and escalating doses (DSM-IV 1994, p. 181).

15. Heroin withdrawal is associated with psychotic symptoms.

False: Heroin withdrawal does not cause psychotic symptoms in otherwise healthy individuals. There have been unconfirmed reports of psychosis in patients with pre-existing CNS disorders including HIV and with ultra-rapid detoxification (Gelder et al 2000, p. 524; Sadock & Sadock 2005, p. 1272).

16. Oral methadone reduces opiate withdrawal symptoms.

True: Methadone is a synthetic opioid analgesic. The duration of action is approximately 24 hours. Therefore, once-daily administration is sufficient to prevent withdrawal symptoms in opiate dependence (Ghodse 2002, p. 102).

17. HIV testing is mandatory in heroin addiction.

False: Clinicians should always seek the patients' consent. They should arrange appropriate pre- and post-test counselling. Do not coerce patients but advise them, especially those who are intravenous drug users and those at risk from other sources (Ghodse 2002, p. 182).

18. Clonidine may be used to treat opiate withdrawal.

True: Clonidine is an α_2 adrenergic agonist which reduces the release of noradrenaline. Opiate withdrawal symptoms are caused partly by noradrenergic overactivity. Clonidine, by blocking noradrenaline release, attenuates the autonomic symptoms of opiate withdrawal. The side-effects of sedation and hypotension limit its use to inpatient treatment settings (Ghodse 2002, p. 247).

19. Naloxone reduces the severity of opiate withdrawal.

False: Naloxone is an opiate antagonist. It displaces opiates by competitive antagonism. Naloxone is used in the treatment of opiate intoxication, e.g. overdose. Due to the relatively short half-life, repeated administration is necessary. Naloxone is also used in accelerated detoxification to precipitate opiate withdrawal that can be treated with neuroleptics, propranolol and atropine. These are inpatient procedures and are done very infrequently (Ghodse 2002, p. 248; Sadock & Sadock 2005, p. 1278).

20. Phencyclidine is an NMDA receptor blocker.

True: The PCP receptor is located in the ion channel of the NMDA-glutamate receptor. Phencyclidine binds to the PCP receptors and, by allosteric modulation, blocks the NMDA receptor complex (Gelder et al 2000, p. 535; Sadock & Sadock 2005, p. 1292; Stahl 2000, p. 387).

21. Most prisoners have substance misuse problems.

True: Prisoners in the UK have the highest rates of illicit drug use. The majority have a history of drug abuse. In one study, dependence on drugs has been reported by 51% of male and 54% of female remand prisoners and 43% and 41% respectively of convicted prisoners (Gelder et al 2006, p. 451).

22. Butane abuse can cause visual hallucinations.

True: Most solvents are central nervous depressants but the apparent initial effect can be stimulation and disinhibition (similar to alcohol). They cause giddiness, ataxia, slurred speech, impaired judgement, dullness, apathy and confusion. Approximately 40% experience hallucinations which are usually visual or tactile. One quarter may develop potentially dangerous delusions, e.g. omnipotence or being able to swim or fly (Ghodse 2002, p. 134; Sadock & Sadock 2005, p. 1252).

23. Solvent abuse can impair cerebellar function.

True: Chronic solvent abuse can cause a variety of neurological problems including headache, hearing loss, paraesthesia with peripheral neuropathy, cerebellar degeneration or reversible cerebellar signs, motor impairment, gait disorders, spasticity, Parkinsonism and memory impairment. MRI and CT scans show diffuse cerebral, cerebellar and brainstem atrophy. Whether these changes may be reversible on abstinence is not yet clear (http://www.drugabuse.gov; Lishman 1997, p. 630; Sadock & Sadock 2005, p. 1251).

24. Anabolic steroids can cause mania.

True: Irritability, aggressiveness, hypomania and mania are associated with anabolic steroid use. The psychiatric effects are dose-related. Mood syndromes are more frequent and more severe with doses above 1000 mg a week (Sadock & Sadock 2005, p. 1325).

25. Confrontation of a person in the pre-contemplation phase about their substance misuse most readily brings about a change to action phase.

False: Motivational interviewing is the preferred approach for patients who are in the pre-contemplation phase of the cycle of change. Motivational interviewing is a client-centred, directive method for enhancing intrinsic motivation to change by exploring and resolving ambivalence. In the spirit of this approach, motivation to change is elicited from the client, and not imposed from without. Coercion, persuasion and constructive confrontation are not in the spirit of motivational interviewing (Chick & Cantwell 1994, p. 132; Johnstone et al 2004, p. 371).

Drug interactions – 1

Judy Chan

	T	F
1. Antacids decrease plasma levels of chlorpromazine.	☐	☐
2. Caffeine antagonizes the anxiolytic effects of benzodiazepines.	☐	☐
3. Carbamazepine reduces serum antipsychotic levels.	☐	☐
4. Cimetidine decreases plasma antidepressant levels.	☐	☐
5. Alcohol and diazepam interact pharmacokinetically.	☐	☐
6. Acamprosate interacts with disulfiram.	☐	☐
7. ACE inhibitors reduce lithium levels.	☐	☐
8. Aminophylline reduces lithium excretion.	☐	☐
9. Consuming alcohol whilst taking metronidazole can cause throbbing headache.	☐	☐
10. Inhalational anaesthetics interact with monoamine oxidase inhibitors (MAOIs).	☐	☐
11. Smoking increases serum antidepressant levels.	☐	☐
12. Tricyclic antidepressants (TCAs) interact with antihypertensive drugs.	☐	☐
13. Alcohol can both decrease and increase the levels of TCAs.	☐	☐
14. TCAs block the depressant effects of alcohol.	☐	☐
15. Adrenaline interacts significantly with TCAs.	☐	☐
16. Barbiturates increase the metabolism of TCAs.	☐	☐
17. Clozapine and carbamazepine should not be co-prescribed.	☐	☐
18. Fluoxetine decreases clozapine levels.	☐	☐
19. Grapefruit juice inhibits cytochrome P450 3A.	☐	☐
20. Chlorothiazide is less likely to cause lithium toxicity than frusemide.	☐	☐
21. Reboxetine inhibits cytochrome P450.	☐	☐
22. SSRIs increase plasma concentrations of carbamazepine.	☐	☐
23. TCAs enhance the effects of chlorpromazine.	☐	☐
24. Clonidine may interact significantly with TCAs.	☐	☐
25. Fluoxetine increases levels of diazepam.	☐	☐

ANSWERS

1. Antacids decrease plasma levels of chlorpromazine.

True: Antacids taken within 2 hours of taking phenothiazines decrease their absorption, reduce their plasma concentrations and hence reduce their therapeutic effects (Kaplan et al 2000, p. 128; King 2004, p. 652).

2. Caffeine antagonizes the anxiolytic effects of benzodiazepines.

True: Caffeine can cause and worsen anxiety and can precipitate panic attacks. Caffeine in high doses antagonizes the anxiolytic effects of benzodiazepines by reducing their receptor binding (Taylor et al 2005, p. 351).

3. Carbamazepine reduces serum antipsychotic levels.

True: Carbamazepine decreases serum concentrations of aripiprazole, clozapine, haloperidol, olanzapine, risperidone and ziprasidone by inducing cytochrome P450 3A4. This effect is particularly important for haloperidol (Sadock & Sadock 2005, p. 2734).

4. Cimetidine decreases plasma antidepressant levels.

False: Cimetidine inhibits cytochrome P450 enzymes CYP 1A2, 2C19 and 3A. This inhibits the metabolism leading to increased plasma levels of tricyclic antidepressants, SSRIs, carbamazepine, valproate and antipsychotics (BNF 2005, Appendix 1; Cookson et al 2002, p. 58; King 2004, pp. 357, 640; Sadock & Sadock 2005, p. 2121).

5. Alcohol and diazepam interact pharmacokinetically.

False: Pharmacokinetic interactions occur when a drug alters the absorption, distribution, metabolism or elimination of a second drug.

In pharmacodynamic interactions, a target action is altered by a second drug operating on the same target receptor. Hence, the interaction between alcohol and diazepam resulting in increased sedation and impaired psychomotor performance is pharmacodynamic (Johnstone et al 2004, p. 303; King 2004, p. 60).

6. Acamprosate interacts with disulfiram.

False: Disulfiram inhibits the enzyme acetaldehyde dehydrogenase resulting in the accumulation of acetaldehyde. Acamprosate (citrated calcium carbamide) is a GABA agonist and glutamate antagonist. Combined treatment with disulfiram and acamprosate may have better outcome than either treatment alone. Acamprosate does not interact with disulfiram (Gelder et al 2000, p. 501).

7. ACE inhibitors reduce lithium levels.

False: Enalapril and other angiotensin-converting enzyme inhibitors increase serum lithium levels by reducing lithium clearance. They increase the risk of lithium toxicity, especially in the elderly.

Thiazide and other diuretics which deplete sodium also raise lithium levels.

Nonsteroidal anti-inflammatory drugs such as indomethacin, and, to a lesser extent, ibuprofen, naproxen, aspirin and sulindac, increase lithium levels.

Osmotic diuretics, acetazolamide, triamterene, methylxanthines and drugs which raise the glomerular filtration rate lower lithium levels (Bazire 2005, p. 322; Kaplan et al 2000, p. 145).

8. Aminophylline reduces lithium excretion.

False: Aminophylline, theophylline and caffeine increase lithium excretion and reduce lithium levels. Aminophylline and theophylline may reduce lithium levels by 20–30%. This effect has been used to treat lithium toxicity (Bazire 2005, p. 326; Kaplan et al 2000, p. 145).

9. Consuming alcohol whilst taking metronidazole can cause throbbing headache.

True: Metronidazole causes a disulfiram-like reaction with alcohol. The symptoms include facial flushing, throbbing headache and palpitations (BNF 2005, 4.10, 5.1.11).

10. Inhalational anaesthetics interact with monoamine oxidase inhibitors (MAOIs).

True: Halothane and enflurane may interact with MAOIs and cause muscle stiffness and hyperpyrexia. MAOIs can interact hazardously with general anaesthetics. Hence, MAOIs should ideally be stopped 2 weeks before surgery. However, general anaesthesia can be attempted in patients on MAOIs in an emergency (BNF 2005, Appendix 1; Stein & Wilkinson 1998, p. 188).

11. Smoking increases serum antidepressant levels.

False: Non-nicotine chemicals, such as aromatic hydrocarbons in tobacco smoke, activate cytochrome P450 enzyme CYP 1A2 and thereby decrease the levels of clomipramine, clozapine, desipramine, doxepin, fluvoxamine, haloperidol, imipramine, nortriptyline, oxazepam and propranolol. The levels of haloperidol, clozapine and fluvoxamine increase 30–40% with abstinence (Cookson et al 2002, p. 58; Sadock & Sadock 2005, p. 1260; Stein & Wilkinson 1998, p. 160).

12. Tricyclic antidepressants (TCAs) interact with antihypertensive drugs.

True: TCAs enhance antihypertensive effect of hydralazine and nitroprusside.

TCAs, however, inhibit the antihypertensive effects of adrenergic neuron blocking agents, e.g. guanethidine, by blocking their uptake into the sympathetic nerve terminal.

TCAs also inhibit the antihypertensive effects of methyldopa and clonidine. The mechanism remains unknown (BNF 2005, Appendix 1; King 2004, p. 210; Stein & Wilkinson 1998, p. 160).

13. Alcohol can both decrease and increase the levels of TCAs.

True: Chronic use of alcohol induces hepatic isoenzymes and may lower tricyclic levels.

Acute ingestion of alcohol can reduce first-pass metabolism by competition, resulting in 2–3 times higher tricyclic levels.

Chronic heavy alcohol consumption can impair hepatic function and elevate blood levels (Johnstone et al 2004, p. 272; King 2004, p. 638; Sadock & Sadock 2005, p. 2963).

14. TCAs block the depressant effects of alcohol.

False: Tricyclic antidepressants enhance the depressant effects of alcohol, including sedation and impairment of psychomotor performance, by the mechanism of summation (Bazire 2005, p. 363; BNF 2005, Appendix 1; King 2004, p. 638).

15. Adrenaline interacts significantly with TCAs.

True: Antidepressants, including TCAs, interact with sympathomimetics like adrenaline to cause hypertension and ventricular arrhythmias by summation (BNF 2005, Appendix 1; King 2004, p. 640).

16. Barbiturates increase the metabolism of TCAs.

True: Barbiturates induce cytochrome P450 CYP 3A4 and, consequently, increase the metabolism and hence reduce the serum levels of amitriptyline, desipramine, protriptyline and nortriptyline by 14–60%. Pentobarbital may affect nortriptyline metabolism within 2 days, both when starting (induction) and on discontinuation. Moreover, tricyclics lower seizure threshold (Bazire 2005, p. 292; Cookson et al 2002, p. 58).

17. Clozapine and carbamazepine should not be co-prescribed.

True: Carbamazepine and phenytoin induce CYP 3A4 and 1A2, and increase the metabolism and decrease plasma levels of clozapine by up to 50%. When carbamazepine is stopped, clozapine levels may double.

Clozapine lowers seizure threshold and hence can compromise the antiepileptic effect of carbamazepine.

Both clozapine and carbamazepine can cause agranulocytosis and the combination is associated with an enhanced risk (Bazire 2005, p. 328; King 2004, p. 650; Sadock & Sadock 2002, p. 1073).

18. Fluoxetine decreases clozapine levels.

False: Fluoxetine inhibits CYP 2D6 markedly and 1A2 and 3A moderately. Clozapine is metabolized by CYP 1A2, 2D6 and 3A4. Therefore, fluoxetine increases clozapine levels. Fluvoxamine causes an even greater increase in clozapine levels (Bazire 2005, p. 284; BNF 2005, Appendix 1; King 2004, p. 635; Sadock & Sadock 2005, p. 2704).

19. Grapefruit juice inhibits cytochrome P450 3A.

True: Grapefruit juice is a powerful inhibitor of CYP 1A2 and 3A4 in the gut mucosa. It increases the plasma levels of buspirone and, possibly, benzodiazepine and sildenafil (BNF 2005, Appendix 1; Cookson et al 2002, p. 58; Sadock & Sadock 2005, pp. 2788, 2889; Stein & Wilkinson 1998, p. 177).

20. Chlorothiazide is less likely to cause lithium toxicity than frusemide.

False: In patients treated with thiazide diuretics and chlorthalidone, the proximal tubules attempt to compensate for sodium loss by increasing the reabsorption of sodium. As the proximal tubule cannot differentiate between sodium and lithium, lithium reabsorption is also increased. This, coupled with fluid loss in diuresis, concentrates lithium in the blood and increases the risk of toxicity. They should be used only when other choices are not available and with strict monitoring.

The risk is much lower with frusemide, a loop diuretic, which inhibits the reabsorption of sodium and lithium in the proximal tubule as well as elsewhere in the nephron.

Potassium sparing diuretics such as spironolactone and triamterene may also increase lithium concentration. The risk is much lower with amiloride which, in fact, may be used to treat lithium-induced polyuria.

Carbonic anhydrase inhibitors such as acetazolamide, osmotic diuretics such as mannitol and urea, and xanthine alkaloids such as caffeine and theophylline all increase the excretion of lithium and hence lower serum lithium levels.

Frusemide may be the safest diuretic with lithium (Bazire 2005, p. 323; Cookson et al 2002, p. 335).

21. Reboxetine inhibits cytochrome P450.

False: Unlike most antidepressants, reboxetine has little inhibitory effect on the cytochrome P450 system (Johnstone et al 2004, p. 280).

22. SSRIs increase plasma concentrations of carbamazepine.

True: Fluoxetine and fluvoxamine inhibit cytochrome P450 enzymes CYP 3A4 and 2C9 respectively and increase the plasma concentration of carbamazepine (Bazire 2005, p. 634; BNF 2005, Appendix 1).

23. TCAs enhance the effects of chlorpromazine.

False: Chlorpromazine increases the level of TCAs by inhibiting CYP 1A2 and 2D6. TCAs do not increase the levels of chlorpromazine (Bazire 2005, p. 292; King 2004, p. 639; Stein & Wilkinson 1998, p. 160).

24. Clonidine may interact significantly with TCAs.

True: Clonidine is an α_2-adrenoceptor agonist. It is used to treat hypertension, migraine and menopausal flushing. TCAs antagonize the hypotensive effects of clonidine (Bazire 2005, p. 293; BNF 2005, Appendix 1; Kaplan et al 2000, p. 34).

25. Fluoxetine increases levels of diazepam.

True: Fluoxetine increases plasma levels of diazepam by inhibiting CYP 2C19 and CYP 3A3/4 (Cookson et al 2002, p. 58; Gelder et al 2006, p. 547; King 2004, p. 452).

Drug interactions – 2

Judy Chan and Kit Wa Chan

	T	F
1. Diclofenac does not increase serum lithium levels.	☐	☐
2. Clinically important interactions occur between diazepam and orphenadrine.	☐	☐
3. Drug interactions may occur at protein binding sites in the plasma.	☐	☐
4. Doxazosin can be used safely with reboxetine.	☐	☐
5. An interaction between disulfiram and warfarin occurs in the liver.	☐	☐
6. Enalapril increases lithium levels.	☐	☐
7. Fluoxetine increases lithium levels.	☐	☐
8. Drug interactions do not occur in the gastrointestinal tract.	☐	☐
9. Together with lithium, haloperidol should not be given at doses higher than 20 mg daily.	☐	☐
10. Patients taking MAOIs should avoid pickled herring.	☐	☐
11. Ibuprofen may reduce lithium levels.	☐	☐
12. Imipramine is incompatible with tyramine rich foodstuffs.	☐	☐
13. Drug interactions do not occur in the kidney.	☐	☐
14. Muscle relaxants interact with MAOIs.	☐	☐
15. Mixing drugs in syringes can cause drug interactions.	☐	☐
16. Interaction by mixing drugs in a syringe is an example of pharmacodynamic drug interaction.	☐	☐
17. MAOIs may interact significantly with TCAs.	☐	☐
18. Methadone may interact significantly with TCAs.	☐	☐
19. TCAs potentiate the pressor effects of noradrenaline.	☐	☐
20. Valproate impairs the efficacy of oral contraceptive drugs.	☐	☐
21. Decreased intestinal absorption of drugs, caused by the anticholinergic effect of amitriptyline, is an example of pharmacodynamic drug interaction.	☐	☐
22. Induction of liver microsomal enzymes is an example of pharmacodynamic drug interaction.	☐	☐

T F

23. Clinically important interactions occur between phenobarbitone and oral contraceptives.

☐ ☐

24. Fluoxetine increases the serum levels of TCAs.

☐ ☐

25. St John's wort increases the levels of warfarin.

☐ ☐

ANSWERS

1. Diclofenac does not increase serum lithium levels.

False: Azapropazone, diclofenac, ibuprofen, indomethacin, mefenamic acid and other NSAIDs reduce the excretion of lithium and raise serum lithium levels by up to 23% and hence increase the risk of toxicity. This is due to inhibition of the renal prostaglandin PGE2, resulting in reduced renal blood flow and reduced lithium clearance. Lithium levels should be monitored frequently when using this combination (Bazire 2005, p. 324; BNF 2005, Appendix 1).

2. Clinically important interactions occur between diazepam and orphenadrine.

False: Antimuscarinic agents may slow down the absorption of benzodiazepines but the amount absorbed remains the same (Bazire 2005, p. 271).

3. Drug interactions may occur at protein binding sites in the plasma.

True: Pharmacokinetic interactions occur when one drug interferes with the disposition of another drug during absorption, distribution or elimination. Many antidepressants, anticonvulsants and warfarin which are highly bound to plasma proteins may displace each other, leading to increased plasma free concentrations of others. Sodium valproate may displace phenytoin from its protein binding sites. SSRIs may displace warfarin, a highly protein bound drug with a narrow therapeutic index (Anderson & Reid 2002, p. 31; Gelder et al 2000, p. 1282; King 2004, p. 67).

4. Doxazosin can be used safely with reboxetine.

True: Doxazosin is an antihypertensive that selectively blocks α_1 receptors. Reboxetine is a potent inhibitor of the noradrenaline transporter. It has a mild sympathomimetic effect and causes only small increases in heart rate and blood pressure. In hypertensive patients whose α_1 receptors are already blocked by doxazosin, even these small increases would not occur (King 2004, p. 215).

5. An interaction between disulfiram and warfarin occurs in the liver.

True: Disulfiram inhibits the metabolism of warfarin. Prothrombin time can rise by about 10%, necessitating reduction in the dose of warfarin (Bazire 2005, p. 356; BNF 2005, Appendix 1).

6. Enalapril increases lithium levels.

True: Enalapril is an angiotensin-converting enzyme inhibitor (ACEI). Lithium should be used with caution in patients receiving NSAIDs, ACEIs and angiotensin 2 antagonists because these drugs may elevate lithium levels. This is due to the inhibition of renal prostaglandin PGE2 resulting in reduced renal blood flow and reduced lithium clearance. Lithium levels should therefore be carefully monitored in patients receiving these drugs, especially in the elderly. ACEIs in combination with lithium may increase the risk of renal failure (Bazire 2005, p. 322; BNF 2005, Appendix 1).

7. Fluoxetine increases lithium levels.

False: Fluoxetine increases the levels of drugs metabolized by CYP 2D6 and, to a lesser extent, those metabolized by CYP 3A4. Lithium is not metabolized in the body. It is eliminated solely by renal clearance. Therefore, lithium levels are unaffected by the co-administration of enzyme inducers or inhibitors.

However, fluoxetine may cause lithium toxicity, without increasing lithium levels. Serotonin syndrome, confusion and seizures have been reported (Bazire 2005, p. 323; BNF 2005, Appendix 1).

8. Drug interactions do not occur in the gastrointestinal tract.

False: Atropine and opiates inhibit gastrointestinal motility, slow absorption, reduce peak concentrations and impair efficacy of analgesics and antibiotics. Metoclopramide stimulates gastric emptying and facilitates absorption of analgesics in the management of acute pain. Charcoal binds with phenobarbitone and TCAs and reduces their absorption in poisoning (King 2004, p. 602).

9. Together with lithium, haloperidol should not be given at doses higher than 20 mg daily.

False: There is no firm evidence that >20 mg haloperidol + lithium combination is specifically associated with increased risk. However, there is no good evidence supporting the use of haloperidol in doses exceeding 20 mg/day either!

A few cases of reversible neurotoxicity have been reported, but these may have been undiagnosed NMS. There have also been unconfirmed reports of encephalopathy, severe EPS, neurotoxicity, irreversible brain damage and increase in lithium-induced neurological adverse effects, etc. When high doses of both drugs are used, there is a risk of missing signs of impending toxicity (Bazire 2005, p. 322; BNF 2005, Appendix 1; Kaplan et al 2000, p. 144).

10. Patients taking MAOIs should avoid pickled herring.

True: Hypertensive crisis results from the direct absorption of pressor amines, e.g. tyramine, phenylethylamine and histamine, formed as part of the bacterial decarboxylation of the amino acid constituents of certain protein-containing foods. Normally these amines are neutralized by MAO in the gut wall. MAOIs inhibit MAO and hence this protective action is lost. This allows the free passage of these enzymes into the systemic circulation. The foods with the highest amount of these amines include pickled herring, yeast extracts, e.g. Marmite, fish and meat extracts, e.g. Bovril, certain vegetable items, e.g. broad bean pods and banana skins, and matured cheese (Gelder et al 2006, p. 550; Johnstone et al 2004, p. 278).

11. Ibuprofen may reduce lithium levels.

False: Lithium should be used with caution in patients receiving NSAIDs, ACE inhibitors, and angiotensin 2 antagonists. They inhibit renal prostaglandin PGE2 resulting in reduced renal blood flow, reduced excretion, elevated lithium levels and lithium toxicity. Lithium levels should therefore be carefully monitored in patients receiving these drugs. ACE inhibitors in combination with lithium may increase the risk of renal failure (King 2004, p. 660).

12. Imipramine is incompatible with tyramine rich foodstuffs.

False: Imipramine does not inhibit MAO and hence it is safe with tyramine rich foodstuffs.

13. Drug interactions do not occur in the kidney.

False: Probenecid was developed to inhibit renal tubular secretion of penicillin. Thiazide diuretics reduce the renal clearance of lithium and can cause toxicity.

14. Muscle relaxants interact with MAOIs.

True: MAOIs decrease plasma pseudocholinesterase activity. Hence, they can prolong muscle relaxation and muscle paralysis with muscle relaxants such as suxamethonium and d-tubocurarine (BNF 2005, Appendix 1; Stein & Wilkinson 1998, p. 188).

15. Mixing drugs in syringes can cause drug interactions.

True: For example, adding soluble insulin to protamine zinc insulin can result in the added insulin binding to the excess protamine, thus reducing the immediate effect of the dose.

16. Interaction by mixing drugs in a syringe is an example of pharmacodynamic drug interaction.

False: Pharmacodynamic interactions occur where two drugs act on the target site of clinical effect. Interaction by mixing in a syringe is an example of pharmaceutical interaction. It is a physiochemical interaction between drugs on a chemical, not on a pharmacological, level. An example is the formation of a complex between thiopentone and suxamethonium, which should not therefore be mixed in the same syringe. These types of interactions are best avoided by giving drugs as bolus injections where appropriate, making up infusions immediately before use and avoiding mixing drugs before administration except where this is known to be safe (Gelder et al 2000, p. 1282).

17. MAOIs may interact significantly with TCAs.

True: The combination of TCAs and irreversible MAOIs can cause serotonin syndrome as well as potentially lethal hypertension and CNS excitation. TCAs should not be given for 2 weeks after stopping MAOIs and MAOIs should not be started until 2 weeks after stopping TCAs (BNF 2005, Appendix 1; King 2004, pp. 193, 630; Gelder et al 2000, p. 1302).

18. Methadone may interact significantly with TCAs.

True: Opioids, alcohol, anxiolytics, hypnotics and over-the-counter cold medications have additive CNS depressant and sedative effects when co-administered with TCAs.

Moreover, amitriptyline and clomipramine increase the bioavailability of morphine and potentiate its analgesic effect. Desipramine blood levels can double with methadone (Bazire 2005, p. 294, 359; BNF 2005, Appendix 1; Kaplan et al 2000, p. 248).

19. TCAs potentiate the pressor effects of noradrenaline.

True: Combination of tricyclic antidepressants and sympathomimetic agents such as noradrenaline can cause hypertension and arrhythmias. The mechanism is summation (Bazire 2005, p. 640; BNF 2005, Appendix 1; Kaplan et al 2000, p. 248).

20. Valproate impairs the efficacy of oral contraceptive drugs.

False: Carbamazepine induces the hepatic microsomal enzymes and thereby lowers the efficacy of several drugs, including oral contraceptives. In contrast, valproate, lithium, lamotrigine, and topiramate have no effect on oral contraceptives. Of note, carbamazepine may also cause false negative pregnancy tests (Bazire 2005, p. 351).

21. Decreased intestinal absorption of drugs, caused by the anticholinergic effect of amitriptyline, is an example of pharmacodynamic drug interaction.

False: Pharmacodynamic interactions occur when two drugs interact at the same site of action. Pharmacokinetic interactions occur when one drug interferes with the disposition of another. Pharmacokinetic interaction may occur at absorption, distribution, metabolism or excretion. Thus decreased absorption is a pharmacokinetic interaction (Gelder et al 2000, p. 1282; King 2004, p. 60).

22. Induction of liver microsomal enzymes is an example of pharmacodynamic drug interaction.

False: Pharmacodynamic interactions occur when two drugs interact at the same site of action. Pharmacokinetic interactions occur when one drug interferes with the disposition of another drug during absorption, distribution or elimination. Induction of liver microsomal enzymes can affect the elimination of some drugs and is therefore a pharmacokinetic interaction (Gelder et al 2000, p. 1282).

23. Clinically important interactions occur between phenobarbitone and oral contraceptives.

True: Phenobarbitone induces the CYP 3A4 enzyme which metabolizes oral contraceptives. This interaction may result in contraceptive failure (Bazire 2005, p. 339).

24. Fluoxetine increases the serum levels of TCAs.

True: The SSRIs inhibit CYP 2D6 and 3A4 in a dose-related way. Fluoxetine, paroxetine and fluvoxamine cause significant inhibition at therapeutic doses. Citalopram and sertraline cause little clinically significant 2D6 inhibition. TCAs are hydroxylated and thus inactivated by 2D6 and 3A4. Hence, SSRIs increase plasma levels of TCAs. Fluoxetine may double or triple tricyclic levels (Bazire 2005, p. 295; Taylor et al 2005, p. 138).

25. St John's wort increases the levels of warfarin.

False: St John's wort (*Hypericum perforatum*) induces hepatic cytochrome P450 enzymes CYP 1A2 and CYP 3A4. This increases the metabolism and reduces the plasma concentrations and efficacy of theophylline, cyclosporine, warfarin, digoxin, the HIV-1 protease inhibitor indinavir, some anaesthetics and oral contraceptives (Bazire 2005, p. 315; King 2004, p. 233).

16 Eating disorders

Eating disorders

Claire Dibben

T F

1. Parental discord has an aetiological role in the genesis of eating disorder.

2. EAT is a self-rated questionnaire.

3. Cholecystokinin in the gastrointestinal tract hinders satiety.

4. Insulin release from the pancreas after a carbohydrate meal reduces the ratio of tryptophan/large amino acids.

5. Paraventricular 5-HT nuclei are responsible for satiety.

6. Leptin level increases in proportion to body mass index.

7. Over 50% of girls in developed countries engage in abnormal eating.

8. Enmeshment is a feature of families of patients with anorexia nervosa.

9. T_4 is increased in anorexia.

10. Anorexia nervosa patients adopt the sick role.

11. In treatment of anorexic patients with severe weight loss, initial weight gain is associated with cognitive improvement.

12. Anorexia can be prevented by education in schools, activities and peer focus group discussions.

13. Family therapy is more effective than individual therapy for younger patients with anorexia nervosa.

14. In anorexia, late onset predicts poor outcome.

15. Vomiting is a positive prognostic factor in anorexia nervosa.

16. In anorexia nervosa, earlier onset is a good prognostic factor.

17. In anorexia the mortality rate is 5% per year.

18. In anorexia family turmoil predicts poor outcome.

19. Short time from onset to presentation is a good prognostic factor for anorexia nervosa.

20. Bulimia nervosa is associated with shoplifting.

21. Menstrual irregularities are frequent in bulimia nervosa.

22. In bulimia there is a risk of seizures.

T   F

23. In bulimia nervosa, cognitive therapy (CBT) and interpersonal therapy (IPT) are equally effective.

☐ ☐

24. Bulimia is associated with increased mortality.

☐ ☐

25. Bulimia is associated with an increased risk of rectal carcinoma.

☐ ☐

ANSWERS

1. Parental discord has an aetiological role in the genesis of eating disorder.

True: Family discord and life events such as parental separation have been associated with the onset of eating disorders. However, no single specific family functioning style appears to be necessary or sufficient for the development of eating disorders. As in most psychiatric disorders, dysfunctional family styles may act as non-specific vulnerability factors and may hamper recovery. Family disturbances seem to increase with the duration of the disorder, suggesting that the disorder causes family disturbance rather than vice versa. However, they are useful for developing working understandings of how certain family patterns may perpetuate the illness (Gelder et al 2006, p. 363; Johnstone et al 2004, p. 494; Sadock & Sadock 2005, p. 2008; Wright et al 2005, p. 222).

2. EAT is a self-rated questionnaire.

True: Eating Attitudes Test is a self-rated questionnaire. Other self-reported questionnaires include Eating Disorders Investigation (EDI) and the Bulimic Investigatory Test, Edinburgh (BITE). Eating Disorders Examination (EDE) is a structured interview. The Morgan–Russell scales assess physical and psychological status (Wright et al 2005, p. 218).

3. Cholecystokinin in the gastrointestinal tract hinders satiety.

False: Cholecystokinin (CCK) is a gut peptide released from the gastrointestinal tract by the local action of digested food that controls meal size in humans and animals. A blunted postprandial CCK release is associated with impaired satiety, e.g. in bulimics. Receptors that initiate CCK's satiating action are located in the proximal small intestine, not in the brain. Activation of these receptors increases the activity of the vagal afferents innervating this site. Transection of the vagal afferent fibres abolishes the satiating action of CCK (Puri & Tyrer 1998, p. 61; Sadock & Sadock 2005, p. 299; Wright et al 2005, p. 232).

4. Insulin release from the pancreas after a carbohydrate meal reduces the ratio of tryptophan/large amino acids.

False: Insulin release leads to an increase in the plasma concentration of tryptophan and a reduction in large neutral amino acid (LNAA) concentrations. This increases the tryptophan/LNAA ratio (Virkkunen & Narvanen 1987).

5. Paraventricular 5-HT nuclei are responsible for satiety.

True: 5-HT inhibits feeding and promotes satiety. Paraventricular, ventromedial and suprachiasmatic nuclei mediate satiety through 5-HT (Gelder et al 2000, p. 840; Wright et al 2005, p. 232).

6. Leptin level increases in proportion to body mass index.

True: Leptin is called the 'satiety hormone'. Leptin is secreted by adipose tissue. Plasma leptin levels are closely correlated with body fat mass and increase in proportion to the body mass index. Leptin is transported across the blood–brain barrier to various brain loci. It acts in the brain to inhibit eating and to stimulate energy expenditure by increasing physical activity (Gelder et al 2000, p. 868; Sadock & Sadock 2005, p. 300).

7. Over 50% of girls in developed countries engage in abnormal eating.

False: In a recent US study, up to 26% of female students and 10% of male students had engaged in abnormal eating or weight control measures over the previous month (Forman-Hoffman 2004).

8. Enmeshment is a feature of families of patients with anorexia nervosa.

True: A specific pattern of family relationships consisting of 'enmeshment, overprotectiveness, rigidity and lack of conflict resolution' was hypothesized to increase the chance of a daughter developing anorexia. However, no single specific family functioning style appears to be necessary or sufficient for the development of eating disorders. These features of family function are not unique to families of anorexics (Gelder et al 2006, p. 363; Johnstone et al 2004, p. 494; Sadock & Sadock 2005, p. 2008).

9. T_4 is increased in anorexia.

False: Thyroxine (T_4) and TSH are usually normal. T_3 is often reduced. TSH response to TRH is blunted (Gelder et al 2000, p. 842; Gelder et al 2006, p. 361; Johnstone et al 2004, p. 492).

10. Anorexia nervosa patients adopt the sick role.

False: Parsons (1951) described the features of *sick role*. They include:

1. Exemption from normal social role responsibilities
2. Right to expect help and care
3. The expectation of a desire to get well and
4. Obligation to seek and cooperate with treatment.

Patients with anorexia nervosa do not adopt the sick role but engage in what Pilowsky (1969) called *abnormal illness behaviour* or dysnosognosia, i.e. persistently pathological modes of experiencing, evaluating and responding to one's own health status despite lucid and accurate appraisal and management options provided by health professionals (Gelder et al 2006, p. 165; Murray et al 1997, pp. 51, 483; Stein & Wilkinson 1998, p. 719;).

11. In treatment of anorexic patients with severe weight loss, initial weight gain is associated with cognitive improvement.

True: Weight restoration results in an improvement in cognitive functioning. Attention improves first, followed by memory, visuospatial functioning and learning (Szmukler et al 1995, p. 205).

12. Anorexia can be prevented by education in schools, activities and peer focus group discussions.

False: There is very little evidence to support this (Pratt & Woolfenden 2002).

13. Family therapy is more effective than individual therapy for younger patients with anorexia nervosa.

True: Family therapy has been shown to be more effective than individual supportive psychotherapy for patients with onset before age 19 years and duration less than 3 years. However, patients with late onset anorexia do better with individual supportive psychotherapy than with family therapy (Gelder et al 2000, p. 849; Johnstone et al 2004, p. 495; Wright et al 2005, p. 224).

14. In anorexia, late onset predicts poor outcome.

True: In anorexia, older age of onset, i.e. above 15 years, is a poor prognostic factor. Other poor prognostic factors include lower minimum weight, longer duration of illness (>6–10 yrs), poor relationship with family, personality difficulties, social problems, premorbid obesity, bulimic behaviour and male gender (Gelder et al 2000, p. 847; Stein & Wilkinson 1998, p. 883; Wright et al 2005, p. 230).

15. Vomiting is a positive prognostic factor in anorexia nervosa.

False: Patients with the bingeing/purging subtype of anorexia have a poorer prognosis. This is consistent with the original description by Russell (1979) of bulimia nervosa as an 'ominous variant' of anorexia nervosa (Wright et al 2005, p. 230).

16. In anorexia nervosa, earlier onset is a good prognostic factor.

True: Those who develop anorexia before the age of 15 years have a better prognosis (Gelder et al 2000, p. 847; Stein & Wilkinson 1998, p. 883; Wright et al 2005, p. 230).

17. In anorexia the mortality rate is 5% per year.

False: The mortality rate in anorexia nervosa is estimated to be 0.59% per year. The mortality is higher amongst those with weight less than 35 kg. The standardized mortality rate is 6 times that of the general population (Stein & Wilkinson 1998, p. 884; Szmukler et al 1995, p. 198; Treasure & Schmidt 2005; Wright et al 2005, p. 230).

18. In anorexia family turmoil predicts poor outcome.

True: Relationship difficulties within the family are a poor prognostic factor (Gelder et al 2000, p. 846; Wright et al 2005, p. 230).

19. Short time from onset to presentation is a good prognostic factor for anorexia nervosa.

True: Favourable prognostic factors include earlier age of onset and shorter interval between onset and treatment (Stein & Wilkinson 1998, p. 883; Treasure & Schmidt, 2005; Wright et al 2005, p. 230).

20. Bulimia nervosa is associated with shoplifting.

True: A minority of bulimia sufferers have 'multi-impulsive behaviours'. They include repeated self-harm, alcohol and drug misuse, sexual promiscuity, shoplifting and other self-damaging behaviours. 10–50% of patients admit to stealing food to binge on (Johnstone et al 2004, p. 496; Sadock & Sadock 2002, p. 747; Wright et al 2005, p. 231).

21. Menstrual irregularities are frequent in bulimia nervosa.

True: Unlike anorexia, amenorrhoea is not necessary for the diagnosis. Up to 60% of bulimics experience loss of ovulation and irregular menstruation or amenorrhoea. An association with polycystic ovaries has also been identified (Gelder et al 2000, p. 859; Johnstone et al 2004, p. 497; Wright et al 2005, p. 220).

22. In bulimia there is a risk of seizures.

True: Generalized seizures are a recognized complication of electrolyte disturbance and large fluid shifts caused by bingeing and vomiting (Johnstone et al 2004, p. 492; Sadock & Sadock 2002, p. 742).

23. In bulimia nervosa, cognitive therapy (CBT) and interpersonal therapy (IPT) are equally effective.

False: At the end of treatment both IPT and CBT result in similar improvement in abstinence from both binge eating and purging. However, at 1 year follow-up, the improvement is better maintained in those who had CBT. CBT is the preferred treatment for bulimia. IPT is an efficacious alternative but may take up to 8–12 months longer to achieve the same results (Hay & Bacaltchuk 2004; NICE).

24. Bulimia is associated with increased mortality.

False: Unlike anorexia the mortality rate is not raised in bulimia (0.3–1.1%). The prognosis is better than for anorexia. The illness runs a relapsing and remitting course with recovery rates between 50 and 70%. At 10-year follow-up about 10% remain bulimic and 15% meet the criteria for an atypical eating disorder (Gelder et al 2000, p. 865; Johnstone et al 2004, p. 493; Stein & Wilkinson 1998, p. 895; Wright et al 2005, p. 235).

25. Bulimia is associated with an increased risk of rectal carcinoma.

False: Bulimia does not increase the risk of rectal carcinoma. Recognized gastrointestinal problems include constipation, cathartic colon, damaged myenteric plexus, gastric and duodenal ulcers, oesophageal erosions, gastric perforation, irritable bowel and pancreatitis (Johnstone et al 2004, p. 492; Sadock & Sadock 2005, p. 2016).

Forensic – 1

Piyal Sen

	T	F
1. An adversarial system is used in Common Law jurisdiction.	☐	☐
2. Common Law is made by the parliament.	☐	☐
3. The criteria for capacity to consent to treatment include that the person retains the information.	☐	☐
4. WHO has included dangerousness in their definition of disability.	☐	☐
5. Risk assessment is subject to the Department of Health guidelines.	☐	☐
6. In civil cases, the medicolegal report is the property of the agency requesting it.	☐	☐
7. 'Fitness to plead' may be raised by the prosecution.	☐	☐
8. Compensation neurosis clears up after settlement in the majority of cases.	☐	☐
9. Delinquency is associated with low IQ.	☐	☐
10. Indecent exposure is the commonest sexual offence by men.	☐	☐
11. Exhibitionists who touch or harass their victims have higher reconviction rates.	☐	☐
12. In sex offenders with learning disability, short-term, intensive, inpatient treatment is the best choice.	☐	☐
13. CBT in learning–disabled sexual offenders involves victim empathy work.	☐	☐
14. People with learning disabilities are more suggestible in an interrogative interview.	☐	☐
15. In the UK, 15% of homicides are followed by suicide.	☐	☐
16. Paedophilia indicates dissocial personality disorder.	☐	☐
17. In the treatment of paedophiles, behaviour change usually occurs only after empathy for victim has developed.	☐	☐
18. Shoplifting is significantly associated with mental illness.	☐	☐
19. Most arsonists are mentally ill.	☐	☐
20. Most cases of arson result in a criminal conviction.	☐	☐
21. The total number of homicides committed by people with schizophrenia has risen over recent years.	☐	☐

T F

22. Most victims are known to their murderers. ☐ ☐

23. Women who commit filicide usually have a history of admissions to psychiatric units. ☐ ☐

24. Mothers who kill their children are often found to have been self-harming. ☐ ☐

25. Those with XYY are more likely to come from families with criminal backgrounds. ☐ ☐

ANSWERS

1. An adversarial system is used in Common Law jurisdiction.

True: The adversarial system is one where the prosecution evidence is pitted against the evidence of the defence and the court determines guilt or innocence. In this system, the evidence of the prosecution is heard first and then the evidence of the defence. This is opposed to the inquisitorial system where the task of the court is to ascertain the facts and arrive at an eventual decision, a model used by inquests and mental health review tribunals.

2. Common Law is made by the parliament.

False: Common Law is based on past judgement of cases. Common Law is influenced by the culture of the home country. In England, the Canon Law of the Christian Church enriched the development of English Common Law in its early stages. This Common Law came to be administered subsequently by the Royal Judges adopting the customs and principles known to them. It then grew by the experience of individual cases, which established the principles. Statutes are Acts of Parliament used to codify parts of the Law, where a myriad of individual case decisions might have made the Law uncertain. Thus, statute often helps to clarify Common Law (Gunn & Taylor 1993, p. 23).

3. The criteria for capacity to consent to treatment include that the person retains the information.

True: Capacity is required for informed consent to be valid. The legal criteria for capacity in British law were laid down in the ruling of Re C. The requirements are that the patient believes the information being given to them, understands that information, is able to recall it and can weigh the pros and cons of various options in the balance. BURP would be an acronym (Fear 2004, p. 194; Johnstone et al 2004, p. 736).

4. WHO has included dangerousness in their definition of disability.

False: Dangerousness is a fluctuating condition and cannot thus be categorized under disability. There is also a wilful aspect to the danger some people pose to others and this again is totally against the spirit of the WHO definition of disability (WHO 2001).

5. Risk assessment is subject to the Department of Health guidelines.

False: Risk assessment depends on four factors, dispositional, clinical, historical and contextual. Every psychiatric unit develops its own strategy of risk assessment based on published scientific research, not based on guidelines from the Department of Health (Gelder et al 2000, p. 2070; Stone et al 2000, p. 264).

6. In civil cases, the medicolegal report is the property of the agency requesting it.

True: In civil cases, the report is the property of the agency requesting it. A report requested by the Court or by the Crown Prosecution Service will be disclosed in open Court to both parties. A report requested by the defence solicitor, on the other hand, may be retained by the solicitor if it does not help his client.

7. 'Fitness to plead' may be raised by the prosecution.

True: Fitness to plead issues may be raised by the defence, the prosecution or the judge. It is a matter that has to be tried in a Crown Court. The plea must be proven on the balance of probabilities (if raised by the defence) or beyond reasonable doubt (if raised by the prosecution). A new jury is empanelled to decide this question.

8. Compensation neurosis clears up after settlement in the majority of cases.

False: More than half of patients fail to return to work after a settlement (Gelder et al 2006, p. 400).

9. Delinquency is associated with low IQ.

True: Delinquency is associated with low IQ even after controlling for family factors and social status. This association may be due to the increased vulnerability to the adverse home and social influences and home background and also the increased likelihood of being apprehended (Gelder et al 2000, p. 1757; Gelder et al 2006, p. 734; Gunn & Taylor 1993, p. 324).

10. Indecent exposure is the commonest sexual offence by men.

True: It is one of the most common of heterosexual offences. The common exhibitionist is a shy, timid and inhibited person, with little confidence in courtship or sexual performance (Gunn & Taylor 1993, p. 547; Stone et al 2000, p. 215).

11. Exhibitionists who touch or harass their victims have higher reconviction rates.

True: Moreover, a further conviction following the first offence of exhibitionism dramatically increases reconviction rates (Gunn & Taylor 1993, p. 547; Stone et al 2000, p. 215).

12. In sex offenders with learning disability, short-term, intensive, inpatient treatment is the best choice.

False: The majority of learning disabled sex offenders are best treated in the community. They can usually be managed quite well with support and supervision where necessary under a probation or guardianship order (Bluglass & Bowden 1990, p. 404).

13. CBT in learning-disabled sexual offenders involves victim empathy work.

True: This would be crucial as learning-disabled sexual offenders often lack full comprehension of the gravity of their offence and its effect on the victim (Chiswick & Cope 1995, p. 74).

14. People with learning disabilities are more suggestible in an interrogative interview.

True: People with learning disabilities have increased suggestibility and hence an increased risk of false confessions. Therefore, they should be interviewed only in the presence of an appropriate adult. Suggestibility can be assessed clinically as well as using formal rating scales.

15. In the UK, 15% of homicides are followed by suicide.

False: In the UK, 10% of homicides are followed by suicide. In the US, homicide followed by suicide represents 1.5% of all suicides and 5% of all homicides. They include:

A. A severely depressed mother killing her children
B. A jealous person killing the spouse (one-fifth kill themselves)
C. Killing of elderly spouses in poor health
D. Multiple murders by a depressed, paranoid or intoxicated person
(Gelder et al 2006, p. 739; Gunn & Taylor 1993, p. 516).

16. Paedophilia indicates dissocial personality disorder.

False: Paedophiles are not inherently antisocial. It is more a disorder of sexual preference.

17. In the treatment of paedophiles, behaviour change usually occurs only after empathy for the victim has developed.

False: In a significant proportion of cases, the behaviour is modified by a combination of environmental manipulation, chemotherapy and close supervision. Often, behaviour change can take place through these measures without the development of victim empathy.

18. Shoplifting is significantly associated with mental illness.

False: Shoplifting is not associated with increased prevalence of mental illness. Occasionally, shoplifting may be associated with eating disorders, mood disorders, schizophrenia, substance misuse or dementia. Pure kleptomania is rare. Most patients with kleptomania have co-morbid depression, anxiety or eating disorders (Gelder et al 2000, p. 2052; Johnstone et al 2004, p. 715; Sadock & Sadock 2005, p. 2044).

19. Most arsonists are mentally ill.

False: Among the highly selected samples examined by psychiatrists, only 20–30% have a mental illness. Alcohol or substance misuse and personality disorders are common. Among those who have a mental illness, schizophrenia or paranoid psychosis are more likely. People with learning disabilities are more likely to commit a fire-setting offence or a sexual offence (Gelder et al 2000, p. 2057; Johnstone et al 2004, p. 715; Stone et al 2000, p. 203).

20. Most cases of arson result in a criminal conviction.

False: Arson is a notoriously difficult offence to detect and also to convict in court (Stone et al 2000, p. 109).

21. The total number of homicides committed by people with schizophrenia has risen over recent years.

False: Taylor & Gunn (1999) reviewed the Home Office statistics in England and Wales from 1957 to 1995 and concluded that the number of homicides by the mentally ill has steadily declined at the rate of 3% per annum since the 1950s.

22. Most victims are known to their murderers.

True: In homicide cases in general, the offender is known to 50% of male victims and 75% of female victims (Stone et al 2000, p. 118).

23. Women who commit filicide usually have a history of admissions to psychiatric units.

False: In D'Orban's study of 89 cases of maternal filicide, only 27% were diagnosed as mentally ill. One had psychotic depression, and 14 had psychosis. Thus, a previous history of admission to psychiatric units would not be a common finding.

24. Mothers who kill their children are often found to have been self-harming.

False: There would be multiple motives for a mother killing her child, including eliminating an unwanted child, mercy killing, psychotic illness or depression, inability to cope with the child, and spouse revenge (Bluglass & Bowden 1990, p. 527).

25. Those with XYY are more likely to come from families with criminal backgrounds.

False: There is no direct connection between XYY and criminality or a criminal background (Bluglass & Bowden 1990, p. 376; Johnstone et al 2004, p. 548).

18 Forensic – 2

Piyal Sen

	T	F
1. Adversarial cases are always tried by jury.	☐	☐
2. The patient has the right to object to a Court of Protection order.	☐	☐
3. Consent to operate on a severely mentally handicapped person may be given by a doctor.	☐	☐
4. In overtly aggressive patients, it is dangerous to interpret the patient's anger.	☐	☐
5. Medicolegal reports requested by the Court should always be revealed to both parties.	☐	☐
6. Regarding medical reports in litigation cases, the psychiatrist is in a contractual relationship with the litigant for the report.	☐	☐
7. Fitness to plead is affected by amnesia for the criminal event.	☐	☐
8. Compensation neurosis is particularly common after accidents involving loss of consciousness.	☐	☐
9. Two-thirds of juvenile offenders have a family history of high crime rate.	☐	☐
10. Indecent exposure is most likely to be directed at teenagers.	☐	☐
11. Aetiological possibilities in a 65-year-old male with a good pre-morbid personality who exposes himself in public for the first time include pneumonia.	☐	☐
12. In sex offenders with learning disabilities the ineffectiveness of preventative work is indicated by the increasing number of hospital orders.	☐	☐
13. People with learning difficulties are more likely to commit serious acts of violence.	☐	☐
14. A full history and mental state examination will in most cases result in disclosure of intra-familial abuse.	☐	☐
15. The accounts of patients who report memories of sexual abuse for the first time during or after psychological therapy are usually reliable.	☐	☐
16. Young girls are twice as likely as young boys to be targeted by paedophiles.	☐	☐
17. Erotomania is the commonest delusion in stalkers.	☐	☐
18. A 50-year-old woman with no previous offences is convicted of shoplifting. It is likely that she was depressed at the time of the offence.	☐	☐

T F

19. Arsonists are over-represented among learning-disabled offenders. ☐ ☐

20. A conviction of arson leads to a compulsory custodial sentence. ☐ ☐

21. Alcohol is frequently associated with crimes of murder. ☐ ☐

22. McNaughton was acquitted of murder on grounds of insanity. ☐ ☐

23. In homicide followed by suicide, there are more likely to be multiple murders. ☐ ☐

24. Mothers who kill their children within 24 h of birth would usually have gone through their pregnancy with denial or dissociation. ☐ ☐

25. XYY is present more often in forensic settings. ☐ ☐

ANSWERS

1. Adversarial cases are always tried by jury.

   False: The adversarial system is adopted in all criminal and civil courts in England. Juries are involved only in Crown Courts, not in Magistrates' Courts (Stone et al 2000, p. 25).

2. The patient has the right to object to a Court of Protection order.

   True: The Court of Protection in England is an office of the Supreme Court. It can take total control over the property and affairs of a mentally incapable person. It appoints a Receiver, who could be a close relative, or a solicitor, or a local authority, to look after the patient's property. There are provisions for the patient or his solicitor to apply to the Court for discharge, with a supporting medical report. The Royal College of Psychiatrists has published guidelines for doctors preparing medical reports for the Court of Protection (Chiswick & Cope 1995, p. 320; Gunn & Taylor 1993, p. 199).

3. Consent to operate on a severely mentally handicapped person may be given by a doctor.

   False: The doctor cannot consent on behalf of a person who lacks the capacity to consent. However, the doctor can take the decision to operate for emergency treatment in order to save the patient's life or to alleviate serious suffering.

4. In overtly aggressive patients, it is dangerous to interpret the patient's anger.

   False: The patient might have set off a maladaptive violent response as a result of an automatic thought. Interpreting the patient's anger could help to arrest that violent response (Bluglass & Bowden 1990, p. 666).

5. Medicolegal reports requested by the Court should always be revealed to both parties.

True: A medicolegal report may be requested from a psychiatrist in criminal or civil cases. The request could come from the Court, from the Crown Prosecution Service or the defending solicitor. The report requested by the Court or by the Crown Prosecution Service will be disclosed in open Court to both parties. A report requested by the defence solicitor, on the other hand, may be retained by the solicitor if it does not help his client.

6. Regarding medical reports in litigation cases, the psychiatrist is in a contractual relationship with the litigant for the report.

False: The psychiatrist has a contractual relationship with the Court and no other body for the purpose of the report.

7. Fitness to plead is affected by amnesia for the criminal event.

False: The test of fitness to plead derives from R vs. Pritchard (1836). The test is of the following:

- To plead with understanding to the indictment,
- To comprehend the course of proceedings to make a proper defence,
- To know that he might challenge a juror,
- To comprehend the details of evidence and
- To be able to instruct legal advisors.

There is no connection with amnesia for the criminal event (Gunn & Taylor 1993, p. 44; Johnstone et al 2004, p. 717; Stone et al 2000, p. 55).

8. Compensation neurosis is particularly common after accidents involving loss of consciousness.

False: The level of psychological damage is more important than the severity of the injury. There is no correlation with the nature and severity of injuries (Gunn & Taylor 1993, p. 415).

9. Two-thirds of juvenile offenders have a family history of high crime rate.

False: There is undoubtedly a family link but the influence is not as high as two-thirds. Other mediating factors like schooling, neighbourhood and life experiences need to be taken into account.

10. Indecent exposure is most likely to be directed at teenagers.

True: The victims are often pubescent or pre-pubescent girls (Gunn & Taylor 1993, p. 547; Stone et al 2000, p. 215).

11. Aetiological possibilities in a 65-year-old male with a good pre-morbid personality who exposes himself in public for the first time include pneumonia.

True: The commonest illnesses in elderly offenders are affective illnesses, dementia, poor physical health and alcoholism. Though rare, this could represent disturbed behaviour in the context of delirium secondary to pneumonia (Gunn & Taylor 1993, p. 325).

12. In sex offenders with learning disabilities the ineffectiveness of preventative work is indicated by the increasing number of hospital orders.

False: Preventative work, e.g. sex education and counselling, is strongly indicated, along with supervision. Hospitalization is indicated only for the rare serious cases (Chiswick & Cope 1995, p. 74).

13. People with learning difficulties are more likely to commit serious acts of violence.

False: There is an association between learning difficulty and sexual offences, particularly exposure in males, and arson. No other crime is closely associated with learning disabilities. There is no specific evidence for increased incidence of murder or other acts of violence (Bouras 1999, p. 233; Gelder et al 2006, p. 735).

14. A full history and mental state examination will in most cases result in disclosure of intra-familial abuse.

False: Not unless there is good rapport and one asks for it specifically. Even then, disclosure is notoriously difficult.

15. The accounts of patients who report memories of sexual abuse for the first time during or after psychological therapy are usually reliable.

True: The incidence of false allegation, even in cases of custody battles, where there is clear evidence of advantage in court from the disclosure, is about 2%.

16. Young girls are twice as likely as young boys to be targeted by paedophiles.

True: According to a MORI survey of the population of Great Britain, the number of women sexually abused before the age of 16 was approximately twice that of men (Bluglass & Bowden 1990, p. 740).

17. Erotomania is the commonest delusion in stalkers.

True: Erotomanic delusions are the commonest in stalkers. However, delusions of jealousy, persecutory delusions, querulant delusions and misidentification syndromes are also encountered. The erotomanic delusions may be due to primary erotomania, or may be a feature of other disorders, such as schizophrenia, bipolar disorder or major depression (Gelder et al 2006, p. 742; Johnstone et al 2004, p. 708).

18. A 50-year-old woman with no previous offences is convicted of shoplifting. It is likely that she was depressed at the time of the offence.

False: Most shoplifting has no association with any mental disorder. Only a minority suffer from psychiatric disorders. They include depressives, those with substance misuse who may steal because of economic necessity, those with eating disorders who steal food impulsively, those with organic mental disorders who are confused, distracted or forgetful and those who may run out of the shop without paying in a panic attack. An association between shoplifting and depression is largely derived from historical literature. Folklore and anecdote point to an association between shoplifting and depression in the elderly, but the evidence is poor (Gelder et al 2000, p. 2052; Johnstone et al 2004, p. 715; Wright et al 2005, p. 469).

19. Arsonists are over-represented among learning-disabled offenders.

True: People with learning difficulties are more likely to commit fire-setting offences or sexual offences. The reasons may include conflicts that are difficult to verbalize, displaced passive aggression, or a sense of power or excitement. Arson is a common index offence among people with learning difficulties in secure hospitals (Gelder et al 2000, p. 2047; Stone et al 2000, p. 203; Johnstone et al 2004, p. 715).

20. A conviction of arson leads to a compulsory custodial sentence.

False: Only a tiny proportion of arsonists receive a psychiatric disposal in court. There is no mandatory sentence (Johnstone et al 2004, p. 715).

21. Alcohol is frequently associated with crimes of murder.

True: In a Scottish sample of 400 individuals charged with murder, 58% of males and 30% of females were intoxicated at the time of the crime. Over a third of the victims also were abusing alcohol (Gelder et al 2000, p. 2047).

22. McNaughton was acquitted of murder on grounds of insanity.

True: A verdict of Not Guilty by Reason of Insanity (NGRI) is based on the McNaughton Rules. This states that 'to establish a defence on the grounds of insanity, it must be clearly proved that at the time of committing the act, the accused party was labouring under such a defect of reason, resulting from disease of the mind, so as not to know the nature and quality of the act he was doing, or if he did know it, that he did not know that what he was doing was wrong' (Gelder et al 2000, p. 2092).

23. In homicide followed by suicide, there are more likely to be multiple murders.

True: Killers who commit suicide are more likely to be responsible for several killings at one time. The majority kill their relatives. Spousal murder–suicide is the commonest type (Gelder et al 2006, p. 739; Gunn & Taylor 1993, p. 516).

24. Mothers who kill their children within 24 h of birth would usually have gone through their pregnancy with denial or dissociation.

False: D'Orban (1979) found that most offenders who attempted to kill children within 24 hours of birth had no demonstrable psychiatric abnormality (Chiswick & Cope 1995, p. 120).

25. XYY is present more often in forensic settings.

False: Up to 3% of patients in maximum security hospitals may have XYY karyotype. This was considered disproportionately high. It was also thought to reflect the dull-normal IQ along with judges taking a more serious view of an offender with above-average height. However, it is now known that the prevalence of XYY karyotype is much higher in the general population than previously thought (Bluglass & Bowden 1990, p. 376; Gelder et al 2000, p. 932; Johnstone et al 2004, p. 548).

Forensic – 3

Piyal Sen

	T	F
1. Adversarial legal systems are inquisitory in nature.	☐	☐
2. A power of attorney is a means whereby one person gives legal authority to another person to manage their affairs.	☐	☐
3. The nearest relative in mental health legislation can be an illegitimate son.	☐	☐
4. A medicolegal report should enhance the case of the party requesting it.	☐	☐
5. In civil cases, the medicolegal report should recommend the damages to be awarded.	☐	☐
6. Those suffering from a severe mental illness are unlikely to be fit to plead.	☐	☐
7. Females have a higher rate of emotional disorders than conduct disorder.	☐	☐
8. The heritability of antisocial behaviour is 0.6–0.8.	☐	☐
9. Indecent exposure may proceed to physical assault.	☐	☐
10. Sexual offending in learning disabilities is usually due to hypersexuality.	☐	☐
11. In sex offenders with learning disabilities, cyproterone acetate is the treatment of choice for males because they are unable to benefit from psychosocial interventions.	☐	☐
12. People with learning disabilities have higher conviction rates than the general population.	☐	☐
13. Recent disclosure of child sexual abuse in a family is an indication for removing the child from the family.	☐	☐
14. Components of treatment planning for sexually abused children include a timetable for expected change.	☐	☐
15. The number of previous convictions is the best indicator of risk of re-offending in paedophilia.	☐	☐
16. In group rape, it is likely that alcohol has been consumed.	☐	☐
17. A woman of 50, with no previous offences, is convicted of shoplifting. It is likely that she needed the articles she stole.	☐	☐
18. Patients with schizophrenia commit arson usually due to their delusions.	☐	☐
19. For arson there is a mandatory custodial sentence or hospital order.	☐	☐

T F

20. Mental illness is uncommon in cases of homicide. ☐ ☐

21. The term 'abnormal homicide' refers to homicides committed when the mental state was abnormal. ☐ ☐

22. Patients with psychoses who kill do so because they are responding to hallucinations or delusions. ☐ ☐

23. Homicide followed by suicide is more likely than not to be associated with a mental illness. ☐ ☐

24. Police attending pubs at closing time reduces crime. ☐ ☐

25. In the prison population, relatively more white people are diagnosed to have psychosis than black people. ☐ ☐

ANSWERS

1. Adversarial legal systems are inquisitory in nature.

False: Adversarial systems are not inquisitory, but accusatory. The evidence of the prosecution is heard first, followed by the evidence of the defence. On the strength of this evidence a decision about guilt in Criminal Courts or responsibility in Civil Courts is made (Stone et al 2000, p. 24).

2. A power of attorney is a means whereby one person gives legal authority to another person to manage their affairs.

True: In making the power of attorney, the donor must have the capacity to give the power. The Enduring Power of Attorney Act, 1985, enables a power of attorney to be continued beyond the failure of the donor's mental capacity. If the donor lacks capacity, the arrangements have to be registered with the Court of Protection.

3. The nearest relative in mental health legislation can be an illegitimate son.

True: A nearest relative means any of the following persons: (a) husband or wife (b) son or daughter (c) father or mother (d) brother or sister (e) grandparent (f) grandchild (g) uncle or aunt (h) nephew or niece. Relatives of whole blood are preferred to relatives of half blood and the elder is preferred to younger relatives. Husband or wife is defined as the person living with the patient as their husband or wife for at least 6 months. In special cases, where a person is not a relative, they can be a relative if the patient has been residing with them for a period of not less than 5 years. Preference would also be given to the relative with whom the patient ordinarily resides or is cared for. The patient's children get priority over his/her parents as nearest relative. An illegitimate child should be treated as a legitimate child of the mother.

4. A medicolegal report should enhance the case of the party requesting it.

False: The foremost duty of the psychiatrist is to the Court and to help the Court in reaching a conclusion on the case. The report should be sufficiently detailed to be able to stand on its own to win the Court's confidence. The report should not necessarily aim at enhancing the case of one party or another, as the status of the expert is that of an independent witness, even though he/she might be instructed by one party.

5. In civil cases, the medicolegal report should recommend the damages to be awarded.

False: While discussing the question of psychological damage, the report should comment on the mental health of the patient before the accident, the mental health immediately after the accident and the mental health at the time of the examination. The report should include the diagnosis and opinions on prognosis and the dysfunction caused by the psychiatric disorder. However, no recommendation on the damages to be ordered should be made, as this is a job for the Court.

6. Those suffering from a severe mental illness are unlikely to be fit to plead.

False: The defendant might be actively psychotic and suffering from a severe mental disorder or mental impairment and yet be fit to plead (Gunn & Taylor 1993, p. 44; Stone et al 2000, p. 55).

7. Females have a higher rate of emotional disorders than conduct disorder.

True: Girls suffer more from emotional disorders, whereas boys suffer more from conduct disorders and mixed disorders of conduct and emotion. The predisposing factors include family discord, parental psychiatric disorder, social disadvantage and inferior quality of schooling. Subsequent disturbed behaviour is also associated with chronic illness, handicap and language delay (Gelder et al 2000, pp. 1689, 1697).

8. The heritability of antisocial behaviour is 0.6–0.8.

False: 0.41–0.5 (Johnstone et al 2004, p. 701).

9. Indecent exposure may proceed to physical assault.

True: A small minority of exhibitionists escalate their offending to commit sexual assaults (Gunn & Taylor 1993, p. 547; Stone et al 2000, p. 215).

10. Sexual offending in learning disabilities is usually due to hypersexuality.

False: It is often due to poor social and relationship skills. It is much more a result of a maturational defect (Bluglass & Bowden 1990, p. 404).

11. In sex offenders with learning disabilities, cyproterone acetate is the treatment of choice for males because they are unable to benefit from psychosocial interventions.

False: Psychosocial interventions, e.g. sex education and counselling, are the treatments of choice for minor offenders. People with learning disabilities are often able to benefit from psychosocial interventions. Sex drive suppressant drugs such as cyproterone acetate can often be an adjunct to management. They may help reduce libido to a level where the individual can better control it. However, they do not substitute for psychosocial interventions (Bluglass & Bowden 1990, p. 414; Chiswick & Cope 1995, p. 74).

12. People with learning disabilities have higher conviction rates than the general population.

False: The prevalence of offending in the population with learning disabilities is low, around 1%. There is over-representation of those with borderline learning disabilities. Surveys of convicted prisoners do not show an over-representation of those with learning disabilities in the UK, but they do in other countries. For example, in Australia, 12–13% of convicted prisoners have learning disabilities (Fraser & Kerr 2003, p. 290).

13. Recent disclosure of child sexual abuse in a family is an indication for removing the child from the family.

False: Every effort is normally made to keep the child within the family. The usual practice is to remove the incest perpetrator from the family environment soon after disclosure so that the initial assessment is not hindered (Bluglass & Bowden 1990, p. 754).

14. Components of treatment planning for sexually abused children include a timetable for expected change.

False: The treatment plan in child sexual abuse includes initial evaluation, disclosure, treatment of the perpetrator, risk assessment, child protection plan, counselling for partner and treatment for the victim. A timetable for expected change is not an essential component. The legal process takes its course in parallel with the treatment.

15. The number of previous convictions is the best indicator of risk of re-offending in paedophilia.

True: The strongest predictor of sexual recidivism in paedophilia is sexual interest in children. A meta-analysis of 61 studies identified antisocial personality disorder, a high number of previous offences, younger age of offending, and being single as predictors of sex offender recidivism (Hanson & Bussiere 1998).

16. In group rape, it is likely that alcohol has been consumed.

True: Gang rapes are characterized by more alcohol and drug involvement, fewer weapons, more night attacks, less victim resistance, and more severe sexual assault outcomes compared with individual rapes. Alcohol is the drug most commonly associated with all kinds of violent and sexual crime, particularly by males. Alcohol consumption has been reported prior to offending in 50% of individual rapes.

17. A woman of 50, with no previous offences, is convicted of shoplifting. It is likely that she needed the articles she stole.

False: In most cases, the shoplifter would have no need for the articles chosen for stealing (Gelder et al 2000, p. 980; Johnstone et al 2004, p. 715; Wright et al 2005, p. 469).

18. Patients with schizophrenia commit arson usually due to their delusions.

False: The relationship between arson and psychiatric abnormality may be direct, where the patient is acting on a delusion or other psychotic phenomena, but may be indirect, reflecting stressors secondary to the illness. The history of previous fire setting and offending, understanding the precipitant to the fire setting and the subject's own account of his fantasies and impulses are important in assessing the risk of recidivism (Johnstone et al 2004, p. 715; Stone et al 2000, p. 109).

19. For arson there is a mandatory custodial sentence or hospital order.

False: There is no mandatory sentence for arson. It depends at least in part on the severity of the crime and the risk of re-offending. However, re-offending rates are very low in those who have served custodial sentences. Arsonists with learning disabilities or mental illness might be more likely to re-offend (Gelder et al 2000, p. 2057).

20. Mental illness is uncommon in cases of homicide.

True: Figures vary for the incidence of mental illness in homicide. However, it seems to be less than 20%. Over the last 30 years, the contribution of mental disorder to homicide has decreased further. The National Confidential Inquiry found only 5% of homicides to be committed by people with schizophrenia.

Of the 1594 people convicted of homicide in England and Wales during 1996–99, 545 (34%) had a mental disorder: most had not attended psychiatric services; 85 (5%) had schizophrenia (lifetime); 164 (10%) had symptoms of mental illness at the time of the offence; 149 (9%) received a diminished responsibility verdict and 111 (7%) a hospital disposal – both were associated with severe mental illness and symptoms of psychosis. Most perpetrators with a history of mental disorder were not acutely ill or under mental health care at the time of the offence (Shaw et al 2006; Stone et al 2000, p. 130; Taylor & Gunn 1999).

21. The term 'abnormal homicide' refers to homicides committed when the mental state was abnormal.

False: Homicides are divided into 'normal' and 'abnormal' based on the legal outcome. Homicide is 'normal' if there is a conviction for murder or manslaughter. Homicide is 'abnormal' if there is a finding of insane murder, suicide murder, diminished responsibility or infanticide (Gelder et al 2006, p. 738).

22. Patients with psychoses who kill do so because they are responding to hallucinations or delusions.

False: Less than half of psychotic offenders describe psychotic motivation, usually delusions, for their offences. Command hallucinations are not particularly associated with murder. There is a motive in most offences.

Of the 1594 people convicted of homicide in England and Wales during 1996–99, 545 (34%) had a mental disorder. However, only 5% had psychotic symptoms and 6% had symptoms of depression at the time of the offence (Gelder et al 2000, p. 2044; Shaw et al 2006).

23. Homicide followed by suicide is more likely than not to be associated with a mental illness.

True: In the UK, homicide is followed by suicide in 10% of cases. A third to a half of all homicides in the UK are 'abnormal' homicides. In most cases the offender had severe depression at the time of the offence. Other causes include jealousy, paranoid disorders and intoxication (Gelder et al 2006, p. 739).

24. Police attending pubs at closing time reduces crime.

True: There is a clustering of offending behaviour at pub closing time, when people come on to the streets with high blood alcohol levels. There is a close relationship between alcohol use and criminal activity. The presence of police at pub closing time will therefore help to reduce the possibility of crime as the police can take preventive action.

25. In the prison population relatively more white people are diagnosed to have psychosis than black people.

False: There is an over-representation of black people among those who are imprisoned, among those who are diagnosed to have psychosis and among the prisoners who are diagnosed to have psychosis. The higher rates of imprisonment might be explained by higher rates of conduct disorder, adolescent-onset criminality and disadvantage within the criminal justice system (Coid et al 2002).

Forensic – 4

Piyal Sen

		T	F
1.	Common Law is based on past judgement of cases.	☐	☐
2.	Dementia excludes testamentary capacity.	☐	☐
3.	Mental health legislation defines the term mental illness.	☐	☐
4.	Perinatal insult increases the risk of violence in later life.	☐	☐
5.	A report to a criminal court may include an opinion on the guilt of the accused.	☐	☐
6.	'Nervous shock' is the legal equivalent of post-traumatic stress disorder.	☐	☐
7.	Being unfit to plead is a common outcome in defendants with mental illness.	☐	☐
8.	Most convicted juveniles are aged 15–16 years.	☐	☐
9.	With non-insane automatism there is a compulsory custodial sentence.	☐	☐
10.	The majority of exhibitionists do not re-offend after a court appearance.	☐	☐
11.	Individual therapy is better than group therapy for the treatment of sexual offences by patients with learning disabilities.	☐	☐
12.	In sex offenders with learning disabilities, understanding the patient's capacity to interpret the world is helpful in assessing dangerousness.	☐	☐
13.	The mean age of offenders with learning disability is higher than that of normal offenders.	☐	☐
14.	Women who are sexually abused by their fathers often disclose to their sisters.	☐	☐
15.	Victims of childhood sexual abuse have a higher incidence of alcohol and drug abuse in later life.	☐	☐
16.	Public exposure is an effective treatment for paedophilia.	☐	☐
17.	In domestic violence women strike first in 20% of cases.	☐	☐
18.	Arson is likely to be repeated if associated with epilepsy.	☐	☐
19.	Men who commit arson do so more for sexual excitement than for fraudulent insurance claims.	☐	☐
20.	Criminal convictions for arson have been on the increase.	☐	☐
21.	30% of homicides are committed by people with mental illness.	☐	☐

T F

22. There is a strong relationship between epilepsy and homicide.

23. A conviction of infanticide leads to a fixed sentence.

24. There is an excess of XYY males in the prison population than can be explained by chance.

25. 25% of prisoners have epilepsy.

ANSWERS

1. Common Law is based on past judgement of cases.

True: The Common Law is often used in the English-speaking world. It is made by judges. It is often based on case law. Common Law has no function if there is applicable statutory law.

2. Dementia excludes testamentary capacity.

False: Testamentary capacity is the capacity to make a valid will, i.e. the person is able to understand the nature of the document, the extent of the property to be disposed of and the claims of other people upon it. One can suffer from dementia and yet retain testamentary capacity. The criteria are legal and not medical. When making an assessment, the person's memory and orientation as well as psychiatric symptoms like hallucinations, delusions and abnormality of mood should be noted (Gunn & Taylor 1993, p. 109).

3. Mental health legislation defines the term mental illness.

False: Mental health legislation does not define the term 'mental illness'. It is a matter for clinical judgement. In practice, psychiatrists use this term to cover a wide range of psychiatric disorders.

4. Perinatal insult increases the risk of violence in later life.

True: Perinatal insult can lead to minimal brain damage which may increase the risk of impulsive and aggressive behaviour later on in life (Stone et al 2000, p. 265).

5. A report to a criminal court may include an opinion on the guilt of the accused.

False: No opinion on the guilt of the accused should be voiced. That is entirely a matter for the court. However, the report can state the intention of the defendant regarding what plea he/she wishes to enter.

6. 'Nervous shock' is the legal equivalent of post-traumatic stress disorder.

False: Psychiatric damage is often referred to by lawyers as 'nervous shock'. Lord Bridge suggested three criteria for nervous shock:

1. The plaintiff must be suffering from a 'positive psychiatric illness'
2. A chain of causation between the negligent act and the psychiatric illness must be clearly established

3. The chain of causation was 'reasonably foreseeable' by the reasonable person. The psychiatrist can express a view on the first of the criteria but would find it difficult to express a definite view on the second and the third. The term PTSD is simply one rather special kind of anxiety state. Serious trauma and threats to life can precipitate many other kinds of psychiatric disorder. Thus, nervous shock is not the legal equivalent of PTSD alone (Gunn & Taylor 1993, p. 102).

7. Being unfit to plead is a common outcome in defendants with mental illness.

False: Despite the large number of recorded crimes and the high prevalence of mental illness in the defendants, the number of cases found unfit to plead and given a restriction order is less than 50 per year (Chiswick & Cope 1995, p. 110; Johnstone et al 2004, p. 718).

8. Most convicted juveniles are aged 15–16 years.

True: Young people aged below 17 are commonly known as juveniles, as stated by the Home Office in The Sentence of the Court (HMSO 1986, Ch. 11). The conviction rates for juvenile offenders continue to rise. The peak age for offending is between 14 and 17 years. Thus, to qualify for the label of juvenile, most convictions will be those between 15 and 16 years (Chick & Cantwell 1994, p. 14).

9. With non-insane automatism there is a compulsory custodial sentence.

False: Subject is found Not Guilty by Reason of Insanity (NGRI). This results in acquittal (Stone et al 2000, p. 61).

10. The majority of exhibitionists do not re-offend after a court appearance.

True: The court appearance itself seems to have a deterrent effect (Gunn & Taylor 1993, p. 547; Stone et al 2000, p. 215).

11. Individual therapy is better than group therapy for the treatment of sexual offences by patients with learning disabilities.

False: Despite significant numbers of offenders with learning disabilities, evidence regarding treatment and its outcome is limited. For sex offenders with learning disabilities, group cognitive behavioural treatments have shown some benefit though most studies were small scale. Moreover, the Prison Sex Offender Treatment Programme tends to exclude people with an IQ of less than 80 (Barron et al 2002; Stone et al 2000, p. 229).

12. In sex offenders with learning disabilities, understanding the patient's capacity to interpret the world is helpful in assessing dangerousness.

True: The capacity to interpret the world will provide some indication of the capacity for self-regulation, which is important to assess in sex offenders with learning disabilities (Bluglass & Bowden 1990, p. 414).

13. The mean age of offenders with learning disability is higher than that of normal offenders.

False: Most people with learning disabilities who are convicted of offences are young males of similar age range to the general offending population (Bouras 1999, p. 232).

14. Women who are sexually abused by their fathers often disclose to their sisters.

False: Disclosure is most likely to the mother. The next most likely person to hear about it would be a trusted outsider, e.g. a friend, older relative or school teacher. Some studies of incest show that a sister who was not the object of the sexual relationship might be more psychologically damaged by the incest and so the abused woman may be less likely to disclose to her (Bluglass & Bowden 1990, p. 754).

15. Victims of childhood sexual abuse have a higher incidence of alcohol and drug abuse in later life.

True: There is an association between childhood sexual abuse and adult personality difficulties and alcohol and drug abuse.

16. Public exposure is an effective treatment for paedophilia.

False: The greatest factor predicting recidivism in paedophilia is the attraction towards children. Public exposure would only serve to drive paedophiles underground and away from help-seeking behaviour.

17. In domestic violence, women strike first in 20% of cases.

False: Women initiate violence in only about 10% of cases. However, the overall incidence of wife-battering and husband-battering is similar. The frequency of aggression classified as homicide, battery, assault with a weapon or rape is greater among males (Sadock & Sadock 2002, p. 151).

18. Arson is likely to be repeated if associated with epilepsy.

False: Recidivism rates are low in arson. There is no known association between epilepsy and arson (Stone et al 2000, p. 108).

19. Men who commit arson do so more for sexual excitement than for fraudulent insurance claims.

False: Insurance fraud is a far commoner reason than sexual excitement for committing arson (Gelder et al 2000, p. 2057; Stone et al 2000, p. 107).

20. Criminal convictions for arson have been on the increase.

False: Arson is a notoriously difficult offence to detect and to convict. Overall, conviction rates continue to be low (Stone et al 2000, p. 108).

21. 30% of homicides are committed by people with mental illness.

True: The 5 year report of the National Confidential Inquiry was published in December 2006.

Of the 2670 people convicted of homicide in England and Wales during 1999–2003, 806 (30%) had a lifetime mental disorder: a half had not attended psychiatric services; 141 (5%) had schizophrenia (lifetime); 261 (10%) had symptoms of mental illness at the time of the offence; 106 (4%) received a diminished responsibility verdict and 154 (6%) a hospital disposal – both were associated with severe mental illness and symptoms of psychosis. Two-thirds of perpetrators with a history of mental disorder were not acutely ill or under mental health care at the time of the offence.

22. There is a strong relationship between epilepsy and homicide.

False: The rates of homicide in patients suffering from epilepsy are the same as the general population (Gelder et al 2000, p. 2047).

23. A conviction of infanticide leads to a fixed sentence.

False: The sentencing guidelines are the same for infanticide and manslaughter and include no fixed sentence.

24. There is an excess of XYY males in the prison population than can be explained by chance.

False: Up to 3% of patients in maximum security hospitals may have an XYY karyotype. In the 1960s this was considered disproportionately high but it is now known that the prevalence of XYY in the general population is higher than was thought at that time. No direct connection between XYY genotype and either aggressive or criminal behaviour has been established though the slightly lower than average IQ seen in this group may predispose to behavioural problems (Bluglass & Bowden 1990, p. 376; Gelder et al 2000, p. 932; Johnstone et al 2004, p. 548).

25. 25% of prisoners have epilepsy.

False: The prevalence of epilepsy in prisoners is approximately 1% (Fazel et al 2002).

Human development

Carla Sharp and K. Martin Beckmann

	T	F
1. Neonates prefer face shapes.	☐	☐
2. The onset of puberty differs by 4–5 years between boys and girls.	☐	☐
3. Adolescent peer culture is largely in opposition to parental values.	☐	☐
4. Maternal ambivalence about the pregnancy may hinder bonding.	☐	☐
5. Indiscriminate attention-seeking in a 6-month-old infant suggests insecure attachment.	☐	☐
6. According to Ainsworth's Strange Situation procedure, a 15-month-old baby not becoming upset when the mother leaves indicates secure attachment.	☐	☐
7. In an 18-month-old child, a puzzled expression when the mother re-enters the room during the Strange Situation procedure is a sign of insecure attachment.	☐	☐
8. Subsequent to psychological trauma, children demonstrate strengthened attachments.	☐	☐
9. Child abuse is associated with increased attachment behaviour.	☐	☐
10. Attachment behaviour depends mainly on parental reinforcement.	☐	☐
11. A child comfortably playing with a stranger in the absence of the mother suggests insecure attachment.	☐	☐
12. Insecure attachment is associated with non-accidental injuries.	☐	☐
13. Secure attachment is easier if the child is adopted rather than institutionalized.	☐	☐
14. Disruptions in childcare have their greatest effects from 9 to 36 months of age.	☐	☐
15. Children with insecure attachment may show disinhibited behaviour.	☐	☐
16. Insecure attachment may be evidenced by the child showing little or no emotion when the attachment figure returns.	☐	☐
17. Those who were securely attached in childhood show better social skills in adulthood.	☐	☐
18. Attachment behaviour precedes object constancy.	☐	☐
19. Object constancy occurs before the onset of stranger anxiety.	☐	☐

T F

20. Object constancy and separation anxiety appear together. ☐ ☐

21. Moral development shows a gender difference. ☐ ☐

22. Piaget's theory of conservation states that a child cannot reverse his action. ☐ ☐

23. In Piaget's model, sensory information is received according to cognitive schemes. ☐ ☐

24. According to Piaget's theory, experiences are stored as personal constructs. ☐ ☐

25. When a child is hospitalized, complete separation causes less disturbance than repeated visiting in the hospital. ☐ ☐

ANSWERS

1. Neonates prefer face shapes.

   True: It has long been known that preference for and tracking of face shapes is present at 4 days. More recently preference for face shapes has been demonstrated in neonates as young as 43 minutes of age. However, neonates cannot discriminate a static face from an equally complex pattern (Gross 2001, p. 235).

2. The onset of puberty differs by 4–5 years between boys and girls.

   False: Age of onset of puberty in boys is between 10 and 14 years (mean = 13).

   Girls enter puberty on average 12–18 months earlier than boys, i.e. between 8 and 13 years (mean = 11). Thus, the mean difference is only 2 years (Gross 2001, p. 534; Sadock & Sadock 2005, p. 3038).

3. Adolescent peer culture is largely in opposition to parental values.

   False: Peer group friendships provide important support, feedback and companionship to adolescents. They become important points of reference in their social development and provide social contexts for shaping day-to-day values. However, parents continue to have a strong influence on their children's identities and values. Adolescents tend to choose peers who share their own values and have similar identities. Thus, peer and friendship groups work in concert with, rather than in opposition to, adult values, attitudes, goals and achievements (Gross 2001, p. 540; Sadock & Sadock 2005, p. 3040).

4. Maternal ambivalence about the pregnancy may hinder bonding.

   True: Bonding refers to the mother's feelings for and relationship to her infant. Bonding is different from attachment, which concerns the infant's relationship with the mother. Bonding consists of feelings aroused by the neonate that result in affectionate, nurturing and protective behaviour. Ambivalence about pregnancy can affect bonding (Gelder et al 2000, p. 1203; Sadock & Sadock 2005, p. 145).

5. Indiscriminate attention-seeking in a 6-month-old infant suggests insecure attachment.

False: Infants show indiscriminate attachment behaviour to any friendly person until age 7–8 months. At around 4–6 months infants start showing increasing differential preference for their mother. Stranger distress and strange place distress develop by 7–9 months. Moreover, at 6 months the infant is too young to have attachment problems (Atkinson et al 2000, p. 89; Sadock & Sadock 2002, p. 141).

6. According to Ainsworth's Strange Situation procedure, a 15-month-old baby not becoming upset when the mother leaves indicates secure attachment.

False: The Strange Situation procedure is a test designed by Mary Ainsworth. It examines the behaviour of children (aged 1 year) and aims to provide information on attachment. The essential steps of the procedure are as follows. Firstly a mother and baby enter a room and the baby is encouraged to play with some toys. Then a stranger enters and plays with the baby. Next, the mother leaves, and the stranger attempts to soothe any distress. The mother returns and the stranger leaves. Then the mother leaves the baby alone before the stranger and then the mother return.

Using this procedure Ainsworth described three attachment styles, anxious-avoidant, anxious-resistant and securely attached. An insecure-disorganized category is often also added. Securely attached children show distress when the mother leaves, seek her out on return and are quickly calmed when they do so. Around 65% of children fall into this category. The exact responses of the different attachment styles to different stages of the test appear in the exam and thus it is an area worth studying in more detail (Atkinson et al 2000, p. 90; Fear 2004, p. 509; Gross 2001, p. 465; Sadock & Sadock 2002, p. 141; Wright et al 2005, p. 58).

7. In an 18-month-old child, a puzzled expression when the mother re-enters the room during the Strange Situation procedure is a sign of insecure attachment.

False: Insecure attachment is evidenced by either ignoring/avoiding the mother on her return (the anxious–avoidant child) or by seeking contact whilst simultaneously showing anger and resisting contact (the anxious–resistant child), or by contradictory approach–avoidance and disorganized behaviour (the disorganized/disoriented child) (Atkinson et al 2000, p. 90; Fear 2004, p. 509; Gelder et al 2000, p. 265; Gross 2001, p. 465).

8. Subsequent to psychological trauma, children demonstrate strengthened attachments.

False: Following psychological trauma, children may show weaker attachments to others. However, children show increased attachment behaviour when under threat (Fear 2004, p. 510; Gross 2001, p. 466).

9. Child abuse is associated with increased attachment behaviour.

True: Abused children often maintain their attachments to their abusive parents and show increased attachment behaviour. When children are hungry, sick, in pain or when rejected by their parents, they show increased attachment behaviour. Whilst there is a positive relationship between child abuse and attachment *behaviour*, child abuse is also associated with an insecure attachment *style* (Sadock & Sadock 2005, p. 3251).

10. Attachment behaviour depends mainly on parental reinforcement.

False: Attachment behaviour depends mainly on parental sensitivity. A sensitive mother is responsive to the child's needs, accepting, cooperative and accessible and promotes secure attachment in the child. By contrast, the insensitive mother interacts according to her own wishes, moods and activities and promotes insecure attachments (Gelder et al 2000, p. 351; Gross 2001, p. 465).

11. A child comfortably playing with a stranger in the absence of the mother suggests insecure attachment.

True: Attachment behaviour peaks at 18 months. Although a secure child will tolerate a stranger, s/he would not be happy. An insecure avoidant child can play as happily with a stranger as with a mother. An insecure resistant–ambivalent child would resist a stranger's efforts to make contact (Atkinson et al 2000, p. 92; Gelder et al 2000, p. 265; Gross 2001, p. 465).

12. Insecure attachment is associated with non-accidental injuries.

True: Disorganized–disoriented attachment is associated with maternal psychopathology, child maltreatment, family violence and poor parental sensitivity to infant cues. Non-accidental injuries indicate abusive care. Physically abused children tend to have insecure and atypical attachment patterns (Sadock & Sadock 2005, pp. 3249, 3415).

13. Secure attachment is easier if the child is adopted rather than institutionalized.

True: Children who have been adopted often develop secure attachments, albeit later. Institutionalized children are much less likely than adopted children to recover from deprivation and to develop secure attachments (Gross 2001, p. 467).

14. Disruptions in childcare have their greatest effects from 9 to 36 months of age.

True: Separation is likely to cause most distress between age 7 months when attachments are beginning to develop and 36 months when most children are secure enough to interact comfortably with other children and adults in the absence of their parents. The maximum distress would be at 12–18 months. This is related to the child's inability to maintain a mental picture of the mother when she is absent; inability to remember that mother did come back previously after brief periods of separation; limited ability to understand explanations such as 'mother will come back soon' and 'grandmother will look after you until then' (Atkinson et al 2000, p. 89; Gelder et al 2000, p. 1692; Gross 2001, p. 468).

15. Children with insecure attachment may show disinhibited behaviour.

True: Insecure attachment is associated with indiscriminate attachment and disinhibited behaviour. In Disinhibited Reactive Attachment Disorder the child participates in diffuse attachments and demonstrates indiscriminate sociability and excessive familiarity with strangers. The onset is before age 5 years. It is associated with 'grossly pathological care' in which there is a disregard for a child's emotional and physical needs, abuse, or frequent changes in caregivers. Since the latter factors are also associated with insecure attachment, it is appropriate to conclude that children with insecure attachment may show disinhibited behaviour (DSM-IV 1994; Sadock & Sadock 2005, p. 1236).

16. Insecure attachment may be evidenced by the child showing little or no emotion when the attachment figure returns.

True: The insecure anxious–avoidant child is indifferent towards the mother. Play is little affected by whether the mother is present or absent. The child shows little distress when the mother leaves, and avoids her on her return (Fear 2004, p. 509; Gross 2001, p. 465; Sadock & Sadock 2005, p. 3428).

17. Those who were securely attached in childhood show better social skills in adulthood.

True: There is continuity of an infant's attachment styles through childhood and adulthood. The early attachment experiences are internalized in 'internal working models', i.e. a mental model of the relations between self and significant others. Childhood attachments become templates for future relationships. Those who had secure attachments expect others to be caring and trustworthy, while those who were neglected or rejected as children grow up expecting others to reject them. Securely attached infants become adults with better self-esteem and positive outlook and are more sociable and cooperative in their relationships (Gelder et al 2000, p. 1692; Gross 2001, p. 465).

18. Attachment behaviour precedes object constancy.

True: The earliest normal attachment behaviours are the reflexes at birth, e.g. rooting, head turning, sucking, swallowing, hand–mouth grasp, digital extension, crying and responsiveness to mother's voice.

Object constancy is Mahler's 6th subphase and lasts from 2 to 5 years. Mahler's subphases are:

1. Normal autism (0–2 months)
2. Symbiosis (2–5 months)
3. Differentiation/Hatching (5–10 months)
4. Practising (10–18 months)
5. Rapprochement (18–24 months)
6. Object constancy (2–5 years) (Sadock & Sadock 2002, p. 141; Sadock & Sadock 2005, p. 729).

19. Object constancy occurs before the onset of stranger anxiety.

False: Stranger anxiety occurs from 7 months till the end of the first year. Object constancy is Mahler's 6th subphase and lasts from 2 to 5 years (Atkinson et al 2000, p. 89; Sadock & Sadock 2002, p. 141).

20. Object constancy and separation anxiety appear together.

False: Object constancy is Mahler's 6th subphase and lasts from 2 to 5 years. Separation anxiety, i.e. distress over separation from a parent, occurs between age 7 months when attachments are beginning to develop, and 36 months when most children are secure enough to interact comfortably with other children and adults in the absence of their parents. The maximum distress would be at 12–18 months (Atkinson et al 2000, p. 89; Gelder et al 2000, p. 1692; Gross 2001, p. 468; Sadock & Sadock 2005, p. 729).

21. Moral development shows a gender difference.

True: Kohlberg's and Piaget's notions of moral development focus on a unified theory of cognitive maturation for both sexes. Others have found no gender differences in moral development in people aged 5–63 years. However, these theories have been criticized as being male biased because they emphasize a masculine style of abstract reasoning. Critics argue that emphasizing the social context of moral development reveals different patterns in moral development. The predominant features of moral reasoning in women are compassion, caring and concern for the integrity and continuation of relationships. Those in men are related to perceptions of justice, rationality and fairness (Atkinson et al 2000, p. 87; Fear 2004, p. 50; Gross 2001, p. 534; Sadock & Sadock 2005, p. 3040).

22. Piaget's theory of conservation states that a child cannot reverse its action.

False: Piaget's concept of conservation refers to the understanding that any quantity such as number, liquid quantity, length, weight, volume, time and substance remains the same despite physical changes in the arrangement of objects. Pre-operational children cannot conserve because their thinking is dominated by the perceptual nature (appearance) of the objects but can reverse when they reach the stage of concrete operations (Fear 2004, p. 48; Gross 2001, p. 494; Sadock & Sadock 2002, p. 136; Sadock & Sadock 2005, p. 530).

23. In Piaget's model, sensory information is received according to cognitive schemes.

True: Piaget's schemes or schemas are the basic units of intelligent behaviour. How the child takes in new sensory information depends on how it fits in with existing schemes. If new experiences can be fitted into what the child can already do, they are assimilated, keeping the child in a comfortable state of equilibrium. If the new information cannot be assimilated into an existing scheme, it leads the child to a less comfortable state of disequilibrium. Hence, s/he must accommodate a scheme to bring him/herself back to equilibrium. This balance of assimilation of and accommodation to new experiences is called adaptation (Gross 2001, p. 491; Sadock & Sadock 2005, p. 529).

24. According to Piaget's theory, experiences are stored as personal constructs.

False: According to Piaget's theory of constructivism, individuals learn by actively discovering what the world is like. Schemes or schemas are the building blocks of intelligent behaviour. They are structures that organize past experience and provide a way of understanding future experiences. Schemes develop in complexity through the process of adaptation, assimilation and accommodation. In contrast, George Kelly's personal construct theory defines personal constructs as the dimensions that individuals use to interpret themselves and their social worlds (Atkinson et al 2000, p. 475; Sadock & Sadock 2002, p. 136).

25. When a child is hospitalized, complete separation causes less disturbance than repeated visiting in the hospital.

False: When a child is hospitalized, prolonged and complete separation from parents causes what René Spitz called hospitalism or anaclitic depression. They become depressed, withdrawn, non-responsive and vulnerable to physical illness, but recover when their mothers return. Hence, parents are usually allowed 24-hour visiting (Sadock & Sadock 2005, p. 2891).

Learning disability – 1

Regi T. Alexander

	T	F
1. The prevalence of learning disability (LD) is 2%.	☐	☐
2. Larger sibships in Social class IV are associated with an increased risk of LD.	☐	☐
3. If a child with LD and an autistic disorder uses few words before the age of 6 years, they are likely to remain mute.	☐	☐
4. Impaired prosody is a feature of Asperger syndrome.	☐	☐
5. Language development is delayed in Asperger syndrome.	☐	☐
6. If a couple has one child with Down's syndrome due to translocation, the risk of a subsequent child with the syndrome is about 1%.	☐	☐
7. Down's syndrome is the most common cause of learning disability.	☐	☐
8. Patients with Down's syndrome have a high risk of vascular dementia.	☐	☐
9. Down's syndrome is associated with hypertension.	☐	☐
10. Language development is normal in Down's syndrome.	☐	☐
11. A defective gene which leads to the Fragile X abnormality has been identified.	☐	☐
12. Fragile X syndrome almost never occurs in females.	☐	☐
13. Survival into adolescence is rare for patients with Hunter's syndrome.	☐	☐
14. Klinefelter syndrome occurs in 1 in 1000 live births.	☐	☐
15. Lesch–Nyhan syndrome is a sex-linked recessive disorder.	☐	☐
16. Metachromatic leucodystrophy is an X-linked recessive condition.	☐	☐
17. If a healthy couple has a baby with phenylketonuria, the chances of the next baby having the same condition are less than 1%.	☐	☐
18. People with Prader–Willi syndrome have an 'elfin' face.	☐	☐
19. Half the patients with Sturge–Weber syndrome may not have mental retardation.	☐	☐
20. Tuberous sclerosis complex may be due to a new mutation.	☐	☐
21. Most patients with Turner's syndrome have learning disabilities.	☐	☐
22. William's syndrome is due to a mutation on chromosome 13.	☐	☐
23. Irritability is a common symptom of depression in LD.	☐	☐

T F

24. Schizophrenia is rare in people with LD.

□□

25. People with learning disability are relatively immune to side-effects of antipsychotics.

□□

ANSWERS

1. The prevalence of learning disability (LD) is 2%.

True: The approximate prevalence of LD in the general population is:

- Mild =1.5 to 2%
- Moderate and severe = 0.5% (range = 0.16–0.73%) and
- Profound = 0.05% (Fraser & Kerr 2003, p. 23; Johnstone et al 2004, p. 529).

2. Larger sibships in Social class IV are associated with an increased risk of LD.

True: Mild LD is over-represented in families from Social classes IV and V and has been associated with larger sibships, room overcrowding, lower income and lower maternal education (Johnstone et al 2004, p. 530).

3. If a child with LD and an autistic disorder uses few words before the age of 6 years, they are likely to remain mute.

True: Children with LD and an autistic spectrum disorder are likely to remain mute if they are using few words before age 6. They may be able to use single words appropriately if they are using words before their 13th birthday. It they use words by 6 and phrases by 12 then they may develop phrase speech (Fraser & Kerr 2003, p. 139).

4. Impaired prosody is a feature of Asperger syndrome.

True: Prosody is the stress, intonation and tone of voice. In Asperger syndrome, expressive and receptive aspects of communication are deficient. They have difficulty in understanding emotional aspects of communication that are communicated through prosody. They are unable to appreciate situational constraints and conventions of discourse and hence often violate them (Fraser & Kerr 2003, p. 147; Harris 2000, p. 226).

5. Language development is delayed in Asperger syndrome.

False: In Asperger syndrome, there is no clinically significant general delay in spoken or receptive language. Abnormalities of speech are more subtle. Prosody (the musicality of speech) is impaired and their speech is over-precise. They may also be insensitive to the social norms surrounding conversation (Fraser & Kerr 2003, p. 147; Gelder et al 2000, p. 1729).

6. If a couple has one child with Down's syndrome due to translocation, the risk of a subsequent child with the syndrome is about 1%.

False: The disorder leading to translocation is often inherited. The risk of occurence in a subsequent child is about 10%. In the case of a trisomy 21, the risk of occurence in a subsequent child is about 1% (Gelder et al 2000, p. 1955; Gelder et al 2006, p. 718).

7. Down's syndrome is the most common cause of learning disability.

True: Down's syndrome is the most common cause of mental retardation. It affects approximately 1 in 1000 live births. Most people with Down's have an IQ between 20 and 55 (moderate to severe learning disability). Only 15% have an IQ above 50 (Gelder et al 2000, p. 1954).

8. Patients with Down's syndrome have a high risk of vascular dementia.

False: Vascular dementia is rare in Down's syndrome. Down's syndrome is considered an 'atheroma free' model. Lower blood pressure, low pulse rate and other protective factors may contribute to the reduced rates of vascular dementia. There may also be less exposure to environmental contributions such as smoking (Fraser & Kerr 2003, p. 268).

9. Down's syndrome is associated with hypertension.

False: The mean blood pressure is 115/75 mmHg. Moreover, environmental contributions such as smoking are also lower (Fraser & Kerr 2003, p. 268).

10. Language development is normal in Down's syndrome.

False: All developments slow down after the first 6 months to 1 year. Language is not an exception to this (Gelder et al 2006, p. 717).

11. A defective gene which leads to the Fragile X abnormality has been identified.

True: The Fragile X mental retardation 1 (FMR-1) gene responsible for Fragile X syndrome is caused by an abnormal nucleotide CGG repeat at a fragile site on the long arm of the X chromosome (Xq27.3) (Gelder et al 2000, p. 1953).

12. Fragile X syndrome almost never occurs in females.

False: The prevalence rates are 1:4000–4500 in men and 1:8000–9000 in women (Johnstone et al 2004, p. 548).

13. Survival into adolescence is rare for patients with Hunter's syndrome.

False: Hunter's syndrome is an X-linked mucopolysaccharide disorder. There are two forms. Type A presents with progressive LD and severe physical disabilities leading to death between 10 and 20 years of age. Type B is a milder form characterized by near normal intelligence and survival into their 60s or 70s. Type B Hunter syndrome is much harder to identify, and might only be recognized when looking at the maternal relatives of a child with Hunter syndrome (Gelder et al 2000, p. 1959; Harris 2000, p. 358).

14. Klinefelter syndrome occurs in 1 in 1000 live births.

True: Klinefelter syndrome (47XXY) occurs in 1:500 to 1:1000 men. 50% of all 47XXY conceptions are lost prenatally. One in 300 spontaneous abortions may be due to 47XXY (Johnstone et al 2004, p. 547).

15. Lesch–Nyhan syndrome is a sex-linked recessive disorder.

True: It is a sex-linked disorder that almost exclusively affects boys. It is caused by a deletion of chromosome 26. It is associated with severe learning disability, chorea, athetosis and severe self-injurious behaviour. They have hypoxanthine phosphoribosyltransferase (HPRT) deficiency resulting in defective purine metabolism (Gelder et al 2000, p. 1956; Johnstone et al 2004, p. 807; Mitchell 2004, p. 454).

16. Metachromatic leucodystrophy is an X-linked recessive condition.

False: Metachromatic leucodystrophy is an autosomal recessive disorder of neural lipid metabolism resulting in the accumulation of galactosyl sulphatide in the affected tissue. There are three forms. The infantile form starts before the age of 3 years and progresses to severe motor and mental retardation. The juvenile form is less common and presents with motor and mental dysfunction. The adult form is the rarest and may present with dementia or psychotic disorder. Metachromatic leucodystrophy and epilepsy are the only two organic brain syndromes that have a higher than chance co-occurrence with schizophrenia (Gelder et al 2000, p. 1592; Lishman 1997, p. 758).

17. If a healthy couple has a baby with phenylketonuria, the chances of the next baby having the same condition are less than 1%.

False: Phenylketonuria is an autosomal recessive disorder. Both parents have to transmit the abnormal gene in order for a child to have the disorder. Siblings of affected probands have a 1 in 4 (25%) risk.

18. People with Prader–Willi syndrome have an 'elfin' face.

False: Williams syndrome has the characteristic 'elfin' face, i.e. broad forehead, medial eyebrow flare, depressed nasal bridge, stellate pattern in the iris, widely spaced teeth, prominent lips, full prominent cheeks, wide mouth, short turned-up nose, long philtrum and flat nasal bridge (Harris 2000, p. 320; Johnstone et al 2004, p. 554).

19. Half the patients with Sturge–Weber syndrome may not have mental retardation.

True: Degree of retardation is variable. Only 50% may be retarded (Craft et al 1985, p.125).

20. Tuberous sclerosis complex may be due to a new mutation.

True: About 60% of tuberous sclerosis complex is due to new mutations leading to dysfunction of hamartin and tuberin (Gelder et al 2000, p. 1958).

21. Most patients with Turner's syndrome have learning disabilities.

False: In general the overall intelligence is normal in Turner's syndrome. There is a 'Turner neurocognitive phenotype' with normal verbal ability but visuomotor and visuospatial difficulties (Fraser & Kerr 2003, p. 89).

22. William's syndrome is due to a mutation on chromosome 13.

False: Williams syndrome is caused by a microdeletion of one elastin allele on the long arm of chromosome 7 (7q11.23) (Gelder et al 2000, p. 1957; Johnstone et al 2004, p. 555).

23. Irritability is a common symptom of depression in LD.

True: People with LD have limited communication skills and limited ability to express their subjective feelings. They are less likely than normals to complain of low mood. Depression in people with LD may manifest with irritability, unexplained temper tantrums or aggression, which are considered 'depressive equivalents' (Gelder et al 2006, p. 710; Johnstone et al 2004, p. 566).

24. Schizophrenia is rare in people with LD.

False: The prevalence of schizophrenia in people with mild and moderate LD is 3% compared to 0.4% in the general population. Schizophrenia has an earlier onset, more poverty of thinking and less elaborate delusions and hallucinations in people with LD compared to the general population.

Kraepelin named dementia praecox arising in people with pre-existing intellectual impairment as *Propfschizophrenie* (Fraser & Kerr 2003, p. 157; Gelder et al 2006, p. 709; Johnstone et al 2004, p. 563).

25. People with learning disability are relatively immune to side-effects of antipsychotics.

False: People with LD have reduced brain and other reserves. This would make them more vulnerable to all forms of stress including pharmacological. They are more likely to have side-effects and toxic effects from antipsychotic drugs. They are also more sensitive to the anticholinergic side-effects and have a high risk of delirium. However, patients with LD are less likely to report adverse effects (Fraser & Kerr 2003, p. 223).

Learning disability – 2

Asif Zia

23

	T	F

1. The prevalence of learning disability is higher among males.

2. Just below half of those with mild learning disability show definite organic factors in the aetiology.

3. A deletion in the maternally derived chromosome 15 causes Angelman syndrome.

4. Asperger syndrome is associated with a general delay in cognitive development.

5. Autistic traits are often associated with Cornelia De Lange syndrome.

6. In Down's syndrome, 50% of chromosomal disjunctions are of paternal origin.

7. Translocation Down's syndromes often have mild learning disability.

8. Down's syndrome is associated with Alzheimer's dementia.

9. In Down's syndrome, the neonate has stiff joints.

10. Fragile X syndrome is the most common inherited cause of LD.

11. Speech is normal in Fragile X syndrome.

12. Galactosaemia is an autosomal dominant condition.

13. Hunter's syndrome can be treated by dietary intervention.

14. Kleinfelter's syndrome is associated with cardiovascular disorders.

15. Lesch–Nyhan syndrome occurs almost exclusively in males.

16. Neurofibromatosis is transmitted by autosomal dominant inheritance.

17. Phenylketonuria is most commonly diagnosed by amniocentesis.

18. Rett syndrome almost exclusively affects girls.

19. Tay–Sachs disease is transmitted by X-linked recessive inheritance.

20. Autistic traits are often associated with tuberous sclerosis complex.

21. Perinatal hypoxia is a common cause of West syndrome.

22. William's syndrome is associated with loquaciousness.

23. Males with XYY tend to have short stature.

T F

24. Delirium is relatively frequent in those with learning disability. ☐ ☐

25. Normalization theory of learning disability means that people with borderline learning disability should be treated like normal individuals. ☐ ☐

ANSWERS

1. The prevalence of learning disability is higher among males.

True: Learning disability is marginally more common in males (Fraser & Kerr 2003, p. 27).

2. Just below half of those with mild learning disability show definite organic factors in the aetiology.

True: Although sociocultural influences are important, biological factors have been underplayed in the past. Up to 45% of those with mild LD may have definite organic factors including subtle chromosomal abnormalities and perinatal insults from toxins such as alcohol. However, physical causes are found in 55–75% of cases of severe LD (Gelder et al 2006, p. 713; Johnstone et al 2004, p. 530).

3. A deletion in the maternally derived chromosome 15 causes Angelman syndrome.

True: About 70% of cases of Angelman syndrome are due to a microdeletion on the long arm of the *maternally* derived chromosome 15 (15q11-13).

About 70% of Prader–Willi syndrome cases are due to a microdeletion at exactly the same point of the *paternally* derived chromosome 15.

The other mechanisms include Uni Parental Disomy (*maternal UPD* for Prader–Willi and *paternal UPD* for Angelman) and imprinting centre errors (Gelder et al 2000, p. 1958; Johnstone et al 2004, pp. 557, 805).

4. Asperger syndrome is associated with a general delay in cognitive development.

False: Both DSM-IV and ICD-10 require normal cognitive function for the diagnosis of Asperger syndrome.

5. Autistic traits are often associated with Cornelia De Lange syndrome.

True: There are a number of similarities between the two syndromes including speech deficits, repetitive and stereotyped behaviour, preference for rigid routines and rigid thinking. The degree of these autistic traits depends on the degree of cognitive disability.

Children with Cornelia De Lange syndrome show characteristic features of hypertricosis, e.g. hirsutism, synophrys and long eyelashes. The facial abnormalities include depressed nasal bridge, ocular abnormalities, prominent philtrum, thin lips, anteverted nostrils, down-turned angle of mouth, bluish tinge around the eyes, widely spaced teeth, high arched palate, low set ears, micrognathia and short neck (Gelder et al 2000, p. 1957).

6. In Down's syndrome, 50% of chromosomal disjunctions are of paternal origin.

False: 75–85% of chromosomal disjunctions are of maternal origin. The extra chromosome in trisomy 21 is maternal in over 90% of cases (Johnstone et al 2004, p. 539).

7. Translocation Down's syndromes often have mild learning disability.

False: In general, the Down's syndrome population has an IQ range of 20–55, i.e. severe to moderate LD. Those with a translocation and Trisomy 21 tend to have moderate to severe intellectual deficits. 1–3% show Mosaicism and may have normal intelligence and achievement (Gelder et al 2006, p. 717).

8. Down's syndrome is associated with Alzheimer's dementia.

True: Prevalence of Alzheimer's increases with age:

- 30–39 years = 2–3%
- 40–49 years = 9–10%
- 50–59 years = 36–40%
- 60–69 years = 55%.

Females have an earlier age of onset than males. The duration of dementia is approximately 6 years (Fraser & Kerr 2003, p. 274).

9. In Down's syndrome, the neonate has stiff joints.

False: Down's syndrome is characterized by hypotonia and hyperextensibility of joints (Gelder et al 2006, p. 717).

10. Fragile X syndrome is the most common inherited cause of LD.

True: Fragile X syndrome affects approximately 1 in 4425 to 6045 males and causes LD in 1 in 8000 females. While Fragile X syndrome is the most common *inherited* cause of LD, Down's syndrome is the most common cause of LD overall (Gelder et al 2000, p. 1953).

11. Speech is normal in Fragile X syndrome.

False: The abnormalities of speech include perseveration of words and phrases, echolalia, palilalia, 'cluttering', narrative speech, comprehension difficulties with high association compounds, productive semantic errors and speech sound substitution difficulties. Syntactic competency and semantic concepts remain intact in Fragile X males (Gelder et al 2000, p. 1954).

12. Galactosaemia is an autosomal dominant condition.

False: Galactosaemia is an autosomal recessive condition caused by the absence of galactose-1-phosphate uridyl transferase. This results in intracellular accumulation of galactose-1-phosphate which is highly toxic. The incidence is 1/60 000 in the UK. Affected infants are normal at birth. On exposure to dietary galactose they develop jaundice, vomiting, diarrhoea, failure to thrive, psychomotor retardation, hepatosplenomegaly, renal disease, cataracts, increased susceptibility to infection, hypoglycaemia, galactosaemia, galactosuria and aminoaciduria (Fanconi syndrome) (www.Gpnotebook.co.uk).

13. Hunter's syndrome can be treated by dietary intervention.

False: Hunter's syndrome is an X-linked mucopolysaccharide disorder. There is no generally accepted effective treatment for mucopolysaccharidoses. Bone marrow transplant has been suggested but remains mostly experimental (Gelder et al 2000, p. 1959; Harris 2000, p. 358).

14. Kleinfelter's syndrome is associated with cardiovascular disorders.

True: Mitral valve prolapse occurs in 55% of patients. Varicose veins occur in 20–40%. The prevalence of venous ulcers is 10–20 times higher than the general population. The risk of deep vein thrombosis and pulmonary embolism is increased (Craft et al 1985, p. 126).

15. Lesch–Nyhan syndrome occurs almost exclusively in males.

True: Lesch–Nyhan syndrome is a sex-linked recessive disorder. It is extremely rare in females. The usual mode of inheritance is from a carrier mother to her son who is affected (Gelder et al 2000, p. 1956; Sadock & Sadock 2005, p. 2053).

16. Neurofibromatosis is transmitted by autosomal dominant inheritance.

True: Neurofibromatosis is an autosomal dominant disorder characterized by café-au-lait spots and tumours arising from neural crest tissue. Neurofibromatosis 1, the commoner form, is characterized by neurofibromas, gliomas and hamartomas of the eye and optic pathways, bone dysplasisa, LD in about 50%, hyperactivity and other behaviour disorders. The gene has been located to chromosome 17.

Neurofibromatosis 2 is characterized by bilateral vestibular schwannomas, other tumours such as meningiomas and ependymomas, and cataracts. The gene has been located to chromosome 22 (Craft et al 1985, p. 114; Gelder et al 2000, p. 1151).

17. Phenylketonuria is most commonly diagnosed by amniocentesis.

False: Phenylketonuria is detected by routine screening of neonates using the Guthrie test or capillary blood phenylalanine estimation. Blood phenylalanine level >20 mg/dL and the presence of phenylpyruvic acid and its metabolites in urine confirm the diagnosis (Gelder et al 2000, p. 1959; Harris 2000, p. 335; Johnstone et al 2004, p. 527).

18. Rett syndrome almost exclusively affects girls.

True: Rett syndrome almost exclusively affects females because the male fetuses tend to die in the womb. 80% of cases are due to sporadic mutations in the gene MECP2 at X q28 (Gelder et al 2000, p. 1955; Johnstone et al 2004, p. 553).

19. Tay–Sachs disease is transmitted by X-linked recessive inheritance.

False: Tay–Sachs disease is an autosomal recessive disorder resulting in increased lipid storage. It is a rare disease except in the Ashkanazi Jews. About 1:30 of them are heterozygous for the gene, compared with 1:300 in other populations. Genetic screening permits preconceptual counselling (Craft et al 1985, p. 95; Fraser & Kerr 2003, p. 37).

20. Autistic traits are often associated with tuberous sclerosis complex.

True: Tuberous sclerosis complex is an autosomal dominant disorder. Symptoms include sleep problems, hyperactivity, aggression, self-injury and a non-compliant obsessiveness. It has a strong association with autism, the prevalence being 200 times more common than in the general population (Fraser & Kerr 2003, p. 89; Gelder et al 2000, p. 1151).

21. Perinatal hypoxia is a common cause of West syndrome.

True: West syndrome consists of the triad of infantile spasms, severe learning disability and hypsarrhythmia. Causes of West syndrome include perinatal hypoxia (the most common), tuberous sclerosis, other congenital brain malformations, Down's syndrome, phenylketonuria, leucodystrophy and various inborn errors of metabolism (Lishman 1997, p. 242).

22. Williams syndrome is associated with loquaciousness.

True: Williams syndrome is associated with loquaciousness (talkativeness or chattiness), good verbal ability and a sociable manner. They tend to approach others spontaneously. This may mask their severe visuospatial and motor deficits. Autistic features are rare (Johnstone et al 2004, p. 555).

23. Males with XYY tend to have short stature.

False: Males with XYY have tall stature and an IQ very slightly below average. They also have behavioural features which may increase the likelihood of antisocial acts (Fraser & Kerr 2003, p. 89; Gelder et al 2000, p. 1861; Johnstone et al 2004, p. 548).

24. Delirium is relatively frequent in those with learning disability.

True: Because of their limited cerebral, cognitive, metabolic and other reserves, people with learning disabilities are predisposed to decompensate and become delirious in the face of a variety of physiological and psychological stressors (Fraser & Kerr 2003, p. 223; Gelder et al 2006, p. 710).

25. Normalization theory of learning disability means that people with borderline learning disability should be treated like normal individuals.

True: Normalization theory is based on the principle that people with learning disabilities should be valued citizens with rights to dignity, growth and development. They should have accommodation and care that provides them with the same lifestyle and opportunities as the rest of the population. It aims to reverse the devaluation of the disabled person and the group while accepting that disability exists. Wolfensberger in 1972 called this 'social role valorization' (Fraser & Kerr 2003, p. 2; Gelder et al 2000, p. 1503).

Learning disability – 3

Regi T. Alexander

	T	F

1. The administrative prevalence of learning disability is approximately double that of its true prevalence. ☐ ☐

2. Placental transmission of the mumps virus can cause learning disability. ☐ ☐

3. In Angelman syndrome paternal disomy is more common than in Prader–Willi syndrome. ☐ ☐

4. Lack of empathy is a characteristic feature of Asperger syndrome. ☐ ☐

5. Cri du chat syndrome is caused by a deletion on the long arm of chromosome 5. ☐ ☐

6. Down's syndrome affects approximately 1% of live births. ☐ ☐

7. Down's syndrome is associated with a loss of acquired milestones. ☐ ☐

8. Hypomania is common in Down's syndrome. ☐ ☐

9. Down's syndrome is associated with hypothyroidism. ☐ ☐

10. Fragile X syndrome is a sex-linked disorder. ☐ ☐

11. Gaze avoidance is characteristic of Fragile X syndrome. ☐ ☐

12. The incidence of galactosaemia is 1:200 000. ☐ ☐

13. Hurler's syndrome can be treated with diet. ☐ ☐

14. Klinefelter syndrome is characterized by a long penis and large testes. ☐ ☐

15. Lesch–Nyhan syndrome can be diagnosed prenatally by sampling amniotic fluid. ☐ ☐

16. Niemann–Pick disease is an autosomal recessive disorder. ☐ ☐

17. Phenylketonuria is treated with a low tryptophan diet. ☐ ☐

18. Rett syndrome is associated with loss of acquired milestones. ☐ ☐

19. Patients with Tay–Sachs disease usually die during childhood. ☐ ☐

20. Most patients with tuberous sclerosis complex have normal intelligence. ☐ ☐

21. Hypsarrhythmia is a feature of West syndrome. ☐ ☐

22. Wilson's disease is an autosomal recessive disorder. ☐ ☐

23. XYY phenotype is associated with low IQ. ☐ ☐

T F

24. The risk of epilepsy in those with profound LD is 100 times that in the general population.

☐ ☐

25. Somatization is common in learning disability.

☐ ☐

ANSWERS

1. The administrative prevalence of learning disability is approximately double that of its true prevalence.

False: Administrative prevalence is defined as 'the numbers for whom services would be required in a community which made provision for all who needed them'. It is roughly half to a third of the true prevalence (Gelder et al 2006, p. 707).

2. Placental transmission of the mumps virus can cause learning disability.

False: Antenatal infection with cytomegalovirus, rubella, toxoplasmosis, herpes simplex and syphilis can cause learning disability as all these agents can cross the placenta (Craft et al 1985, p. 133; Gelder et al 2006, p. 714).

3. In Angelman syndrome paternal disomy is more common than in Prader–Willi syndrome.

True: In Prader–Willi syndrome, around 70% have a microdeletion of the *paternally* derived chromosome 15, about 28% have a *maternal* disomy and the rest have imprinting centre mutations or are carriers of a chromosomal translocation.

In Angelman syndrome, about 70% have a microdeletion of the *maternally* derived chromosome 15, about 5% have a *paternal* disomy, 3% have an imprinting centre mutation and 5% have a mutation in the UBE3A gene. The others have no identifiable defects on chromosome 15 and the locus may be elsewhere on the genome.

Thus in those where uniparental disomy is the cause of the syndrome, Prader–Willi is associated with a maternal disomy and Angelman with a paternal disomy (Gelder et al 2000, p. 1958; Johnstone et al 2004, p. 557).

4. Lack of empathy is a characteristic feature of Asperger syndrome.

True: (Gelder et al 2000, p. 1729).

5. Cri du chat syndrome is caused by a deletion on the long arm of chromosome 5.

False: Cri du chat syndrome is caused by a deletion on the short arm of chromosome 5, i.e. 5p15.3 and 5p15.2. It is the commonest human deletion syndrome. It accounts for around 1% of the profoundly learning disabled population. Severe learning disability, microcephaly and a high-pitched cat-like cry are prominent features. Patients may survive to adulthood (Gelder et al 2000, p. 1960).

6. Down's syndrome affects approximately 1% of live births.

False: Down's syndrome affects approximately 1 in 1000 live births. The incidence increases with maternal age as follows:

- 15–29 years = 1 in 1500 live births
- 30–34 years = 1 in 800
- 35–39 years = 1 in 270
- 40–44 years = 1 in 100
- > 45 years = 1 in 25–50
- Overall = 1 in 400 (Gelder et al 2000, p. 1954).

7. Down's syndrome is associated with a loss of acquired milestones.

False: There is no loss of skills. Milestones develop fairly quickly in the first year and then more slowly (Gelder et al 2006, p. 717).

8. Hypomania is common in Down's syndrome.

False: Bipolar affective disorder (BPAD) is not common in Down's syndrome. However, previous reports that BPAD does not occur at all in Down's syndrome have been proved wrong. The frequency and clinical features of BPAD in Down's syndrome are the same as in non-Down's syndrome learning disability (Fraser & Kerr 2003, p. 279; Johnstone et al 2004, p. 544).

9. Down's syndrome is associated with hypothyroidism.

True: Autoimmune thyroid dysfunction, especially hypothyroidism, is common in Down's syndrome. Hypothyroidism occurs in 20% of adolescents and adults with Down's syndrome. Hypothyroidism is a differential diagnosis in behavioural disturbance, depression and dementia in Down's syndrome (Johnstone et al 2004, p. 542).

10. Fragile X syndrome is a sex-linked disorder.

True: Fragile X syndrome is an X-linked disorder. It shows an X-linked dominant inheritance with incomplete penetrance. It is the most common LD syndrome caused by mutation of a single gene. It is the most common inherited cause of LD. It accounts for 50% of all cases of X-linked LD (Craft et al 1985, p. 123; Gelder et al 2000, p. 1953).

11. Gaze avoidance is characteristic of Fragile X syndrome.

True: Gaze avoidance is shared by Fragile X syndrome as well as autism. It may be a manifestation of defective non-verbal communication (Gelder et al 2000, p. 1954; Johnstone et al 2004, p. 552).

12. The incidence of galactosaemia is 1:200 000.

False: One per 30 000 live births in the UK and one per 62 000 births in the USA (Craft et al 1985, p. 97; Sadock & Sadock 2002, p. 1172).

13. Hurler's syndrome can be treated with diet.

False: Hurler's syndrome is an autosomal recessive mucopolysaccharide disorder. There is no generally accepted effective treatment for mucopolysaccharidoses. Allogenic bone marrow transplantation is being investigated (Gelder et al 2000, p. 1959; Harris 2000, p. 358).

14. Klinefelter syndrome is characterized by a long penis and large testes.

False: XXY karyotype and male hypogonadism are the key features of Klinefelter syndrome. Diagnosis often occurs at puberty with varying development of secondary sexual characteristics, small testes or infertility. Even though the adults are usually around 4 cm taller than average, the length of the penis is normal or moderately short. Testes are normal until puberty but thereafter small and firm (Craft et al 1985, p. 126; Johnstone et al 2004, p. 547).

15. Lesch–Nyhan syndrome can be diagnosed prenatally by sampling amniotic fluid.

True: Many fetal disorders – cytogenetic, biochemical, molecular and neural tube defects – can be diagnosed prenatally at 15–18 weeks of gestation by amniocentesis. Lesch–Nyhan syndrome can be diagnosed prenatally with amniocentesis or chorionic villus sampling.

16. Niemann–Pick disease is an autosomal recessive disorder.

True: Niemann–Pick disease is a group of four autosomal recessive disorders. Types A and B result in accumulation of sphingomyelin. Types C and D have defective neuronal cholesterol transport.

17. Phenylketonuria is treated with a low tryptophan diet.

False: Phenylketonuria is caused by the deficiency of phenylalanine hyroxylase, which converts phenylalanine to tyrosine. Phenylalanine hydroxylase deficiency results in the accumulation of phenylalanine to toxic levels causing severe LD, epilepsy and microcephaly. Elimination of phenylalanine from the diet from birth drastically reduces the severity of LD (Fraser & Kerr 2003, p. 36; Gelder et al 2000, p. 1960; Johnstone et al 2004, p. 527).

18. Rett syndrome is associated with loss of acquired milestones.

True: The affected girls develop normally for 6–28 months. Thereafter, there is deterioration in speech and motor abilities. Abnormal involuntary stereotyped movements, particularly involving the hands and fingers, e.g. hand flapping and hand wringing, appear later (Gelder et al 2000, p. 1955; Johnstone et al 2004, p. 552).

19. Patients with Tay–Sachs disease usually die during childhood.

True: Tay–Sachs disease is an autosomal recessive disorder resulting in increased lipid storage. The features include progressive blindness and deafness, spasticity, cherry red macular spot and mental retardation. There are several different clinical forms. The commonest is the infantile form. Death occurs most commonly between 2 and 4 years (Craft et al 1985, pp. 37, 95; Fraser & Kerr 2003, p. 37; Gelder et al 2006, p. 715).

20. Most patients with tuberous sclerosis complex have normal intelligence.

False: One-third have average intelligence. Two-thirds have mild to severe LD (Craft et al 1985, p. 114; Gelder et al 2000, p. 1958).

21. Hypsarrhythmia is a feature of West syndrome.

True: West syndrome consists of the triad of infantile spasms, severe LD and hypsarrhythmia. Hypsarrhythmia is an EEG pattern of a chaotic mixture of high amplitude slow waves with variable spikes and sharp waves. Onset is in infancy (Lishman 1997, p. 242).

22. Wilson's disease is an autosomal recessive disorder.

True: Wilson's disease or hepatolenticular degeneration is a rare, autosomal recessive disorder of copper metabolism. The pathogenesis is the absence or dysfunction of the copper-transporting P-type ATPase coded on chromosome 13q14. It causes liver dysfunction, personality and cognitive changes, tremor, dysarthria and wing-beating tremor, i.e. arms beat up and down at the shoulders (Johnstone et al 2004, p. 336; Mitchell 2004, p. 171).

23. XYY phenotype is associated with low IQ.

True: The IQ may be very slightly lower than normal. They also have behavioural features that increase the likelihood of antisocial acts (Gelder et al 2000, p. 1861; Johnstone et al 2004, p. 548).

24. The risk of epilepsy in those with profound LD is 100 times that in the general population.

True: The risk of active epilepsy in various IQ groups is as follows:

- Normal = 0.5%
- IQ 50–70 = 4%
- IQ 20–50 = 30%
- IQ below 20 = 50%.

Severe, intractable epilepsy can cause LD. Non-epileptic seizures are more common in LD than in the general population. In addition, patients with true epilepsy are the most likely to have non-epileptic seizures (Johnstone et al 2004, p. 571).

25. Somatization is common in learning disability.

True: People with mild LD have a higher prevalence of brooding, somatization and sleep disturbances than the general population, especially when depressed or anxious (Johnstone et al 2004, p. 566).

Learning disability – 4

Asif Zia

T F

1. Less than half of those with learning disability (LD) have mild LD.

2. Birth injuries account for over 40% of mental retardation.

3. Angelman syndrome is associated with a cheerful disposition.

4. Patients with Asperger syndrome have a narrower repertoire of emotional facial expression.

5. Di George syndrome is caused by a deletion on chromosome 21q11.

6. Down's syndrome is associated with grand mal seizures.

7. The overall prevalence of mental disorders is lower in Down's syndrome than in the general population.

8. Children with Down's syndrome are very capable at mimicry.

9. Up to half of the people with Down's syndrome have pathology affecting heart valves.

10. Fragile X syndrome is caused by a CAG repeat on the X chromosome.

11. Cryptorchidism is common in Fragile X syndrome.

12. Dietary alteration can reduce the incidence of low IQ in Hartnup disease.

13. In patients with Hurler's syndrome, survival into the 20s is common.

14. Klein–Levin syndrome is associated with hypersexuality.

15. Infants with Lesch–Nyhan syndrome have hypertonia.

16. Phenylketonuria occurs in 1 in 20 000 live births.

17. Most cases of Prader–Willi syndrome are caused by a chromosome 15 deletion of paternal origin.

18. In Rett syndrome the IQ is usually less than 35.

19. Patients with Trisomy 13 and Trisomy 18 usually survive to adulthood.

20. Tuberous sclerosis complex is associated with seizures.

21. Wilson's disease is caused by defective absorption of copper.

22. Psychiatric morbidity is higher in those with LD than in the general population.

23. Obsessive compulsive disorder is less frequent in those with LD than in the general population.

T F

24. Challenging behaviour occurs in 40% of people with learning disability. ☐ ☐

25. Naltrexone is used in managing self-harm in learning disability. ☐ ☐

ANSWERS

1. Less than half of those with learning disability (LD) have mild LD.

False: Among people with LD, 85% have mild, 10% have moderate, 3–4% have severe and 1–2% have profound LD. Thus, there are 5 to 6 mildly learning disabled people for every person with a more severe degree of learning disability (Gelder et al 2006, p. 708).

2. Birth injuries account for over 40% of mental retardation.

False: Clinically recognizable birth injuries account for about 10% of LD (Gelder et al 2006, p. 717).

3. Angelman syndrome is associated with a cheerful disposition.

True: Also known as 'Happy puppet syndrome', Angelman syndrome is characterized by severe mental retardation, jerky limb movements, gait abnormalities, inappropriate bouts of laughter unrelated to prevailing affect or environment, epilepsy and a happy disposition (Gelder et al 2000, p. 1958; Johnstone et al 2004, p. 805).

4. Patients with Asperger syndrome have a narrower repertoire of emotional facial expression.

True: Patients with autistic spectrum disorders may have a limited range of facial expression. They lack the 'spontaneous seeking of shared enjoyment', for example, showing and sharing. Their problems in emotional and social expression are paralleled by difficulties in recognizing and responding appropriately to the emotional expressions of others (Gelder et al 2000, p. 1725).

5. Di George syndrome is caused by a deletion on chromosome 21q11.

False: Both velocardiofacial syndrome and its more severe form the Di George syndrome are caused by a microdeletion on chromosome 22 (del (22) (q11.2q11.2)) (Johnstone et al 2004, p. 556).

6. Down's syndrome is associated with grand mal seizures.

True: In Down's syndrome the frequency of seizures is 10%. Most have grand mal seizures (Fraser & Kerr 2003, p. 272).

7. The overall prevalence of mental disorders is lower in Down's syndrome than in the general population.

False: Overall prevalence is higher, but the epidemiological profile is different. For example, Alzheimer's dementia is more common while alcohol and drug misuse are less common (Fraser & Kerr 2003, p. 274).

8. Children with Down's syndrome are very capable at mimicry.

False: The earlier descriptions of being very capable of mimicry, affectionate, music loving, easily amused, etc. were based on anecdotes and case reports. They have not been systematically validated (Craft et al 1985, p. 119; Gelder et al 2000, p. 1955).

9. Up to half of the people with Down's syndrome have pathology affecting heart valves.

True: Mitral valve prolapse, tricuspid valve prolapse and pulmonary valve fenestrations are the most common (Fraser & Kerr 2003, p. 268).

10. Fragile X syndrome is caused by a CAG repeat on the X chromosome.

False: Fragile X syndrome is caused by abnormal nucleotide CGG repeats at a fragile site on the long arm of the X chromosome (Xq27.3). In Fragile X syndrome, CGG repeats range from 230 to over 1000 while normal individuals have an average of 30 (6–54) (Gelder et al 2000, p. 1953).

11. Cryptorchidism is common in Fragile X syndrome.

False: Cryptorchidism, i.e. undescended testes, is rare. Macro-orchidism, i.e. enlarged testes, is present in 90% of adults with Fragile X syndrome (Craft et al 1985, p. 122; Johnstone et al 2004, p. 551).

12. Dietary alteration can reduce the incidence of low IQ in Hartnup disease.

True: Hartnup disease is a rare inborn error of metabolism with nicotinic acid deficiency due to the reduced availability of its precursor tryptophan. Cases may be asymptomatic or present with a photosensitive skin rash, cerebellar ataxia and other neurological or psychiatric disturbances. Mental retardation occurs in some patients. A high protein diet can alter the deficient transport of neutral amino acids in most patients. In patients with symptomatic disease, daily diet supplementation with nicotinamide or nicotinic acid reduces the severity of symptoms (Lishman 1997, p. 573).

13. In patients with Hurler's syndrome, survival into the 20s is common.

True: The overall prognosis is poor. However, survival into the 20s is common (Gelder et al 2000, p. 1959).

14. Klein–Levin syndrome is associated with hypersexuality.

True: Klein–Levin syndrome usually occurs in male adolescents. They have periods of excessive sleepiness, overeating, hypersexuality and disturbed behaviour alternating with periods of normality. The frequency of episodes is once every 1–6 months and the duration is 1 day to a few weeks (Gelder et al 2000, p. 1803; Johnstone et al 2004, p. 782).

15. Infants with Lesch–Nyhan syndrome have hypertonia.

True: Attacks of hypertonia develop within a few weeks of birth followed by choreoathetosis, spasticity, ataxia and dystonia. Other features include severe mental retardation, microcephaly and epilepsy in about 50% (Gelder et al 2000, p. 1956; Mitchell 2004, p. 454).

16. Phenylketonuria occurs in 1 in 20 000 live births.

True: Phenylketonuria occurs in 1 in 5000 to 20000 live births. It is an autosomal recessive condition caused by an error of amino acid metabolism. It is the most frequent and the most studied inborn error of metabolism (Fraser & Kerr 2003, p. 37; Gelder et al 2000, p. 1959; Johnstone et al 2004, p. 527).

17. Most cases of Prader–Willi syndrome are caused by a chromosome 15 deletion of paternal origin.

True: Prader–Willi syndrome is a genetically heterogeneous disorder. About 70% of cases are caused by a deletion on chromosome 15 (q11q13) of paternal origin. It can also be caused by inheriting two chromosome 15s from the mother (maternal disomy) or by a paternal gene mutation (Gelder et al 2000, p. 1956; Johnstone et al 2004, p. 557).

18. In Rett syndrome the IQ is usually less than 35.

True: Patients with Rett syndrome usually have severe or profound LD. This would correspond to an IQ score below 35 (Gelder et al 2000, p. 1955; Johnstone et al 2004, p. 553).

19. Patients with Trisomy 13 and Trisomy 18 usually survive to adulthood.

False: All patients with Patau's syndrome (Trisomy 13) have severe LD, and most have microcephaly, congenital heart defects, marked hypertonia and myoclonic spasms. More than 50% die within the first month and only 5% survive beyond 3 years of age.

Edward syndrome (Trisomy 18) is associated with severe LD and epilepsy and often with congenital heart abnormalities. Only 10% survive beyond the first year (Craft et al 1985, p. 123; Johnstone et al 2004, p. 536).

20. Tuberous sclerosis complex is associated with seizures.

True: Seizures occur in 60–80% of patients. Seizures of any type can occur. Infantile spasms are common in those with learning disability. Mild to severe LD is present in two-thirds (Gelder et al 2000, p. 1151; http://www.ninds.nih.gov).

21. Wilson's disease is caused by defective absorption of copper.

False: Wilson's disease or hepatolenticular degeneration is an autosomal recessive disorder of copper metabolism. The absence or dysfunction of the copper-transporting P-type ATPase coded on chromosome 13q14 results in deficiency of ceruloplasmin, impaired transport of copper from the liver to the biliary system and faulty excretion of copper. No abnormalities in copper absorption have been described (Craft et al 1985, p. 99; Gelder et al 2000, p. 1161; Mitchell 2004, p. 171).

22. Psychiatric morbidity is higher in those with LD than in the general population.

True: Psychiatric morbidity is higher in those with LD than in the general population. The lower the IQ, the greater the problems and the more difficulty assessing and managing them (Gelder et al 2006, p. 709; Johnstone et al 2004, p. 563).

23. Obsessive compulsive disorder is less frequent in those with LD than in the general population.

False: OCD is more common in LD. However, the diagnosis of OCD can be difficult because many patients may not have sufficient communication skills to reveal the presence of obsessive thoughts. Moreover, many patients with LD have repetitive and stereotyped behaviours that may be difficult to distinguish from OCD (Gelder et al 2000, p. 1968; Gelder et al 2006, p. 709).

24. Challenging behaviour occurs in 40% of people with learning disability.

False: Challenging behaviour occurs in 20% of children and adolescents and 15% of adults with LD (Gelder et al 2006, p. 709).

25. Naltrexone is used in managing self-harm in learning disability.

True: Naltrexone is an opioid antagonist. It has been used for rapid outpatient opiate detoxification in combination with clonidine; to aid relapse prevention in alcohol, opiate, cocaine and nicotine dependence; and in the treatment of eating disorders, obesity and pathological gambling. Naltrexone has also been used in the treatment of self-injurious behaviour in learning disability. The efficacy of naltrexone in most of these conditions remains unclear (Bouras 1999, p. 298; Fraser & Kerr 2003, p. 234; Sadock & Sadock 2005, p. 2877).

26 Learning disability – 5

Regi T. Alexander

	T	F
1. Low IQ occurs in subsequent generations.	☐	☐
2. Maternal smoking during pregnancy is associated with mental retardation in her children.	☐	☐
3. Asperger syndrome is more common in males than in females.	☐	☐
4. There is more than chance association between Asperger syndrome and Gilles de la Tourette syndrome.	☐	☐
5. Translocation accounts for 95% of Down's syndrome.	☐	☐
6. The prevalence of epilepsy in Down's syndrome varies with age.	☐	☐
7. Autistic features are rare in Down's syndrome.	☐	☐
8. Down's syndrome is associated with both conduction and sensorineural deafness.	☐	☐
9. Sleep apnoea and recurrent respiratory infections are common in Down's syndrome.	☐	☐
10. In Fragile X syndrome, the fragile fragment occurs on the short arm of the X chromosome.	☐	☐
11. Female carriers of Fragile X syndrome have more cognitive impairment than males.	☐	☐
12. In Heller's disease the development is normal in the first 2 years of life.	☐	☐
13. Most patients with Klinefelter syndrome have moderate LD.	☐	☐
14. Lennox–Gestaut syndrome is usually associated with LD.	☐	☐
15. Lesch–Nyhan syndrome can be successfully treated with diet.	☐	☐
16. Phenylketonuria is an autosomal dominant condition.	☐	☐
17. Temper tantrums are a feature of Prader–Willi syndrome.	☐	☐
18. Sturge–Weber syndrome is transmitted by dominant inheritance.	☐	☐
19. Tuberous sclerosis complex (TSC) is transmitted through a single recessive gene.	☐	☐
20. Café au lait spots are seen in tuberous sclerosis complex.	☐	☐
21. Onset after West's syndrome is a poor prognostic indicator in Lennox–Gestaut syndrome.	☐	☐

T F

22. Episodes of delirium are a feature of Wilson's disease. ☐ ☐

23. People with LD are more likely to present with complaints of low mood when depressed. ☐ ☐

24. Personality disorders can be diagnosed in those with LD. ☐ ☐

25. Children with profound LD and behavioural problems usually benefit from behavioural therapy. ☐ ☐

ANSWERS

1. Low IQ occurs in subsequent generations.

True: While moderate to severe learning disabilities are mainly due to chromosomal anomalies, severe genetic misendowments and brain damage, only a small proportion of cases of mild learning disabilities are caused by these factors. Assortative mating would also tend to exacerbate the tendency for low IQ to occur in subsequent generations (Craft et al 1985, p. 84).

2. Maternal smoking during pregnancy is associated with mental retardation in her children.

True: Maternal smoking is a risk factor for low infant birthweight, which is a risk factor for LD. Maternal smoking may independently affect fetal neurological development (Johnstone et al 2004, p. 533).

3. Asperger syndrome is more common in males than in females.

True: Both epidemiological and clinical studies report a male: female ratio of 3.5–4:1 for children with autism. However, this ratio varies with the IQ level. Females with autism who have IQs in the normal range are 50 times less common than males. The male:female ratio for Asperger syndrome appears to be closer to 9:1 (Fraser & Kerr 2003, p. 119; Gelder et al 2000, p. 1730).

4. There is more than chance association between Asperger syndrome and Gilles de la Tourette syndrome.

True: The prevalence of Tourette syndrome in children with autistic spectrum disorders is 4.3–6.5%. This is higher than in the general population. The prevalence of Tourette syndrome is 4 per 10 000 in male adolescents and as high as 49 per 10 000 in American schoolchildren with behaviour disturbances (Fraser & Kerr 2003, p. 125; Gelder et al 2000, p. 1149)

5. Translocation accounts for 95% of Down's syndrome.

False: Trisomy 21 accounts for 94% of cases. The cause is unknown. The risk of recurrence is 1%.

Translocation accounts for 3–5%. Translocation is familial. It can be identified at birth and used for genetic counselling. The risk of recurrence is 10%.

Mosaicism is found in 1–3%. They may have normal intelligence (Fraser & Kerr 2003, p. 33; Gelder et al 2000, p. 1955; Gelder et al 2006, p. 718).

6. The prevalence of epilepsy in Down's syndrome varies with age.

True: There are three peaks, i.e. early infancy, the third decade and with the development of Alzheimer's over the age of 40 years. The prevalence of epilepsy in Down's syndrome is 10% overall, 40% in those over 40 and 80% in those with Alzheimer's disease.

7. Autistic features are rare in Down's syndrome.

False: The prevalence of childhood autism in the general population is 2–5 per 10 000. The estimates of the prevalence of autistic features in Down's syndrome vs. in those with an equivalent degree of LD from other causes vary, e.g. 5% vs. 10%, 11% vs. 7%. The definition of autism and the exclusion of other disorders such as behavioural phenotypes, OCD and depression that account for autistic spectrum behaviours influence prevalence estimates. Though these factors make an exact estimate of the frequency of autistic features difficult it is true that such features are not rare in Down's syndrome (Fraser & Kerr 2003, p. 280).

8. Down's syndrome is associated with both conduction and sensorineural deafness.

True: Most children with Down's syndrome have unilateral or bilateral hearing impairment. The high prevalence of conduction deafness especially in children may be caused by glue ear. Otitis media affects many children with Down's syndrome and may be exacerbated by the structural anomalies of the ear. The hearing impairment in children is compounded by the later onset of sensorineural deafness. Thus, there is a high prevalence of both conduction and sensorineural hearing loss in adults with Down's syndrome (Fraser & Kerr 2003, p. 269; Johnstone et al 2004, p. 542).

9. Sleep apnoea and recurrent respiratory infections are common in Down's syndrome.

True: The narrowed hypopharynx increases the risk of sleep apnoea. Immune system defects increase the vulnerability to infections, particularly recurrent respiratory infections. Infection, especially pneumonia, is still the leading cause of death in Down's syndrome (Gelder et al 2000, p. 1955; Johnstone et al 2004, p. 541).

10. In Fragile X syndrome, the fragile fragment occurs on the short arm of the X chromosome.

False: Fragile X syndrome is caused by abnormal nucleotide CGG repeats at a fragile site on the long arm of the X chromosome (Xq27.3). In Fragile X syndrome, CGG repeats range from 230 to over 1000 while normal individuals have an average of 30 (6–54) (Gelder et al 2000, p. 1953).

11. Female carriers of Fragile X syndrome have more cognitive impairment than males.

False: Most female carriers have normal intelligence. However, 30–50% have mild LD (Craft et al 1985, p. 123; Gelder et al 2000, p. 1954).

12. In Heller's disease the development is normal in the first 2 years of life.

True: Heller's disease or childhood disintegrative disorder starts after normal development, usually for 2 years. Like autism, there is loss of cognitive and social skills. In addition, there is decline in motor skills and bowel and bladder control (Gelder et al 2006, p. 675).

13. Most patients with Klinefelter syndrome have moderate LD.

False: The average IQ in Klinefelter syndrome (47XXY) is 90. Many have mild LD. Most have IQ above 60. Some have normal or above average intelligence (Johnstone et al 2004, p. 547; Sadock & Sadock 2002, p. 733).

14. Lennox–Gestaut syndrome is usually associated with LD.

True: Lennox–Gestaut syndrome typically starts between ages 1 and 8 years. 60% have evidence of pre-existing brain damage and LD. They have frequent, severe intractable tonic, atonic, myoclonic and atypical absence seizures. They have bilateral slow spike and wave complexes on the EEG (Gelder et al 2000, p. 1787; Lishman 1997, p. 242).

15. Lesch–Nyhan syndrome can be successfully treated with diet.

False: The overall prognosis of Lesch–Nyhan syndrome is poor. Most affected subjects die by early adulthood. Treatment is symptomatic. Gout can be treated with allopurinol. Kidney stones may be treated with lithotripsy. There is no standard treatment for the neurological symptoms. Carbidopa, levodopa, diazepam, phenobarbital or haloperidol may be used. There is no effective dietary treatment (Gelder et al 2000, p. 1956).

16. Phenylketonuria is an autosomal dominant condition.

False: Phenylketonuria is an autosomal recessive condition caused by an error of amino acid metabolism (Fraser & Kerr 2003, p. 37; Gelder et al 2000, p. 1959; Johnstone et al 2004, p. 527).

17. Temper tantrums are a feature of Prader–Willi syndrome.

True: Patients with Prader–Willi syndrome are described as pleasant and good tempered. However, they can manifest severe behavioural problems associated with hyperphagia and self-injurious behaviour in addition to temper tantrums (Gelder et al 2000, p. 1957).

18. Sturge–Weber syndrome is transmitted by dominant inheritance.

False: Sturg–Weber syndrome (encephalotrigeminal angiomatosis) is a congenital, non-familial disorder of unknown incidence and cause. It occurs sporadically with no particular pattern of inheritance. Clinical features include a congenital facial birthmark (port wine stain), neurological abnormalities (brain angiomas and epilepsy), glaucoma and buphthalmos (Craft et al 1985, p. 110; http://www.sturge-weber.com; http://www.sturgeweber.org.uk).

19. Tuberous sclerosis complex (TSC) is transmitted through a single recessive gene.

False: TSC is due to spontaneous mutations (60%) or is inherited as an autosomal dominant disorder (40%). Two disease-determining genes have been identified: TSC1 and TSC2. TSC1 is on chromosome 9 (9q34) and encodes for the protein hamartin. TSC1 is less likely to cause mental retardation. TSC2 is on chromosome 16 (16p13.3) and encodes for the protein tuberin. About 60% of TSC is due to new mutations leading to dysfunction of hamartin and tuberin (Gelder et al 2000, p. 1958).

20. Café au lait spots are seen in tuberous sclerosis complex.

True: The first clue to diagnosis may be white patches on the skin, i.e. hypomelanotic macules. Skin lesions in TSC include facial angiofibroma, adenoma sebaceum, white ash leaf-shaped macules, shagreen patches, depigmented naevi, subcutaneous nodules and café au lait spots (Gelder et al 2000, p. 1958).

21. Onset after West's syndrome is a poor prognostic indicator in Lennox–Gestaut syndrome.

True: West syndrome consists of the triad of infantile spasms, severe LD and hypsarrythmia. Lennox–Gestaut syndrome usually starts between ages 1 and 8 years. They have severe intractable epilepsy and bilateral slow spike and wave complexes on the EEG.

Poor prognostic indicators in Lennox–Gestaut syndrome include onset before age 3 years, greater frequency of seizures and status seizures, onset after West syndrome and more slow wave and focal abnormalities on the EEG (Gelder et al 2000, p. 1787; Lishman 1997, p. 242).

22. Episodes of delirium are a feature of Wilson's disease.

True: Cognitive impairment increases with time. Fluctuating levels of consciousness with episodes of delirium occur. Delirium is more likely in the later stages and may be related to liver failure and seizures (Lishman 1997, p. 665; Mitchell 2004, p. 173).

23. People with LD are more likely to present with complaints of low mood when depressed.

False: People with LD may have limited communication skills and limited ability to express their subjective feelings. They are less likely than normal people to complain of low mood. Those with mild LD show similar symptoms to those with normal IQ, but with more loss of confidence and tearfulness. With lower IQ somatic symptoms such as changes in sleep, appetite, weight, energy and activity levels may indicate depression. Behavioural changes including psychomotor agitation, social withdrawal, increased self-harm, irritability, aggression, wandering and worsening of existing behavioural problems are also more common in those with LD and co-morbid depression (Bouras 1999, p. 179; Fraser & Kerr 2003, p. 159; Johnstone et al 2004, p. 566).

24. Personality disorders can be diagnosed in those with LD.

True: Personality disorders may be diagnosable, particularly in those with mild to moderate LD. Features such as dependence, passiveness and temperament may be features of LD, personality or both. A diagnosis of personality disorder may lead to exclusion from some services and, hence, many clinicians tend to withhold the diagnosis (Gelder et al 2006, p. 710; Johnstone et al 2004, p. 566).

25. Children with profound LD and behavioural problems usually benefit from behavioural therapy.

True: Behavioural therapy, for example behaviour modification and operant conditioning techniques, is used effectively in a variety of difficult and disruptive behaviours in people with LD. Parents and teachers are taught to apply consistent rewards and consequences for adaptive and maladaptive behaviours. Behavioural therapy approaches based on detailed behaviour analysis of the antecedents and consequences of difficult behaviour are also effective.

Positive behavioural interventions are most effective for affective symptoms, e.g. depression and anxiety, and for social skills deficits.

Punishment procedures, e.g. extinction, disapproval, time-out, overcorrection are effective in destructive, aggressive and self-injurious behaviours.

Behavioural therapy has 65–75% success rate in stereotypic behaviours, psychophysiological symptoms and non-compliance. Behavioural therapy has 45–65% success rate in destructive behaviours. Inappropriate social interactions have only 35–45% success rate with behavioural therapy (Fraser & Kerr 2003, p. 103; Harris 2000, p. 520).

27 Mood disorders – 1

Chris O'Loughlin

T F

1. Depression is less common in the recently unemployed with support.

2. Bipolar II disorder is more common in higher socio-economic groups.

3. Rapid cycling mood disorder is more common in women.

4. The gap in inception rates for depression in males and females increases with age.

5. The age of onset of bipolar affective disorder in females is earlier than in males.

6. Schizoaffective disorder was described by Kraepelin as a mixed affective state.

7. People from lower social classes are more likely than those from middle social classes to develop depression following a life event.

8. Poverty doubles the depression risk in women.

9. Hypomania differs from mania by the absence of psychotic symptoms.

10. Heritability for bipolar disorder is 45%.

11. The first-degree relatives of patients with bipolar affective disorder have a higher risk of developing schizoaffective disorder.

12. Relatives of patients with depression have increased genetic risk for alcoholism.

13. Genetic linkage studies of BPAD have shown that a susceptibility gene on chromosome 18 occurs in some families.

14. A disturbance in REM sleep often precedes the onset of depression.

15. ACTH secretion is increased in depression.

16. Salivary cortisol falls more than plasma cortisol in the dexamethasone suppression test.

17. Long-term caffeine use causes dexamethasone non-suppression.

18. TSH response to TRH is blunted in depression.

19. Melatonin changes have consistently been shown to cause depression.

20. In seasonal affective disorder there is clear evidence of disruption of melatonin circadian rhythms.

21. Tryptophan-induced prolactin release is increased in depression.

T F

22. In depression, people are as likely to recall negative words about themselves as about other people. ☐ ☐

23. Use of a light box for seasonal affective disorder is equally effective when used in the morning or the evening. ☐ ☐

24. As the age of a person with BPAD increases, episodes of depression decrease in frequency, and episodes of mania increase in frequency. ☐ ☐

25. Delusions in depression predict poor response to ECT. ☐ ☐

ANSWERS

1. Depression is less common in the recently unemployed with support.

True: Depression is significantly more common in the recently unemployed. However, interventions focused on enhancing the sense of mastery through the acquisition of job-search and problem-solving skills, and on inoculation against setbacks, benefit the re-employment and mental health outcomes of the high-risk subjects (Vinokur et al 1995).

2. Bipolar II disorder is more common in higher socio-economic groups.

True: Bipolar II patients tend to belong to higher social classes. They are relatively over-represented among better educated, socially active and creative people. However, bipolar I disorder is associated with lower social status (Murray et al 1997, p. 322; Sadock & Sadock 2005, p. 1580).

3. Rapid cycling mood disorder is more common in women.

True: Rapid cycling is defined as four or more mood episodes per year. Rapid cycling occurs in 10–20% of individuals with bipolar disorder. Even though bipolar disorder has equal sex incidence, women comprise 70–90% of those with rapid cycling. Rapid cycling is associated with female gender, borderline hypothyroidism, menopause, temporal lobe dysrhythmias, alcohol, minor tranquillizer, stimulant or caffeine abuse, long-term aggressive antidepressant drug use and being of middle or upper social class (DSM-IV-TR; Sadock & Sadock 2005, p. 1639).

4. The gap in inception rates for depression in males and females increases with age.

False: Females are at higher risk of depression than men at all ages after puberty. Prior to puberty there is an excess of depression in boys. However, the difference may be smaller in the elderly than in younger adults (Gelder et al 2000, p. 1622).

5. The age of onset of bipolar affective disorder in females is earlier than in males.

False: The mean age of onset for BPAD is 21 years in hospital studies and 17 years in community studies. There is no sex difference in the age of onset (Gelder et al 2006, pp. 230, 245; Sadock & Sadock 2005, p. 1579).

6. Schizoaffective disorder was described by Kraepelin as a mixed affective state.

False: Following Kraepelin's separation of dementia praecox and manic depressive disorder, in 1933 he added schizoaffective disorders under the rubric of schizophrenia. Kraepelin described six mixed affective states based on the level of mood, and psychic and motor activity: Depressive or anxious mania, Excited depression, Mania with poverty of thought, Manic stupor, Depression with flight of ideas, and Inhibited mania. Thus schizoaffective disorder is not one of Kraepelin's mixed affective states (Johnstone et al 2004, p. 397; Sato et al 2002; Sims 2004, p. 322).

7. People from lower social classes are more likely than those from middle social classes to develop depression following a life event.

True: Individuals with lower educational and social achievement have higher vulnerability for affective disorders. The social causation hypothesis suggests that the stress associated with lower social position, e.g. exposure to adversity and lack of resources to cope with difficulties, contributes to affective disorders. The social selection hypothesis suggests that genetically predisposed persons drift down to or fail to rise out of such positions. However, the effect of poverty may be substantially reduced when controlling for the degree of isolation from friends and family (Gelder et al 2000, p. 706; Murali & Oyebode 2004).

8. Poverty doubles the depression risk in women.

True: Low socio-economic status is associated with high prevalence of mood disorders (Murali & Oyebode 2004).

9. Hypomania differs from mania by the absence of psychotic symptoms.

True: The ICD-10 explicitly states that hypomania should not be diagnosed if the change in mood is accompanied by delusions or hallucinations. If these are present the diagnosis is one of mania with psychotic symptoms. The other major distinction ICD-10 makes between hypomania and mania is that, whilst hypomania is associated with some interference with personal functioning and daily living, mania is associated with *severe* interference.

DSM-IV distinguishes mania from hypomania by the presence of marked impairment in social functioning, need for hospitalization, or the presence of psychotic symptoms.

10. Heritability for bipolar disorder is 45%.

False: Heritability is the relative influence of genetic factors. Heritability estimate for bipolar disorder is 48–80% (Gelder et al 2006, p. 98; Johnstone et al 2004, p. 431).

11. The first-degree relatives of patients with bipolar affective disorder have a higher risk of developing schizoaffective disorder.

True: The first-degree relatives of patients with schizoaffective disorder, BPAD and unipolar depression have a higher than average risk of developing unipolar depression, BPAD and schizoaffective disorder in that order of frequency (Gelder et al 2006, p. 231; Johnstone et al 2004, p. 430).

12. Relatives of patients with depression have increased genetic risk for alcoholism.

True: Significant genetic correlations (from +0.4 to +0.6) between major depression and alcoholism in women have been demonstrated. The correlations are higher when using narrower criteria for alcoholism. The co-morbidity in women results from genetic factors that influence the risk of both disorders (Johnstone et al 2004, p. 431).

13. Genetic linkage studies of BPAD have shown that a susceptibility gene on chromosome 18 occurs in some families.

True: Several regions on chromosome 18 may be linked to BPAD. Other chromosomes of interest include 9, 10, 13, 14 and 22 (Gelder et al 2000, p. 703; Sadock & Sadock 2005, p. 1590).

14. A disturbance in REM sleep often precedes the onset of depression.

True: Shortened REM latency is considered a trait marker in depression. It occurs in dysthymia, borderline personality disorder, as well as among clinically well offspring of adults with major depression (Sadock & Sadock 2005, p. 1570).

15. ACTH secretion is increased in depression.

True: In depression there is increased cortisol production; increased release of hypothalamic beta-endorphin and a pulsatile increase in adrenocorticotrophin (ACTH) (Gelder et al 2000, p. 715; Johnstone et al 2004, p. 437).

16. Salivary cortisol falls more than plasma cortisol in the dexamethasone suppression test.

False: In the dexamethasone suppression test, salivary and plasma cortisol fall at similar rates. Salivary cortisol is related to unbound plasma cortisol. It is approximately 5% of the total cortisol and the part that is biologically active (Cook et al 1986).

17. Long-term caffeine use causes dexamethasone non-suppression.

False: Acute caffeine administration increases cortisol and causes dexamethasone non-suppression in normal humans. Chronic caffeine use is unlikely to be a major factor in dysregulation of the HPA axis in depression (Lee et al 1988).

18. TSH response to TRH is blunted in depression.

True: The TSH response to TRH is blunted in 20–30% of patients with depression. The clinical significance of this remains unclear (Gelder et al 2000, p. 715; Sadock & Sadock 2005, p. 1600).

19. Melatonin changes have consistently been shown to cause depression.

False: Some, but not all, studies suggest melatonin secretion is decreased in depressed patients. There is no evidence of a phase shift or of disorders of circadian rhythm in depression.

20. In seasonal affective disorder there is clear evidence of disruption of melatonin circadian rhythms.

False: Seasonal affective disorder has been difficult to ascribe to any underlying biochemical abnormality including melatonin disruption (Gelder et al 2000, p. 1352; Johnstone et al 2004, p. 428).

21. Tryptophan-induced prolactin release is increased in depression.

False: Serotonin is a prolactin releasing factor while dopamine is a prolactin release-inhibiting factor. Most studies have found normal basal and circadian prolactin levels in depression. Many studies have shown a blunted prolactin response to various 5-HT agonists (Sadock & Sadock 2005, p. 1600).

22. In depression, people are as likely to recall negative words about themselves as about other people.

False: Bradley & Matthews (1983) tested the negative self-schema model of depression using recall measures for self- and other person-referent positive and negative adjectives. Compared to non-psychiatric controls, depressed patients recalled more negative than positive self-referent adjectives. However, their negative bias in recall applied only to self-referent negative adjectives. They showed a normal positive recall bias towards other-referent adjectives.

23. Use of a light box for seasonal affective disorder is equally effective when used in the morning or the evening.

False: Morning phototherapy is more effective in most patients compared to midday or evening phototherapy for winter depression. However, others claim that there is no difference in benefits between exposure to bright light over dim light or early morning exposure over midday exposure (Gelder et al 2006, p. 572; Johnstone et al 2004, p. 428).

24. As the age of a person with BPAD increases, episodes of depression decrease in frequency, and episodes of mania increase in frequency.

False: The frequency of episodes and the pattern of remissions and relapses are both very variable. Depressive episodes tend to become more frequent and longer lasting and remissions become shorter after middle age. Manic episodes become less frequent. However, after middle age, there may be an increase of newly diagnosed bipolar patients, often with neurological problems (ICD-10 1992; Jacoby & Oppenheimer 2002, p. 684).

25. Delusions in depression predict poor response to ECT.

False: The therapeutic effects of ECT are greatest in severe depressions, especially those with marked weight loss, early morning wakening, retardation and delusions. In trials of ECT versus simulated ECT, delusions appear to distinguish patients who respond to ECT from those who respond to placebo treatments (Gelder et al 2006, pp. 249, 258).

Mood disorders – 2

Salbu Krishnan

	T	F

1. The incidence of depression has decreased in the Western world in the last two decades.

2. Prevalence of mania in old age is 5%.

3. The difference between prevalence among males and females, of depression, narrows after age 65 years.

4. The age of onset of bipolar affective disorder is 5–10 years earlier than unipolar depression.

5. The genetic link between alcohol dependence and depression is determined by gender.

6. Obstetric complications are a risk factor for bipolar disorder.

7. Exit life events are more common than entry life events in depression.

8. Life events are no less likely to precede depression in the elderly than in adults.

9. Childhood sexual abuse doubles the risk of depression in adult men.

10. Women who terminate their pregnancies due to fetal abnormalities are more likely to become depressed than those who suffer spontaneous abortions.

11. The concordance of BPAD in monozygotic twins is approximately 60%.

12. The chance of the monozygotic twin of a proband with bipolar disorder developing schizophrenia is 3–5%.

13. Patients suffering from the first episode of depression in old age are more likely to have a family history of depression.

14. REM sleep is reduced in depression.

15. Delta waves in the EEG are increased in depression.

16. In depression blunted cortisol suppression and blunted response to TRH combined gives a diagnostic sensitivity of 80%.

17. There is usually a greater fall of cortisol following dexamethasone administration in depression than in normal volunteers.

18. Growth hormone response to clonidine is decreased in depression.

19. TSH response to TRH is normal in euthyroid depressed patients.

T F

20. Melatonin secretion increases in the winter.

21. Platelet 5-HT binding is decreased in depression.

22. Vanillylmandelic acid (VMA) is significant in studies of depression.

23. Mania is associated with depressive symptoms more often in the elderly.

24. There is a familial component to response to antidepressant medication in BPAD.

25. After an episode of mania, more than 80% of individuals will have at least one further episode of either mania or depression.

ANSWERS

1. The incidence of depression has decreased in the Western world in the last two decades.

False: The risk of major depression has been increasing in the Western world in recent decades. Moreover, there has been a shift forward in the age of onset and lifetime risk. This may be related to social changes including family relationships and the frequency of life events.

However, the observed increase may be due to artefacts of memory, higher subjective awareness, better definitions and better methods of identification (Johnstone et al 2004, p. 429; Sadock & Sadock 2005, p. 1581).

2. Prevalence of mania in old age is 5%.

False: Mania is rare in older people. The community prevalence falls from 1.4% in younger adults to 0.1% in the over 65s. In the ECA study of 20 000 people, the 1-month prevalence of mania was 0.4–0.8% in 18–44-year-olds and 0.2% in 45–64-year-olds. No cases were identified in those aged above 64 years (Copeland et al 2002, p. 478; Gelder et al 2000, p. 1650).

3. The difference between prevalence among males and females, of depression, narrows after age 65 years.

True: Overall, depression is lower in the elderly. Females are at higher risk but the size of the gender difference is smaller in the elderly compared to the young (Gelder et al 2000, p. 1622).

4. The age of onset of bipolar affective disorder is 5–10 years earlier than unipolar depression.

True: The mean age of onset for BPAD is 17–21 years and for unipolar depression is 27 years (Gelder et al 2006, p. 230; Sadock & Sadock 2005, p. 1579).

5. The genetic link between alcohol dependence and depression is determined by gender.

True: Significant genetic correlations (from +0.4 to +0.6) between major depression and alcoholism in women have been demonstrated. The correlations are higher when using narrower criteria for alcoholism. The co-morbidity in women results from genetic factors that influence the risk of both disorders (Johnstone et al 2004, p. 431).

6. Obstetric complications are a risk factor for bipolar disorder.

False: Following the positive findings of a relationship between obstetric complications and schizophrenia, a similar study investigated the relationship with affective psychoses, including mania, but found no association (Bain et al 2000).

7. Exit life events are more common than entry life events in depression.

True: Though not a strong association (Paykel 1992, p. 2003).

8. Life events are no less likely to precede depression in the elderly than in adults.

True: Murphy (1982) found that the rate of life events in the year preceding the onset of depression was similar for adults across the age range. However, the elderly tend to present with more medical problems. There was at least one severe life event in 48% of elderly people with depression compared to 23% of a control group. They included death of a loved one, life-threatening illness in someone close, major financial problems and enforced removal from one's home (Butler & Pitt 1998, p. 112; Gelder et al 2000, p. 1622; Jacoby & Oppenheimer 2002, p. 644; Murphy 1982; Paykel 1992, p. 224).

9. Childhood sexual abuse doubles the risk of depression in adult men.

False: Childhood sexual abuse doubles the risk of depression in females, but not in men (Spataro et al 2004).

10. Women who terminate their pregnancies due to fetal abnormalities are more likely to become depressed than those who suffer spontaneous abortions.

False: Grief and depressive symptoms in women who terminate pregnancies for fetal anomalies and those who experience spontaneous perinatal loss are comparable (Zeanah et al 1993).

11. The concordance of BPAD in monozygotic twins is approximately 60%.

True: The concordance rate in twin genetic studies is the rate of concurrence of an index trait or disorder that occurs in one member also occurring in the co-twin. The concordance rate in BPAD is approximately 60% (range = 58–92%) in monozygotic and 20% (range 14–35%) in dizygotic twin pairs (Johnstone et al 2004, p. 430; Sadock & Sadock 2005, p. 1583).

12. The chance of the monozygotic twin of a proband with bipolar disorder developing schizophrenia is 3–5%.

False: There is substantial overlap between genetic loci identified for schizophrenia and bipolar disorders. Chromosome 13q has been of particular interest. Recent twin studies suggest that the chance of the monozygotic twin of a proband with bipolar disorder developing schizophrenia is 5–15% (Cardno et al 2002; Johnstone et al 2004, p. 162; Sadock & Sadock 2005, p. 1591).

13. Patients suffering from the first episode of depression in old age are more likely to have a family history of depression.

False: Genetic factors have their greatest influence in younger ages. They are causally much less important in affective disorder starting in late life, while physical illness is significant in 60–75% of cases. The risk to first-degree relatives of probands with depressive disorder of late onset is $\frac{1}{3}$ to $\frac{1}{2}$ of those of early onset. However, up to a third of those with late-onset depression may have a family history of depression (Butler & Pitt 1998, p. 127; Gelder et al 2006, p. 512; Jacoby & Oppenheimer 2002, p. 637; Johnstone et al 2004, p. 646; Stein & Wilkinson 1998, p. 61).

14. REM sleep is reduced in depression.

False: In depression there is decreased REM-latency, i.e. the time from the onset of sleep to the onset of REM sleep is reduced. Moreover, there is increased REM density and increased total REM sleep (Sadock & Sadock 2005, p. 1601).

15. Delta waves in the EEG are increased in depression.

False: Delta waves occur in deep, non-REM sleep or slow wave sleep. The length of slow wave sleep is reduced in depression (Johnstone et al 2004, p. 437; Sadock & Sadock 2005, p. 1601).

16. In depression, blunted cortisol suppression and blunted response to TRH combined gives a diagnostic sensitivity of 80%.

False: The sensitivity of DST is approximately 60% and of TRH–TSH is approximately 25%. Neither test alone or in combination is of sufficient sensitivity or specificity to be of clinical use (Gelder et al 2000, p. 714; Johnstone et al 2004, p. 436; Puri & Hall 2004, p. 274).

17. There is usually a greater fall of cortisol following dexamethasone administration in depression than in normal volunteers.

False: Normal subjects have suppressed plasma cortisol levels throughout the following day after a dose of 1–2 mg of dexamethasone. A high proportion of severely depressed patients do not show this suppression effect and continue to produce normal/elevated levels of cortisol. However, the specificity and sensitivity are not sufficiently high to be used as a diagnostic test (Gelder et al 2000, p. 714; Murray et al 1997, p. 329).

18. Growth hormone response to clonidine is decreased in depression.

True: Growth hormone is secreted from the anterior pituitary on stimulation by noradrenaline and dopamine. Growth hormone response to both the noradrenaline reuptake inhibitor desipramine and the noradrenaline α_2-adrenoceptor agonist clonidine is blunted in depression (Gelder et al 2006, p. 241; Sadock & Sadock 2005, p. 1600)

19. TSH response to TRH is normal in euthyroid depressed patients.

False: Blunted thyroid-stimulating hormone (TSH) response to thyrotropin-releasing hormone (TRH) occurs in 20–30% of patients with major depression. This does not normalize on remission of depression. They have an increased risk of relapse despite maintenance antidepressant therapy.

On the other hand, 5–10% of depressed patients have elevated basal TSH levels and an increased TSH response to TRH (Gelder et al 2006, p. 241; Sadock & Sadock 2005, p. 1600).

20. Melatonin secretion increases in the winter.

True: Melatonin secretion is inhibited by light. Melatonin secretion occurs particularly at night, with increased secretion hypothesized in the longer winter nights (Gelder et al 2000, p. 1352; Johnstone et al 2004, p. 428).

21. Platelet 5-HT binding is decreased in depression.

True: Platelet membranes contain secondary carrier systems for the uptake of 5-HT. It is generally agreed that 5-HT binding is reduced in depression compared to healthy controls (Paykel 1992, p. 224).

22. Vanillylmandelic acid (VMA) is significant in studies of depression.

True: VMA is the major metabolite of adrenaline and noradrenaline (NE) in the periphery, while MHPG is the CNS metabolite. In depression, decreased central NE activity is evidenced by decreased urinary MHPG. However, a subgroup of depressed patients has elevated circulating levels of NE and its metabolites including VMA. This may suggest a dissociation of NE activity in the median forebrain bundle and the sympathomedullary systems (Anderson & Reid 2002, p. 19; Sadock & Sadock 2005, p. 1598).

23. Mania is associated with depressive symptoms more often in the elderly.

False: In the 60s and 70s it was reported that the elderly manic patients had more depressive features, mood incongruent persecutory delusions, hostility and resentment, but less flight of ideas and infectious euphoria. Recent prospective studies have found no such differences except for more severe illness in the young (Copeland et al 2002, p. 479; Gelder et al 2000, p. 1650).

24. There is a familial component to response to antidepressant medication in BPAD.

True: Pharmacogenetics is the study of genetic variations in pharmacodynamic and pharmacokinetic factors. Serotonin transporter variants have been associated with the likelihood of antidepressant response to SSRIs and also with the susceptibility to develop antidepressant-induced mania in bipolar disorder (King 2004, p. 51).

25. After an episode of mania, more than 80% of individuals will have at least one further episode of either mania or depression.

True: 90% of patients with mania experience a further episode of mood disturbance (Gelder et al 2006, p. 245).

29 Neuropsychiatry – 1

Rudi Kritzinger

T F

1. Alexia with agraphia is associated with anomia.

2. In bilingual patients, the first language is most affected in aphasia.

3. Wernicke's area is supplied by the anterior cerebral artery.

4. Early CJD is associated with specific EEG changes.

5. Methionine homozygosity of the polymorphic residue at codon 129 is associated with nvCJD.

6. Alpha waves increase on eye opening.

7. Epileptic automatisms usually last 5 to 15 minutes.

8. Interictal psychosis in complex partial seizures is almost always associated with non-dominant focus.

9. Seizures lasting more than 30 minutes indicate non-epileptic rather than true seizure.

10. Methylenetetrahydrofolate reductase gene polymorphism is a risk factor for hyperhomocysteinaemia.

11. Polymerase chain reaction involves dissolving DNA at 95°C.

12. Apathy is a common feature of patients with penetrating head injury to the right frontal cortex, even at 5 years follow-up.

13. Increased sensitivity to neuroleptics is a complication of HIV infection.

14. The suicide rate in HIV is 10% higher than expected.

15. The EEG shows exaggerated spikes in Huntington's disease.

16. Episodic memory is usually impaired in semantic dementia.

17. Euphoria in multiple sclerosis is associated with cognitive impairment.

18. ECT is contraindicated in the treatment of depression in multiple sclerosis.

19. Non-dominant parietal lobe lesions lead to apraxia.

20. Prosopagnosia means impaired recognition of previously well-known faces.

21. Galvanic skin conductance is increased in anxiety disorders.

22. Slow wave sleep is decreased in the elderly.

23. Alcohol can precipitate sleepwalking.

T F

24. Tau protein is essential for microtubule formation.

☐☐

25. Persecutory delusions are more common than hallucinations in hypothyroidism.

☐☐

ANSWERS

1. Alexia with agraphia is associated with anomia.

True: Anomic aphasia often co-occurs with alexia and agraphia. The neuropathology often involves the left angular gyrus or the left temporal pole (Yudofsky & Hales 2002, p. 572).

2. In bilingual patients, the first language is most affected in aphasia.

False: In aphasia the acquired or second language tends to be more severely affected than the mother tongue.

3. Wernicke's area is supplied by the anterior cerebral artery.

False: Wernicke's area is supplied by the middle temporal artery which is a cortical branch of the middle cerebral artery (Fitzgerald 1996, p. 45).

4. Early CJD is associated with specific EEG changes.

False: Although the EEG is almost always abnormal, the changes are usually variable and non-specific, especially in the early stages. Initially, there may only be local or diffuse slowing. This may progress to paroxysmal sharp waves or slow spike and wave discharges. A characteristic pattern of 1–2 Hz periodic simple, biphasic, triphasic or polyspike sharp wave complexes on a slow background with loss of alpha rhythm occurs in 70–90% of cases late in the illness (Lishman 1997, p. 478; Mitchell 2004, p. 180; Sadock & Sadock 2005, p. 469; Wright et al 2005, p. 386).

5. Methionine homozygosity of the polymorphic residue at codon 129 is associated with nvCJD.

True: There are many differences between CJD and nvCJD. nvCJD affects a younger age group than sporadic CJD. nvCJD is more commonly associated with a non-specific psychiatric prodrome of anxiety and depression and is therefore more likely to present to psychiatrists. Ataxia occurs relatively earlier in the course of nvCJD and myoclonus later. In nvCJD, the EEG lacks the characteristic 1–2 Hz sharp waves of CJD and histopathology shows increased plaque formation. nvCJD is strongly associated with methionine homozygosity at codon 129 where a met–val polymorphism is seen (Lishman 1997, p. 476).

6. Alpha waves increase on eye opening.

False: The alpha rhythm has a frequency range of 8–14 Hz. It is best recorded over the occipital and parietal region. It occurs during wakefulness on eye closure and attenuates on eye opening (Yudofsky & Hales 2002, p. 45).

7. Epileptic automatisms usually last 5 to 15 minutes.

False: An epileptic automatism is a state of clouding of consciousness which occurs during or immediately after a seizure. During an automatism the individual retains control of posture and muscle tone and performs movements and actions without being aware of what is happening. They are usually brief, lasting a few seconds to a few minutes. In Knox's 1968 series 80% lasted less than 5 minutes and another 12% less than 15 minutes (Lishman 1997, p. 253).

8. Interictal psychosis in complex partial seizures is almost always associated with non-dominant focus.

False: Visual hallucinations and interpretative illusions of familiarity derive more commonly from the right than the left temporal lobe. However, interictal psychosis may be linked with dominant temporal lobe seizures (Lishman 1997, p. 251; Mitchell 2004, p. 119).

9. Seizures lasting more than 30 minutes indicate non-epileptic rather than true seizure.

False: Non-epileptic seizures (NES) are notoriously difficult to distinguish from epileptic seizures. The diagnosis of NES depends not only on the duration of the seizure but also on other clinical characteristics. NES can follow a generalized tonic clonic seizure. A generalized tonic clonic seizure lasting more than 30 minutes could represent status epilepticus and should be taken seriously. Associations of NES include: more common in females; psychosocial disturbance; consciousness retained in the presence of bilateral jerking; resistance to examination; vocalization, pelvic thrusting, gaze aversion and normal pupillary reflexes during convulsion; normal pupillary, deep tendon and plantar reflexes immediately after a convulsion.

10. Methylenetetrahydrofolate reductase gene polymorphism is a risk factor for hyperhomocysteinaemia.

True: Hyperhomocysteinaemia is a risk factor for coronary artery disease, stroke, vascular dementia and Alzheimer's disease. Methylenetetrahydrofolate reductase regulates homocysteine levels by converting it to methionine. Hence, methylenetetrahydrofolate reductase genotype influences the levels of homocysteine (Jacoby & Oppenheimer 2002, p. 523; Sadock & Sadock 2005, p. 3741).

11. Polymerase chain reaction involves dissolving DNA at 95°C.

True: Polymerase chain reaction is a laboratory technique for rapid amplification of DNA sequences. First, two oligonucleotide primers which flank the gene of interest are created. The DNA is heat treated in order to separate the two strands ready for replication. The DNA primers and DNA polymerase are incubated and replication of the original DNA sequence occurs. Because of the need to heat the DNA to separate the two strands, a special heat resistant DNA polymerase from a thermophilic bacterium is used. At the end of the first cycle two double stranded DNA molecules of the gene of interest are produced. The cycle is then repeated resulting in exponential growth in the number of copies of the gene with each cycle. Each replication takes about 5 minutes. This process is automated. Thus, genes can be amplified a billion fold using this technique (Alberts et al 2000, p. 508).

12. Apathy is a common feature of patients with penetrating head injury to the right frontal cortex, even at 5 years follow-up.

True: Damage to the dorsolateral prefrontal cortex, on either side, causes slowness, apathy and perseveration (Yudofsky & Hales 2002, p. 634).

13. Increased sensitivity to neuroleptics is a complication of HIV infection.

True: In general, late stage HIV patients, especially those with AIDS dementia complex, are far more sensitive to the therapeutic effects, but even more so to the side-effects and toxic effects of antipsychotic drugs. Extrapyramidal side-effects, tardive dyskinesia and neuroleptic malignant syndrome are all more common in patients with AIDS, especially AIDS dementia complex. They are also more sensitive to anticholinergic side-effects and have a high risk of delirium (Gelder et al 2000, p. 1170; Mitchell 2004, p. 382; Sadock & Sadock 2005, p. 438).

14. The suicide rate in HIV is 10% higher than expected.

True: The figures are conflicting. However, the suicide rates are significantly greater than in the general population. The risk is particularly raised in the first 6 months after diagnosis and also in the late stages of HIV infection (symptomatic AIDS) (Lishman 1997, p. 331; Mitchell 2004, p. 457).

15. The EEG shows exaggerated spikes in Huntington's disease.

False: The EEG in Huntington's disease shows loss of alpha rhythms. There may be generalized low voltage fast activity or random slow activity. As the disease progresses the EEG may become completely flat. These changes are not ubiquitous. Normal traces may be achieved even in advanced disease (Lishman 1997, p. 470; Mitchell 2004, p. 161; Yudofsky & Hales 2002, p. 964).

16. Episodic memory is usually impaired in semantic dementia.

False: Semantic dementia is a form of presenile dementia presenting as a selective loss of semantic knowledge, i.e. factual information and vocabulary. Episodic memory is memory for events. Three classic causes of episodic memory loss evident from an inability to retain new material for more than a few minutes are Korsakoff's syndrome, transient global amnesia and hippocampal damage from herpes simplex encephalitis. The latter may also result in a semantic memory deficit. Other causes of semantic memory dysfunction include Picks' disease, Alzheimer's disease, head injury and vascular lesions (Hodges 1994, p. 16; Lishman 1997, p. 753; Mitchell 2004, p. 69).

17. Euphoria in multiple sclerosis is associated with cognitive impairment.

True: Euphoria is a manifestation of advanced multiple sclerosis, commensurate with extensive cerebral damage. Euphoria has been associated with greater physical disability and cognitive impairment, progressive disease course, enlarged ventricles on CT scan, frontal lesions and more widespread lesions on

MRI. Lesion load and cognitive impairment are more strongly associated with high mood than with low mood. First onset mania in multiple sclerosis is likely to reflect new brain lesions (Feinstein 1999, p. 59; Lishman 1997, p. 694; Mitchell 2004, p. 144).

18. ECT is contraindicated in the treatment of depression in multiple sclerosis.

False: ECT is not contraindicated in MS. However, ECT can cause neurological deterioration in 20% of patients with active disease. Ideally, an MRI should be done to aid decision-making. Active disease, i.e. white matter plaques on MRI, would indicate a higher risk of deterioration. In the presence of active disease, ECT should be used only in emergencies or if pharmacotherapy fails (Feinstein 1999, p. 44).

19. Non-dominant parietal lobe lesions lead to apraxia.

True: *Ideomotor apraxia* refers to the inability of a patient with intact comprehension and motor system to carry out a motor action when instructed to do so, but at other times they may carry out this action spontaneously. Patients have difficulty with selection, sequencing and spatial orientation of movement in gestures, demonstrating the use of imagined items and imitating gestures. Lesions are usually found in the left parietal or frontal lobes.

Ideational apraxia refers to a patient's inability to carry out a complex sequence of coordinated movements, for example lighting a cigarette, although in contrast to ideomotor apraxia, the patient can carry out the separate components of the action. Corpus callosum or generalized lesions are normally associated with this deficit.

Dressing apraxia is not an apraxia in the sense that it is not a motor disorder but rather seems to be related to visuospatial difficulties. Localized lesions in the right posterior parietal lobe can lead to this problem, but more often it is seen with generalized lesions to the right hemisphere.

Constructional apraxia refers to the inability to copy two-dimensional shapes and figures, and is a defect of visual analysis and visuomotor ability. It is more often seen in lesions of the right hemisphere, particularly if the parietal lobe is affected. It can however arise with right- or left-sided damage. Left-sided lesions often lead to oversimplified copying, whereas right-sided lesions may lead to gross distortions in spatial arrangement (Hodges 1994, p. 70; Mitchell 2004, p. 74).

20. Prosopagnosia means impaired recognition of previously well-known faces.

True: Prosopagnosia is the inability to recognize the identities of previously well-known faces and the inability to learn new ones. Exposure to the voice of the unrecognized individual will elicit prompt recognition. It is associated with damage to the temporo-occipital junction or bilateral damage to the ventral aspect of the occipital lobes (Mitchell 2004, p. 75; Yudofsky & Hales 2002, p. 82).

21. Galvanic skin conductance is increased in anxiety disorders.

True: The electrodermal system is under the sole control of the sympathetic nervous system rather than under a dynamic balance between sympathetic and parasympathetic systems. Sympathetic activation may be tonic or phasic.

Activation increases sweating and hence increases conductance. Anxiety causes increased tonic activity. Depression may decrease skin conductance. Relaxation decreases skin conductance (Sadock & Sadock 2005, p. 1729).

22. Slow wave sleep is decreased in the elderly.

True: Young children show the highest proportion of slow wave sleep. This declines with age until slow wave sleep may disappear altogether after age 60 years. Sleep also becomes more fragmented with age and shows increased latency to sleep onset, increased nighttime arousals and daytime napping. REM sleep is preserved in the normal elderly but may be severely disrupted in Alzheimer's disease (Sadock & Sadock 2005, p. 283).

23. Alcohol can precipitate sleepwalking.

True: Sleepwalking represents partial arousal from the deep non-REM stages of sleep. It occurs most often during the first third of the night when stages 3 and 4 predominate.

Conditions that increase slow wave sleep, such as sleep deprivation, shift work or alcohol consumption may increase the frequency of sleepwalking (Lishman 1997, p. 736).

24. Tau protein is essential for microtubule formation.

True: Tau protein in its physiological state is essential for the formation and stability of microtubules. Abnormal phosphorylated tau is found in neurofibrillary tangles (Lishman 1997, p. 422).

25. Persecutory delusions are more common than hallucinations in hypothyroidism.

False: Both delusions and auditory and visual hallucinations are common in hypothyroidism (Lishman 1997, p. 512).

30 Neuropsychiatry – 2

Fernando Lazaro-Perlado

T F

1. Alexia without agraphia occurs in anterior cerebral artery lesions. ☐ ☐

2. Patients with Broca's aphasia use short phrases. ☐ ☐

3. Pathological blushing is also known as Binswanger's disease. ☐ ☐

4. The EEG is normal in 20–40% of people in the very early stages of CJD. ☐ ☐

5. CJD can cause dementia with myoclonus. ☐ ☐

6. Alpha waves on the EEG are maximal over the frontal region. ☐ ☐

7. The EEG during epileptic automatisms typically shows 8–14-Hz spikes. ☐ ☐

8. Flexibilitas cerea can occur after encephalitis. ☐ ☐

9. Exons are excluded during splicing. ☐ ☐

10. Polymerase chain reaction requires a thermostable DNA polymerase. ☐ ☐

11. Disinhibition is a common long-term consequence of a penetrating parietal lobe injury. ☐ ☐

12. 'AIDS panic' is a recognized symptom in seronegative individuals. ☐ ☐

13. AIDS patients with euphoria have a poorer prognosis. ☐ ☐

14. Anticipation phenomenon occurs in Huntington's disease. ☐ ☐

15. In Alzheimer's disease the memory degradation curve starts off gradually and then becomes progressively steeper. ☐ ☐

16. Cognitive impairment is a feature of longstanding multiple sclerosis. ☐ ☐

17. Narcolepsy with cataplexy occurs in 3 per 10 000 of the population. ☐ ☐

18. Parietal lobe damage causes nominal aphasia. ☐ ☐

19. Pathological laughing and crying occurs in response to specific stimuli. ☐ ☐

20. In prosopagnosia, the patient can recognize individuals only from non-facial characteristics. ☐ ☐

21. In systemic lupus erythematosis, depression has slow onset. ☐ ☐

22. Hypersomnia with apnoea is commonest between ages 40 and 60 years. ☐ ☐

23. In adults, night terrors can be related to relationship difficulties. ☐ ☐

24. Nominal aphasia occurs in non-dominant temporal lobe lesions. ☐ ☐

T   F

25. Pimozide is markedly superior to haloperidol in treating motor tics in Tourette syndrome.

☐ ☐

ANSWERS

1. Alexia without agraphia occurs in anterior cerebral artery lesions.

False: Alexia without agraphia usually accompanies infarction of the left occipital lobe following occlusion of the left posterior cerebral artery. Patients are able to comprehend words spelt aloud and also to write but they are quite unable to read. They cannot read even their own writing (Hodges 1994, p. 61; Lishman 1997, p. 19).

2. Patients with Broca's aphasia use short phrases.

True: In Broca's aphasia spontaneous speech is sparse, slow, non-fluent, effortful, dysarthric, dysprosodic, short in phrase length and agrammatical in the presence of relatively preserved comprehension, abnormal repetition and naming, and disturbed reading and writing (Mitchell 2004, p. 72; Yudofsky & Hales 2002, p. 568).

3. Pathological blushing is also known as Binswanger's disease.

False: Pathological fear of blushing is called erythrophobia. Binswanger's disease is a subcortical vascular dementia affecting the deep white matter of the brain (Lishman 1997, p. 458; Mitchell 2004, p. 46).

4. The EEG is normal in 20–40% of people in the very early stages of CJD.

False: Although the EEG is almost always abnormal, the changes are usually variable and non-specific, especially in the early stages. Initially there may only be local or diffuse slowing. This may progress to paroxysmal sharp waves or slow spike and wave discharges. A characteristic pattern of 1–2-Hz periodic simple, biphasic, triphasic or polyspike sharp wave complexes on a slow background with loss of alpha rhythm occurs in 70–90% of cases late in the illness (Lishman 1997, p. 478; Sadock & Sadock 2005, p. 469).

5. CJD can cause dementia with myoclonus.

True: Myoclonus is a muscular jerk that may be localized or diffuse. The differential diagnosis of dementia with myoclonus includes CJD, late stages of dialysis dementia, AIDS dementia and Alzheimer's disease.

CJD is a rare cause of dementia and in its classical form myoclonus is often present. Parkinsonism and choreoathetoid movements may also be seen. New variant CJD may show similar movement disorders but is also accompanied by sensory problems including painful neuropathy (Mitchell 2004, p. 16; Wright et al 2005, p. 387).

6. Alpha waves on the EEG are maximal over the frontal region.

False: The alpha rhythm is best recorded over the occipital and parietal region. It occurs during wakefulness on eye closure and attenuates on eye opening (Yudofsky & Hales 2002, p. 45).

7. The EEG during epileptic automatisms typically shows 8–14-Hz spikes.

False: During epileptic automatisms consciousness is clouded but not completely lost. Hence, seizure activity may not be immediately obvious. Stereotyped movements (e.g. lip smacking) may occur. More complex behaviour is seen more rarely. The EEG shows initial low voltage theta waves and later, bilateral delta waves (Wright et al 2005, p. 395).

8. Flexibilitas cereas can occur after encephalitis.

True: Flexibilitas cereas or waxy flexibility was associated with encephalitis lethargica. Although an aetiological agent was never identified, the onset and course of the disease was consistent with encephalitis (Lishman 1997, p. 349).

9. Exons are excluded during splicing.

False: Exons are the coding regions. At no point are they excluded. The process of replication involves transcription of DNA to mRNA, splicing out of introns and then translation of mRNA to protein (Puri & Tyrer 1998, p. 171).

10. Polymerase chain reaction requires a thermostable DNA polymerase.

True: During the polymerase chain reaction the double helix of DNA needs to be separated to allow replication of a DNA sequence. This separation is facilitated by heating the DNA. A special thermostable DNA polymerase which will not be denatured by heat is therefore required (Alberts et al 2000, p. 508).

11. Disinhibition is a common long-term consequence of a penetrating parietal lobe injury.

False: Disinhibition is more typical after frontal lesions, especially those involving the orbito-frontal areas (Mitchell 2004, p. 136).

12. 'AIDS panic' is a recognized symptom in seronegative individuals.

True: Individuals may present themselves for testing in states of severe distress and alarm. This is called AIDS anxiety or AIDS panic (Lishman 1997, p. 331).

13. AIDS patients with euphoria have a poorer prognosis.

True: The prevalence of manic syndromes in AIDS patients is more than 10 times that in the general population. AIDS mania is a secondary mania consequent to brain HIV involvement. This is associated with late stage HIV infection, cognitive impairment and absence of previous episodes or family history of bipolar affective disorder. AIDS mania is usually quite severe in its presentation and the course is often chronic rather than episodic. They may develop a delusion that their HIV has been cured and this can interfere with treatment. They are also more sensitive to the side-effects of psychotropic medication (Gelder et al 2000, p. 1170; Mitchell 2004, p. 189; Sadock & Sadock 2005, p. 437).

14. Anticipation phenomenon occurs in Huntington's disease.

True: Anticipation phenomenon means that each successive generation tends to develop Huntington's disease at an earlier age than the previous one. This is more marked with paternal inheritance. The paternally derived gene may be more unstable than those from the maternal line and this leads to an expanded number of repeats in the next generation. This in turn leads to earlier clinical manifestation (Yudofsky & Hales 2002, p. 332).

15. In Alzheimer's disease the memory degradation curve starts off gradually and then becomes progressively steeper.

True: In the early phases, memory decline is almost imperceptible, but gradually accelerates to an average of 3 points or more on the MMSE per year (Mitchell 2004, p. 427).

16. Cognitive impairment is a feature of longstanding multiple sclerosis.

True: Cognitive impairment is present in 40% of community samples and 50–60% of clinic attenders. It may present early in the illness and becomes more common as the disease progresses. Neuropsychological deficits may be evident even before the full diagnosis of multiple sclerosis is made, for example when the only symptoms are those of optic neuritis (Gelder et al 2006, p. 353; Lishman 1997, p. 693; Mitchell 2004, p. 145).

17. Narcolepsy with cataplexy occurs in 3 per 10 000 of the population.

False: Narcolepsy is characterized by a tetrad of symptoms:

1. Excessive daytime sleepiness
2. Cataplexy
3. Sleep paralysis and
4. Hypnagogic hallucinations.

The prevalence of narcolepsy is between 3 and 6 per 100 000. Cataplexy is the temporary loss of muscle tone precipitated by emotions such as anger and laughter. The severity of cataplexy ranges widely from transient weakness of the knees to total paralysis while the patient is fully conscious. Usually the patient is unable to speak and may fall to the floor. Episodes may last from several seconds to minutes. Cataplexy occurs only in 60–70% of those with narcolepsy. Hence, the prevalence of narcolepsy with catalepsy would be approximately 0.3 per 10 000 (Fear 2004, p. 328).

18. Parietal lobe damage causes nominal aphasia.

True: Nominal dysphasia, amnesic aphasia or anomic aphasia, is the commonest form of aphasia, but the least well understood. It involves difficulties in evoking names at will. Mild forms of nominal aphasia may be caused by diffuse brain dysfunction due to toxic or degenerative conditions. Nominal aphasia may also be caused by focal brain lesions, especially by dominant temporo-parietal lesions in the neighbourhood of the angular gyrus. Nominal aphasia is often associated with acalculia and other components of Gerstmann syndrome (Lishman 1997, p. 52).

19. Pathological laughing and crying occurs in response to specific stimuli.

False: Poeck in 1969 described the features of pathological laughing and crying as:
- Response to non-specific stimuli
- Absence of an association between affective change and the expressed emotion
- Absence of voluntary control of facial expression and
- Absence of corresponding change in mood exceeding the period of crying or laughing (Feinstein 1999, p. 68).

20. In prosopagnosia, the patient can recognize individuals only from non-facial characteristics.

True: Prosopagnosia is the inability to recognize the identities of previously well-known faces and to learn new ones. Exposure to the voice of the unrecognized individual will elicit prompt recognition. It is associated with damage to the temporo-occipital junction or bilateral damage to the ventral aspect of the occipital lobes (Yudofsky & Hales 2002, p. 81).

21. In systemic lupus erythematosis, depression has slow onset.

True: In systemic lupus erythematosis, depression starts gradually, lasts several weeks or months and resolves slowly (Lishman 1997, p. 420).

22. Hypersomnia with apnoea is commonest between ages 40 and 60 years.

True: Most cases of obstructive sleep apnoea occur in males after the age of 40. Central sleep apnoea can affect all age groups (Lishman 1997, p. 730).

23. In adults, night terrors can be related to relationship difficulties.

True: Night terror is characterized by a sudden incomplete arousal from sleep with intense fearfulness. The individual typically sits in bed, is unresponsive to stimuli, and if awakened is confused or disorientated. There is often amnesia for the episode. These episodes arise from slow wave sleep. Psychopathology is seldom associated with night terrors in children. However, adults with night terrors often have psychiatric problems or a history of traumatic experiences. The frequency ranges from less than once per month to almost every night (Yudofsky & Hales 2002, p. 717).

24. Nominal aphasia occurs in non-dominant temporal lobe lesions.

False: Nominal aphasia refers to difficulties with language function manifest as problems with word finding and naming. Temporal lobe damage can affect semantic memory. Difficulty with vocabulary may result in severe anomia and semantic dementia. Such deficits are most commonly associated with dominant lobe lesions. Non-dominant lesions impair appreciation of music. Dominant lobe lesions are also associated with Wernicke's dysphasia (Hodges 1994, p. 44).

25. Pimozide is markedly superior to haloperidol in treating motor tics in Tourette syndrome.

False: Haloperidol, sulpiride and pimozide are the most commonly used, but there is no good evidence that suggests any particular drug has superior efficacy (Mitchell 2004, p. 359).

31 | Neuropsychiatry – 3

Ben Underwood

	T	F

1. Dyslexia is a characteristic feature of Gerstmann syndrome.

2. Difficulty in reading and writing is a feature of Wernicke's aphasia.

3. Carbon monoxide poisoning can cause amnesic confabulatory syndrome.

4. CJD is associated with triphasic waves on the EEG in 80% of cases.

5. A normal CSF reading includes 5 neutrophils per mL.

6. Barbiturates increase fast activity on the EEG.

7. Epilepsy-related automatisms are a common cause of homicide.

8. Dorsolateral prefrontal cortex lesions cause apathy.

9. Genes code for introns, exons and tRNA.

10. The polymerase used in a polymerase chain reaction (PCR) is heat stable.

11. In post-concussion syndrome the symptoms most rapidly improve after the first 6 months.

12. Schizophreniform psychosis is recognized in HIV.

13. Huntington's disease is associated with CAG repeats.

14. In Huntington's disease the unaffected siblings have a higher than average rate of criminal behaviour.

15. Implicit memory is preserved in Korsakoff's syndrome.

16. Psychotic disorder in the context of multiple sclerosis has a poor outcome.

17. Narcolepsy is associated with loss of muscle tone in clear consciousness.

18. Left–right disorientation is a feature of left parietal lobe lesions.

19. Fluoxetine is effective in the treatment of pathological laughing/crying.

20. Prosopagnosia can result from a penetrating right-sided head injury.

21. Neuropsychiatric symptoms occur in most patients with systemic lupus erythematosis.

22. The treatment of choice for hypersomnia associated with severe apnoea is tracheostomy.

23. Night terror in adults is associated with depression.

24. Depression is rare in hyperthyroidism.

T F

25. Vitamin B12 deficiency commonly causes dementia in the elderly.

ANSWERS

1. Dyslexia is a characteristic feature of Gerstmann syndrome.

False: Gerstmann syndrome results from damage to the left angular gyrus or less commonly the dominant parietal lobe. The characteristic features are dysgraphia, dyscalculia, right–left disorientation and finger agnosia (Lishman 1997, p. 65; Mitchell 2004, p. 84; Yudofsky & Hales 2002, p. 573).

2. Difficulty in reading and writing is a feature of Wernicke's aphasia.

True: Fluent or Wernicke's aphasia is characterized by a fluent verbal output with normal word count, phrase length, effort, articulation and prosody. There is difficulty in repetition and in word finding. The verbal output is often empty of content words. Paraphrasic substitutions and neologisms are common. Extreme and unintelligible fluent aphasia is called jargon aphasia. Reading and writing are usually impaired. Patients produce paraphrasic and disjointed written text (Hodges 1994, p. 57; Mitchell 2004, p. 72; Yudofsky & Hales 2002, p. 568).

3. Carbon monoxide poisoning can cause amnesic confabulatory syndrome.

True: Amnesia is common. It is often the last symptom to resolve. Delirium is an early symptom and classical Korsakoff syndrome is sometimes seen. Memory and executive problems occur in most patients (Lishman 1997, p. 550; Mitchell 2004, p. 249).

4. CJD is associated with triphasic waves on the EEG in 80% of cases.

True: A characteristic pattern of 1–2-Hz periodic simple, biphasic, triphasic or complex polyspike sharp wave complexes on a slow background with loss of alpha rhythm occus in 70–90% of cases late in the illness.

Although the EEG is almost always abnormal, the changes are usually variable and non-specific in the early stages. Moreover, nvCJD does not show these characteristic EEG changes (Lishman 1997, p. 478; Mitchell 2004, p. 180; Sadock & Sadock 2005, p. 469; Wright et al 2005, p. 386).

5. A normal CSF reading includes 5 neutrophils per mL.

False: Normal CSF should contain less than 5 white cells per mL, and usually no neutrophils (Lindsay & Bone 2004, p. 56).

6. Barbiturates increase fast activity on the EEG.

True: Barbiturates increase beta (fast) activity, particularly in the frontal regions. This effect is opposite to that of alcohol (Sadock & Sadock 2005, p. 185).

7. Epilepsy-related automatisms are a common cause of homicide.

False: Epileptic automatism is an extremely rare cause of serious violence (Gelder et al 2000, p. 2050; Sadock & Sadock 2005, p. 385).

8. Dorsolateral prefrontal cortex lesions cause apathy.

True: Apathy has been associated with damage to the orbitofrontal, dorsomedial and dorsolateral prefrontal cortex, the basal ganglia, the thalamus and the internal capsule (Fitzgerald 1996, p. 237; Hodges 1994, p. 23; Lindsay & Bone 2004, p. 109; Mitchell 2004, p. 442; Sadock & Sadock 2005, p. 325).

9. Genes code for introns, exons and tRNA.

True: A gene is that segment of DNA which codes for a single protein or for a single stretch of RNA if it is not one which undergoes translation (e.g. genes for tRNA). This includes coding (exon) and non-coding (intron) segments. The gene is transcribed into mRNA before the non-coding regions are spliced out. The remaining mRNA is then translated into protein. The mRNA is divided into codons, i.e. triplets of nucleotides which code for specific amino acids. This triplet code is 'read' by a separate molecule of RNA, the tRNA, which has a single amino acid bound to it. The tRNA also has a triplet code (the anticodon) with which it matches the codon on the mRNA. At the ribosome the tRNA molecules line up on the mRNA by matching their anticodons with the mRNA codons and the amino acids they carry are joined in the correct sequence to form a protein. A separate strech of DNA codes for the tRNA molecules (Alberts et al 2000, p. 6).

10. The polymerase used in a polymerase chain reaction (PCR) is heat stable.

True: PCR is a technique used to amplify DNA. Firstly a mix is prepared containing buffers, nucleotides, short primers and a DNA thermostable polymerase (Taq) isolated from the thermophilic bacterium *Thermus aquaticus*. This mix is added to the sample DNA. It is then placed in a machine to automate the next part of the process. This first involves heating the sample to separate the two strands of DNA. This allows the primers to attach to the DNA and start a process of localized replication using the nucleotides and the DNA polymerase. The machine lets the sample cool before starting a new cycle. Each cycle doubles the amount of the DNA of interest that is present providing exponential growth. After a few hours this usually results in enough DNA to analyse further – for instance to run on a gel to identify a polymorphism in an individual. The polymerase has to be heat stable to avoid being denatured during the heating process (Alberts et al 2000, p. 508).

11. In post-concussion syndrome the symptoms most rapidly improve after the first 6 months.

False: Post-concussion syndrome presents in some patients after mild traumatic brain injury (post-traumatic amnesia <24 hours, loss of consciousness <20 min). It consists of a number of somatic, perceptual, cognitive and emotional symptoms. Most individuals recover usually within 6 months. In some cases it persists longer, with little improvement over time (Mitchell 2004, p. 138; Yudofsky & Hales 2002, p. 641)

12. Schizophreniform psychosis is recognized in HIV.

True: Various psychotic disorders, i.e. depressive, manic, paranoid and schizophrenic, may arise in patients who already show physical manifestations of ARC or AIDS or the psychosis may first draw attention to the disease (Lishman 1997, p. 331; Yudofsky & Hales 2002, p. 798). However, others believe that there is no evidence that HIV infection causes schizophrenia (Mitchell 2004, p. 190; Sadock & Sadock 2005, p. 438)

13. Huntington's disease is associated with CAG repeats.

True: Huntington's disease is an autosomal dominant neurodegenerative disorder with motor, cognitive and psychiatric symptoms. It is caused by a CAG trinucleotide repeat expansion mutation in exon 1 of the Huntington gene on the short arm of chromosome 4. As CAG encodes for glutamine, the mutation results in a protein with excess glutamine residues. Repeats of more than 35 CAGs are associated with disease. The longer the repeat length beyond 35, the earlier the onset of the disease. This at least partially explains the anticipation phenomenon, i.e. the disease becomes manifest at earlier ages in successive generations, as repeats tend to increase in length during parental transmission. This phenomenon may be more common in mutations inherited from the paternal line (Lishman 1997, p. 466; Mitchell 2004, p. 161; Sadock & Sadock 2005, p. 414).

14. In Huntington's disease the unaffected siblings have a higher than average rate of criminal behaviour.

True: Conduct disorder and criminal behaviour are not uncommon in the offspring of Huntington's disease patients, even in those not carrying the genetic mutation. Environmental factors, limbic-basal-cortex disruptions and being brought up by an affected parent may be contributory (Yudofsky & Hales 2002, p. 930).

15. Implicit memory is preserved in Korsakoff's syndrome.

True: The diencephalic structures involved in memory include the mamillary bodies, medial dorsal thalamic nuclei, internal medullary lamina and the mamillothalamic tracts. They support the role of the hippocampi. Hippocampi are involved in explicit (declarative) memory. They are not involved in implicit (procedural) memory, e.g. the non-conscious, automatic performance of previously learned skills such as driving a car.

In Korsakoff's syndrome, anterograde memory is most severely affected. New learning is impaired. Disturbance of time sense and confabulation occur. Immediate memory span is well preserved, and beyond a variable retrograde gap remote memories are well preserved. Implicit memory is well preserved. They can learn to mirror write even though they do not remember having been asked to perform the task before (Lishman 1997, p. 30; Mitchell 2004, p. 234).

16. Psychotic disorder in the context of multiple sclerosis has a poor outcome.

False: Psychotic disorders in the context of multiple sclerosis are rare, but have a good prognosis with remission rates over 90% (Feinstein 1999, p. 80).

17. Narcolepsy is associated with loss of muscle tone in clear consciousness.

True: Narcolepsy is characterized by excessive daytime sleepiness, cataplexy, sleep paralysis and hypnagogic hallucinations.

Cataplexy is the temporary loss of muscle tone precipitated by emotions such as anger and laughter while the patient is fully conscious. Cataplexy occurs in 60–70% of those with narcolepsy (Mitchell 2004, p. 224; Yudofsky & Hales 2002, p. 715).

18. Left–right disorientation is a feature of left parietal lobe lesion.

True: Left–right disorientation suggests a dominant parietal lesion. Gerstmann syndrome refers to the presence of dyscalculia, dysgraphia, finger agnosia and left–right confusion (Lindsay & Bone 2004, p. 111; Mitchell 2004, p. 84).

19. Fluoxetine is effective in the treatment of pathological laughing/crying.

True: Although the evidence is empirical, small doses of fluoxetine have been tried with success. Rapid improvement has been achieved without unpleasant side-effects. Other drugs used with some success are amitriptyline, levodopa, and amantadine. Dopamine agonists should be reserved for cases that have not responded to either fluoxetine or amitriptyline (Feinstein 1999, p. 76; Mitchell 2004, p. 320).

20. Prosopagnosia can result from a penetrating right-sided head injury.

True: Prosopagnosia results from bilateral or non-dominant parieto-occipital lesions (Lishman 1997, p. 18; Mitchell 2004, p. 75).

21. Neuropsychiatric symptoms occur in most patients with systemic lupus erythematosis.

True: Neuropsychiatric manifestations occur in up to 60% of patients with systemic lupus erythematosis. They include acute and chronic organic reactions, schizophrenic and affective psychoses, changes in personality, neurotic symptoms, seizures, cranial nerve palsies, peripheral neuropathy, movement disorders and intracranial ischaemic events (Lishman 1997, p. 419; Mitchell 2004, p. 219).

22. The treatment of choice for hypersomnia associated with severe apnoea is tracheostomy.

False: In sleep apnoea, the treatment of choice is usually nasal continuous positive airway pressure (nCPAP) (Lindsay & Bone 2004, p. 106).

23. Night terror in adults is associated with depression.

True: Sleep terrors are sudden and brief episodes of panic and confusion with intense autonomic activation. They are most common between ages 5 and

7 years. Thereafter they become increasingly uncommon. They are more common in males. They are often associated with sleepwalking, sleep talking, confusional arousals and Gilles de la Tourette syndrome. Night terror persisting after age 20 years is often associated with anxiety, depression and phobias (Schneerson 2000, p. 142).

24. Depression is rare in hyperthyroidism.

False: Up to a third of hyperthyroid patients would meet criteria for major depressive episodes. Moreover, the symptoms of hyperthyroidism such as anxiety, fatigue, insomnia, lability, dysphoria, poor attention span and weight loss overlap with those of depression (Lishman 1997, p. 508; Sadock & Sadock 2005, p. 2154).

25. Vitamin B12 deficiency commonly causes dementia in the elderly.

False: The prevalence of vitamin B12 deficiency in the elderly is 15–44%. However, the prevalence of reversible vitamin B12 deficiency as the primary aetiology in dementia is less than 1% (Sadock & Sadock 2005, p. 1091).

32

Neuropsychiatry – 4

Rudi Kritzinger

T F

1. A frontal lesion is the likely cause of dyslexia without agraphia.

2. In receptive aphasia speech can be fluent.

3. Acute confusional states due to carbon monoxide poisoning may last 2–3 weeks.

4. Most patients with CJD have abnormalities on CT brain scan.

5. Normal CSF glucose is 1–4 mmol per litre.

6. Benzodiazepines increase beta waves on the EEG.

7. Primary generalized epilepsy is usually associated with an aura.

8. Absence seizures in combination with generalized tonic-clonic seizures (GTCS) are associated with an increased risk of psychosis.

9. The prefrontal cortex is involved in the control of attention.

10. Autosomal dominant diseases usually show incomplete penetrance.

11. Restriction fragment length polymorphisms (RFLPs) are inherited in a Mendelian fashion.

12. Herpes virus encephalitis is associated with progressive memory loss.

13. Psychosis in HIV is associated with a poor outcome.

14. Huntington's disease is caused by a CAG repeat of greater than 35.

15. The anterior thalamus is affected in Huntington's disease.

16. The primacy effect is a feature of declarative memory.

17. Pathological laughing and crying is found in the early stages of multiple sclerosis.

18. Narcolepsy is associated with sudden onset REM sleep.

19. Neglect is a characteristic feature of right-sided parietal lobe lesion.

20. The planum temporale is located close to the auditory cortex.

21. If there is a left-sided hemiplegia, there is increased likelihood of a reading disorder.

22. Serotonin inhibits REM sleep.

23. Obstructive sleep apnoea is more common in ages 40–60 years.

T F

24. Depression may present with similar features to hyperthyroidism.

☐ ☐

25. Pantothenic acid deficiency causes dementia.

☐ ☐

ANSWERS

1. A frontal lesion is the likely cause of dyslexia without agraphia.

False: Pure alexia (without agraphia) results from lesions to the dominant occipital cortex (Mitchell 2004, p. 89).

2. In receptive aphasia, speech can be fluent.

True: Receptive aphasia (Wernicke's aphasia, primary sensory aphasia) implies a difficulty in understanding language. The difficulty in comprehension may range from a partial difficulty to a total inability to understand spoken language.

However, the faulty speech is produced fluently and without effort. Normal rhythm, inflexion and articulation are preserved (Lishman 1997, p. 51; Mitchell 2004, p. 72; Yudofsky & Hales 2002, p. 568).

3. Acute confusional states due to carbon monoxide poisoning may last 2–3 weeks.

True: Following carbon monoxide poisoning 20% of patients suffer prolonged delirium lasting several hours to several weeks (Lishman 1997, p. 550; Mitchell 2004, p. 248).

4. Most patients with CJD have abnormalities on CT brain scan.

False: CT brain scans may be normal, even in late stages of CJD and when the dementia is well advanced. CT may show cortical atrophy and ventricular enlargement, but it is usually mild (Lishman 1997, p. 478).

5. Normal CSF glucose is 1– 4 mmol per litre.

False: The CSF glucose is between 40% and 60% of the blood glucose level which should be taken at the same time as the lumbar puncture. 1 mmol/L is abnormally low unless the patient has a very low blood glucose level. Normal values for CSF are:
- Glucose = 2.8–4.2 mmol/L
- Protein = 0.15–0.45 g/L
- Opening pressure = 70–180 mm CSF.

6. Benzodiazepines increase beta waves on the EEG.

True: Benzodiazepines, even in small doses, always generate significant diffuse beta activity. If a particular region does not exhibit the expected benzodiazepine-induced beta activity, that area may be considered dysfunctional (Sadock & Sadock 2005, p. 183).

7. Primary generalized epilepsy is usually associated with an aura.

False: Aura is that part of the seizure which occurs before consciousness is lost and for which memory is retained. Simple partial seizures that become complex or possible secondary generalized are called auras. In primary generalized seizures consciousness is lost at the onset of the seizure and hence these are not associated with aura (Fitzgerald 1996, p. 259; Lishman 1997, p. 249; Sadock & Sadock 2005, p. 379).

8. Absence seizures in combination with generalized tonic-clonic seizures (GTCS) are associated with an increased risk of psychosis.

True: Absence seizures + GTCS in combination carry a 10% risk of psychosis, in contrast with 1% in myoclonic jerks + GTCS and 3% in juvenile myoclonic epilepsy + GTCS (Trimble & Schmitz 2002, p. 42).

9. The prefrontal cortex is involved in the control of attention.

True: Attention is an integrated and multimodal cognitive function. The anatomical substrates include the reticular activating system, prefrontal cortex, posterior parietal regions and temporal lobes (Hodges 1994, p. 2).

10. Autosomal dominant diseases usually show incomplete penetrance.

False: Autosomal dominant diseases are usually transmitted from generation to generation. Incomplete penetrance refers to cases where the phenotype is not transmitted to the next generation. The disease 'skips' a generation because despite having the dominant gene the phenotype is not expressed. This may be due to environmental or transmissible modifiers of gene expression. Polydactyly is an example of a condition with incomplete penetrance. Even people with the dominant allele can have a normal number of fingers and toes (Sadock & Sadock 2005, p. 239).

11. Restriction fragment length polymorphisms (RFLPs) are inherited in a Mendelian fashion.

True: DNA can be digested by restriction endonucleases. Endonucleases are bacterial enzymes which cleave DNA at specific sites. Identification of these sites allows a 'map' of the genome to be created with the restriction sites being marker points. Random base changes between individuals may alter these cleavage sites. These polymorphisms are called RFLPs. RFLPs are usually inherited in a Mendelian fashion and thus can be used as a marker to track a gene or chromosomal location of interest in a pedigree (Puri & Tyrer 1998, p. 193).

12. Herpes virus encephalitis is associated with progressive memory loss.

True: Although due to rapid destruction of the temporal lobe and thus similarly rapid memory loss, progression can occur. This progression still tends to be faster than memory loss associated with neurodegenerative conditions (Mitchell 2004, p. 201).

13. Psychosis in HIV is associated with a poor outcome.

True: Patients who develop first-onset psychosis after the diagnosis of AIDS have a higher than expected mortality rate (Mitchell 2004, p. 191).

14. Huntington's disease is caused by a CAG repeat of greater than 35.

True: Huntington's disease is caused by a CAG trinucleotide repeat expansion in exon 1 of the Huntingtin gene on the short arm of chromosome 4. As CAG encodes for glutamine, the mutation results in a protein with excess glutamine residues. Repeats of more than 35 CAGs are associated with disease. The longer the repeat length beyond 35, the earlier the onset of the disease (Lishman 1997, p. 466; Mitchell 2004, p. 161; Sadock & Sadock 2005, p. 414).

15. The anterior thalamus is affected in Huntington's disease.

False: Though ultimately almost all areas of the brain are affected in late stage Huntington's disease (HD), the anterior thalamus is not an area which is characteristically associated with HD. The striatum is the first area to show changes and pathology then spreads laterally to the putamen and globus pallidus (Mitchell 2004, pp. 46, 358; Yudofsky & Hales 2002, p. 926).

16. The primacy effect is a feature of declarative memory.

True: Declarative memory is a form of long-term memory for facts. The primacy effect explains why we can recall the first items from a long list more easily. This is because they have been transferred to the long-term memory. The most recent items from a list are also recalled more easily (recency effect) as these are presumably still in the short-term memory (Gross 2001, p. 249).

17. Pathological laughing and crying is found in the early stages of multiple sclerosis.

False: Pathological laughing and crying occurs in 10% of multiple sclerosis sufferers. It is associated with longer duration and progressive course of the illness, more physical disabilities, greater intellectual impairment and more extensive brain involvement (Feinstein 1999, p. 72).

18. Narcolepsy is associated with sudden onset REM sleep.

True: Narcolepsy is characterized by the tetrad of excessive daytime sleepiness, cataplexy, sleep paralysis and hypnagogic hallucinations. Narcolepsy is an REM sleep intrusion syndrome, possibly resulting from dysfunction in the REM sleep generator gating mechanisms. REM sleep occurs soon after sleep onset, both at night and during daytime naps (Mitchell 2004, p. 224; Yudofsky & Hales 2002, p. 715).

19. Neglect is a characteristic feature of right-sided parietal lobe lesion.

True: In patients with extensive non-dominant (right) hemisphere damage, there is often 'anosodiaphoria', i.e. indifference about left-sided weakness.

Occasionally there may be 'anosognosia', i.e. complete denial that any impairment exists (Lindsay & Bone 2004, p. 111; Mitchell 2004, p. 85).

20. The planum temporale is located close to the auditory cortex.

True: The planum temporale is a part of the superior temporal cortex. It is located close to the primary auditory cortex. It is associated with receptive language functions. It is larger in the left hemisphere than the right. Reversed asymmetry, i.e. larger planum temporale on the right, has been associated with dyslexia (Sadock & Sadock 2005, p. 15).

21. If there is a left-sided hemiplegia, there is increased likelihood of a reading disorder.

False: Reading, writing and language are localized dominant, i.e. left hemisphere, functions in most people. Reading disorders are called dyslexias.

Pure alexia (alexia without agraphia) is associated with left occipital lesions.

In surface dyslexias the patient relies on decoding words letter by letter. Errors are made in reading irregular words where the normal letter sound is replaced by another (e.g. mauve). Surface dyslexias occur in left temporo-parietal strokes and dementias.

Extensive left hemisphere damage results in deep dyslexia where the patient reads by recognizing whole words and their meaning – they are unable to read non-words such as 'gorth'.

Though dyslexia may also result from neglect (not reading one half of a word) in right parietal lesions, the majority of dyslexias result from left hemispheric lesions. If these lesions were large enough to also include the motor cortex then they would result in contralateral (right) hemiplegia, not left-sided hemiplegia (Hodges 1994, pp. 44, 61).

22. Serotonin inhibits REM sleep.

True: Acetylcholine promotes REM sleep. Serotonergic input from the dorsal raphé nuclei has an inhibitory effect on the cholinergic neurons. Thus, serotonin inhibits REM sleep (Yudofsky & Hales 2002, p. 60).

23. Obstructive sleep apnoea is more common in ages 40–60 years.

True: The prevalence of obstructive sleep apnoea increases during adult life, reaching a peak at around 40–60 years. Thereafter it becomes less common, probably because of the reduction in chest wall muscle activity during sleep which lessens the negative intrapharyngeal pressure (Schneerson 2000, p. 195).

24. Depression may present with similar features to hyperthyroidism.

True: Both hyperthyroidism and depression share symptoms such as anxiety, fatigue, insomnia, lability, dysphoria, poor attention span and weight loss. Moreover, up to a third of hyperthyroid patients would meet the criteria for a diagnosis of major depressive episode (Lishman 1997, p. 508; Sadock & Sadock 2005, p. 2154).

25. Pantothenic acid deficiency causes dementia.

False: Sensory neuropathy is the only neurological or psychiatric disorder that has been attributed to pantothenic acid deficiency (Lishman 1997, p. 571).

Neuropsychiatry – 5

Fernando Lazaro-Perlado

	T	F

1. The amygdala has a role in visuo-spatial function.

2. The area implicated in dyslexia is supplied by the anterior cerebral artery.

3. Carbon monoxide poisoning is rarely associated with long-term sequelae.

4. Spongiform degeneration in CJD is due to neuronal loss.

5. A normal CSF pressure is 70–180 mm.

6. Metabolic disorders often increase alpha waves on the EEG.

7. Death by suicide occurs in 1.4% of patients with epilepsy.

8. Alternative psychosis with forced normalization of the EEG is a subtype of ictal psychosis.

9. Verbal recall is affected in right frontal lesions.

10. Linkage analysis can be used to study genetic disorders in families.

11. The transcriptome is a collection of RNA transcripts.

12. HIV enters the brain in the late stage of the illness.

13. Progressive memory loss is seen in HIV encephalitis.

14. The age of onset of Huntington's disease is associated with the number of trinucleotide repeats.

15. In Huntington's disease the degree of atrophy of the caudate nucleus is the best indicator of cognitive dysfunction.

16. Procedural memory is not affected in Korsakoff's syndrome.

17. Lethargy in multiple sclerosis is often due to a depressive disorder.

18. Iomazenil is used as a ligand for benzodiazepine receptors.

19. The planum temporale is located in the anterior part of the inferior temporal gyrus.

20. Difficulties with spatial recognition are more likely to occur in lesions with right-sided hemiplegia than left-sided.

21. Stage 4 sleep occurs more frequently in the second half of the night.

22. Sleep apnoea is seen in left ventricular failure.

23. Superior oblique muscle paralysis results in an inability to see inwards and downwards.

T F

24. The EEG in hypothyroidism shows reduced alpha waves. ☐ ☐

25. White matter hyperintensities are most commonly periventricular. ☐ ☐

ANSWERS

1. The amygdala has a role in visuo-spatial function.

False: The amygdala has a complex range of functions centring on emotions, emotionally conditioned behaviour and establishing links between emotional value and memories. It has no role in visuo-spatial function (Sadock & Sadock 2005, p. 1749).

2. The area implicated in dyslexia is supplied by the anterior cerebral artery.

True: Two areas have been implicated in dyslexia:

1. The inferior frontal gyrus/superior temporal cortex (peri sylvian area) which is supplied by the middle cerebral artery and
2. The splenium of the corpus callosum which is supplied by the anterior cerebral artery (Lishman 1997, p. 47).

3. Carbon monoxide poisoning is rarely associated with long-term sequelae.

False: Delayed neuropsychiatric symptoms occur in 10–30% of victims. They include personality changes, cognitive impairment, Parkinsonism, incontinence, dementia, and psychosis. Recovery within one year occurs in 50–75% of cases. Approximately 11% have gross sequelae. The level of consciousness on admission to hospital correlates with neuropsychiatric sequelae (Lishman 1997, p. 552; Mitchell 2004, p. 249).

4. Spongiform degeneration in CJD is due to neuronal loss.

False: The characteristic spongiform appearance of the brain in CJD is due to vacuolation of glial cells and not due to neuronal loss (Lishman 1997, p. 478).

5. A normal CSF pressure is 70–180 mm.

True: The normal values for CSF are:

- Glucose = 2.8–4.2 mmol/L
- Protein = 0.15–0.45 g/L
- Opening pressure = 70–180 mm CSF.

6. Metabolic disorders often increase alpha waves on the EEG.

False: Metabolic disorders cause EEG abnormalities. Initial changes include slowing of alpha rhythms with diminution in voltage. Later there is progressive slowing and disorganization with runs of theta activity. In metabolic coma, regular high voltage delta activity appears, sometimes bilaterally synchronous and sometimes more random in distribution. In deep coma, the EEG becomes flat and featureless (Lishman 1997, p. 130).

7. Death by suicide occurs in 1.4% of patients with epilepsy.

False: 5% of patients with epilepsy commit suicide compared with 1.4% of the general population (Trimble & Schmitz 2002, p. 107).

8. Alternative psychosis with forced normalization of the EEG is a subtype of ictal psychosis.

False: The terms alternative psychosis and forced paradoxical normalization refer to the antagonism between psychosis and seizures or EEG discharges. They are a group of inter-ictal psychoses that appear after spontaneous or, more often, drug-induced disappearance of clinical and subclinical seizure manifestations (Trimble & Schmitz 2002, p. 45).

9. Verbal recall is affected in right frontal lesions.

False: Verbal recall is affected mostly in left frontal lesions.

10. Linkage analysis can be used to study genetic disorders in families.

True: Linkage analysis is a technique which localizes disease genes on chromosomes. It relies on the fact that genes which are close together on a chromosome are more likely to be inherited together. The further apart they are then the more likely that they will be split by recombination during meiosis. The recombination fraction (θ) can be calculated and converted to centimorgans (cM) with a θ value of 0.01 corresponding to 1 cM. For low values of θ this approximates to a distance of around 1000 kb and this relation holds for values of up to around 30 cM.

Where it is difficult to use genes as a known location, other markers such as restriction fragment length polymorphisms (RFLPs) or single nucleotide polymorphisms (SNPs) are used. Linkage analysis was employed to localize the genes for Huntington's disease and cystic fibrosis.

Association studies look for association between a phenotype and a genetic marker. This may be a specific allele of a candidate gene. Candidate genes are those where variation has a biologically plausible reason to cause the phenotype, e.g. dopamine transporter and schizophrenia. Alternatively, association between known genetic markers and the phenotype may be studied to implicate a chromosomal region (Puri & Tyler 1998, p.194).

11. The transcriptome is a collection of RNA transcripts.

True: Genomics is the study of entire genomes. The genome is the sum total of the genetic material, i.e. DNA within the organism. Transcription of DNA into RNA is the basic mechanism by which cells mediate their growth, function and metabolism.

The transcriptome is the sum total of RNAs transcribed.

The proteome is the collection of translated proteins.

The metabolome or metabonome is the collection of breakdown products of enzymatic activity (Sadock & Sadock 2005, p. 115).

12. HIV enters the brain in the late stage of the illness.

False: The nervous system is a prime target for the HI virus and is affected early in the illness. Abnormalities are found in the CSF in a large proportion of asymptomatic HIV positive individuals (Lishman 1997, p. 319; Mitchell 2004, p. 182).

13. Progressive memory loss is seen in HIV encephalitis.

True: HIV encephalitis typically presents as delirium, but occasionally directly as dementia. Delirium is seen in about 10% of patients who are HIV positive and in 25–50% of hospitalized patients with AIDS. Delirium may be the most common single neuropsychiatric complication in AIDS (Mitchell 2004, p. 186).

14. The age of onset of Huntington's disease is associated with the number of trinucleotide repeats.

True: The CAG repeat size and the age of onset are inversely correlated. However, for a given repeat size, there is a wide range of onset ages. CAG repeat lengths are also associated with the age of onset of psychiatric symptoms (Mitchell 2004, p. 161; Yudofsky & Hales 2002, p. 333).

15. In Huntington's disease the degree of atrophy of the caudate nucleus is the best indicator of cognitive dysfunction.

True: In Huntington's disease, cognitive dysfunction including intelligence, memory and visuospatial deficits correlates with the degree of atrophy of the caudate nucleus. Moreover, impairments in executive functions correlate more robustly with caudate nucleus atrophy than with frontal atrophy (Yudofsky & Hales 2002, p. 926).

16. Procedural memory is not affected in Korsakoff's syndrome.

True: The diencephalic structures involved in memory include the mamillary bodies, medial dorsal thalamic nuclei, internal medullary lamina and the mamillothalamic tracts. They support the role of the hippocampi. The hippocampi are involved in explicit (declarative) memory, e.g. memory for facts such as who the Prime Minister is. They are not involved in implicit (procedural) memory, e.g. the non-conscious, automatic performance of previously learned skills such as driving a car.

In Korsakoff's syndrome, anterograde memory is most severely affected. New learning is impaired. Disturbance of time sense and confabulation occur. Immediate memory span is well preserved, and beyond a variable retrograde gap remote memories are well preserved. Implicit (procedural) memory is well preserved. They can learn to mirror write even though they do not remember having been asked to perform the task before (Lishman 1997, p. 30; Mitchell 2004, p. 234).

17. Lethargy in multiple sclerosis is often due to a depressive disorder.

True: Fatigue in multiple sclerosis is caused by the direct effects of multiple sclerosis itself and by depression in approximately equal measure. Fatigue can be episodic or persistent in a third of multiple sclerosis patients. The fatigue is central rather than peripheral in origin (Feinstein 1999, p. 30; Mitchell 2004, p. 144).

18. Iomazenil is used as a ligand for benzodiazepine receptors.

True: [^{123}I]Iomazenil and [^{125}I]Iomazenil are specific ligands for benzodiazepine receptors. They are used to study benzodiazepine receptors and epileptic foci.

19. The planum temporale is located in the anterior part of the inferior temporal gyrus.

False: The planum temporale or the temporal plane is located in the superior part of the temporal lobe near the auditory cortex. It is the upper surface of the Wernicke's area. It is associated with language function (Fitzgerald 1996, p. 11; Sadock & Sadock 2005, p. 15).

20. Difficulties with spatial recognition are more likely to occur in lesions with right-sided hemiplegia than left-sided.

False: Although not fully lateralized, neglect phenomena and visuospatial deficits are more common with right hemisphere lesions (by implication left hemiplegia) (Gelder et al 2006, p. 324; Hodges 1994, p. 73).

21. Stage 4 sleep occurs more frequently in the second half of the night.

False: Sleep is divided into REM sleep and non-REM sleep. NREM sleep is itself divided into stages 1–4. Sleep progesses through stages 1–4 and then enters REM sleep. NREM and REM sleep then alternate through the night in 90–110-minute cycles. In successive cycles the amount of NREM sleep decreases and the amount of REM sleep increases. The proportion of stages of sleep in a healthy young adult are: stage 1 = 5%; stage 2 = 25–50%; stage 3 = 20–25%; stage 4 = 20–25%; REM = 25%. Stage 1 is at the beginning of sleep, stages 3 & 4 predominate in the first third and REM in the last third of sleep (Fear 2004, p. 327; Sadock & Sadock 2005, p. 282).

22. Sleep apnoea is seen in left ventricular failure.

True: Sleep apnoea is cessation of breathing for 10 seconds or more. It is caused by airway obstruction, central changes in ventilatory control, metabolic factors or heart failure. It may be accompanied by oxygen desaturation and cardiac arrhythmias (Yudofsky & Hales 2002, p. 713).

Features of obstructive sleep apnoea include excessive daytime sleepiness, loud snoring with frequent awakenings, awakening with choking and/or gasping for breath, morning dry mouth and witnessed apnoea.

Predisposing factors include male gender, middle age, obesity, micrognathia or retrognathia and nasal pharyngeal abnormalities, hypothyroidism and acromegaly.

Other features and co-morbidities include sleep choking, morning headaches, nocturnal sweating, sleepwalking, sleep talking, nocturia, enuresis, impotence, memory impairment, impaired quality of life, depression, hearing loss, automatic behaviour, hypertension, polycythemia, and right-sided heart failure (Yudofsky & Hales 2002, p. 713).

23. Superior oblique muscle paralysis results in an inability to see inwards and downwards.

True: The superior oblique muscle is supplied by the fourth cranial nerve, the trochlear. Paralysis of this nerve results in an inability to see inwards and downwards. Isolated nerve damage can occur as a result of closed head injury. Alternatively, the muscle can be directly affected in dysthyroid eye disease or myasthenia. Patients may complain of diplopia when looking downwards – for instance going down stairs. In contrast, in third nerve lesions the affected eye looks down and out due to unopposed actions of lateral rectus and superior oblique, as well as showing ptosis and pupillary dilatation (Lindsay & Bone 2004, p. 145).

24. The EEG in hypothyroidism shows reduced alpha waves.

True: Hypothyroidism is associated with low voltage, decreased alpha activity and generalized beta activity (Stern & Engel 2004, p. 98).

25. White matter hyperintensities are most commonly periventricular.

True: White matter lesions (WMLs) are conventionally divided into those around the ventricular system, i.e. periventricular lesions or PVLs and those elsewhere, i.e. deep white matter lesions, DWMLs or leukoaraiosis. Severe DWMLs and large PVLs may be associated with neurological dysfunction. PVLs may be more common in Alzheimer's disease than in elderly controls or depressed patients. Large PVLs are related to cognitive impairment and gait abnormalities. Small PVLs are probably clinically insignificant. The association of both periventricular and subcortical WMLs with subjective memory complaints and mild cognitive impairment has been replicated (Mitchell 2004, p. 45; Sadock & Sadock 2005, p. 3619).

34 Neuropsychiatry – 6

Ben Underwood and Michael Spencer

	T	F

1. Anosognosia is more likely to be associated with right than with left limb hemiplegia.

2. The hippocampus is supplied by the anterior cerebral artery.

3. In chronic fatigue syndrome, patients who attribute their symptoms to exclusively physical causes have a better prognosis.

4. Prion protein on tonsillar biopsy is highly specific for variant CJD.

5. Reverse calendar test performance is unimpaired in delirium tremens.

6. Delirium is associated with theta waves on the EEG.

7. The EEG during absence seizures is diagnostic.

8. Prolactin levels return to normal within 60 minutes following a non-epileptic seizure.

9. Social judgement and decision-making are spared in lesions of the ventromedial frontal cortex.

10. The proteome is the total number of expressed proteins.

11. Head injury associated with amnesia lasting less than 24 hours is more likely to be associated with epilepsy.

12. HIV disease progression is measured by CD4 counts.

13. HIV infection is a predisposing factor for Alzheimer's disease.

14. In dementia associated with Huntington's disease, amnesia is similar for all decades of life.

15. The globus pallidus is part of the limbic system.

16. The recency effect is preserved in diencephalic amnesia.

17. Irritability in multiple sclerosis is often due to a depressive disorder.

18. Paralysis of vertical gaze is characteristically seen in normal pressure hydrocephalus.

19. Lewy bodies are found in Parkinson's disease.

20. Hallucinations occur in acute intermittent porphyria.

21. The serial sevens test can provoke a catastrophic reaction in patients with dementia.

T F

22. Delta waves are maximal in the second half of sleep.

23. Somnambulism occurs in sleep stages 3 and 4.

24. Depressive symptoms are less common after breast conserving surgery than radical mastectomy for cancer of the breast.

25. Hypothyroidism can cause hirsutism.

ANSWERS

1. Anosognosia is more likely to be associated with right than with left limb hemiplegia.

False: Anosognosia is the lack of awareness of disease. It usually results from non-dominant parietal lobe lesion. It is usually associated with unilateral neglect and left hemiplegia (Lishman 1997, p. 18; Mitchell 2004, p. 85).

2. The hippocampus is supplied by the anterior cerebral artery.

False: The hippocampus receives its blood supply from the anterior temporal artery which is a branch of the posterior cerebral artery.

The anterior cerebral artery supplies the frontal pole and medial surface of the hemisphere (Fitzgerald 1996, p. 231).

3. In chronic fatigue syndrome, patients who attribute their symptoms to exclusively physical causes have a better prognosis.

False: Patients with chronic fatigue syndrome often ascribe their problem to an underlying physical cause and may be reluctant to accept a psychiatric element. Those who attribute their symptoms to exclusively physical causes have a worse prognosis (Gelder et al 2000, p. 1116).

4. Prion protein on tonsillar biopsy is highly specific for new variant CJD.

True: In nv-CJD, prion protein can be found in peripheral lymphoreticular tissues, e.g. tonsils, lymph nodes, spleen and Peyer's patches, as well as in the dorsal root and trigeminal ganglia. This is unique to nv-CJD. A negative biopsy does not rule out the possibility of nv-CJD (Sadock & Sadock 2005, p. 477).

5. Reverse calendar test performance is unimpaired in delirium tremens.

False: All cognitive domains, i.e. orientation, attention, memory, visuospatial abilities and executive functions are affected in delirium. Tests of attention, concentration and memory such as the reverse calendar test are quick bedside tests which are often impaired in delirium (Mitchell 2004, p. 233; Yudofsky & Hales 2002, p. 536).

6. Delirium is associated with theta waves on the EEG.

True: The EEG is very sensitive to delirium. The characteristic change is generalized slowing including the appearance of theta waves. An important exception to this is delirium tremens which is characterized by increased low-voltage fast activity (Yudofsky & Hales 2002, p. 539).

7. The EEG during absence seizures is diagnostic.

True: Absence or petit mal seizures occur primarily in children. They are primary generalized seizures associated with loss of consciousness from the start and without significant motor features. The EEG during seizures shows generalized synchronous 3–4-Hz spike and slow waves (Yudofsky & Hales 2002, p. 675).

8. Prolactin levels return to normal within 60 minutes following a non-epileptic seizure.

False: There is usually an abrupt 3–4-fold rise in plasma prolactin level within 15–20 minutes of a generalized tonic-clonic seizure. The prolactin level returns to normal within 60 minutes. Recurrent seizures and greater frequency of seizures decrease the prolactin response. Prolactin levels are not raised following non-epileptic seizures. Post-ictal prolactin level is not reliable in differentiating between true and non-ictal seizures because only about 50% of complex partial seizures give a measurable stress hormone response (Gelder et al 2006, p. 348; Mitchell 2004, p. 124; Yudofsky & Hales 2002, p. 677).

9. Social judgement and decision-making are spared in lesions of the ventromedial frontal cortex.

False: The prefrontal cortex projects to subcortical structures in a series of distinct closed loops. Disruption of any of these produces a pattern of discrete deficits. However, these clinical syndromes seldom present as neatly in clinical practice as pathological lesions seldom respect anatomy. The syndromes are:

1. Dorsolateral prefrontal cortex. Damage here may be caused by trauma, stroke or damage to the subcortical structures, e.g. Parkinson's disease. It presents with damaged executive function manifest as poor problem solving and difficulties with working memory.
2. Dorsomedial prefrontal cortex. Lesions may be due to stroke or tumours. This presents with apathy, poor motivation and problems with initiation of action. Akinetic mutism is the most extreme form. Attention is a cognitive function distributed beyond one anatomical region but the cingulate cortex has been implicated in scanning and animal models. This may be the mechanism for the efficacy of cingulotomy in OCD if OCD is conceptualized as a disorder of excessive attention.
3. Orbito-frontal cortex. Damage is often secondary to trauma and damage to sense of smell is a related clinical sign. Otherwise bedside neuropsychological tests may be normal. This syndrome presents with change in personality. Most commonly this involves impulsivity, disinhibition, emotional lability, poor judgement and lack of insight.

The mnemonic 'Don't Let Exam Demons Marr Any Opportunity For Passing' can be used to help remember this. The initial letters spell DLEDMAOFP. Dorso Lateral – Executive function. Dorso Medial – Akinetic mutism (also apathy and attention). Orbito Frontal – Personality change.

Although clinical lesions seldom fall neatly into these categories, it is the orbito-frontal and dorsolateral syndromes which are generally associated with social judgement and decision-making respectively (Lindsay & Bone 2004, p. 109; Mitchell 2004, p. 77; Sadock & Sadock 2005, p. 325).

10. The proteome is the total number of expressed proteins.

True: The proteome is the total number of proteins produced by the genome. There are many more proteins expressed than there are genes as there is variability in transcription, translation and post-translational modification (Pennington et al 2005).

11. Head injury associated with amnesia lasting less than 24 hours is more likely to be associated with epilepsy.

False: Annergers et al reported that post-traumatic epilepsy with repeated seizures necessitating anticonvulsant medication occurs in approximately 12%, 2% and 1% of patients with severe, moderate and mild head injuries respectively within 5 years of the injury. Risk factors for post-traumatic epilepsy include severe injury, depressed skull fractures, penetrating wounds, chronic alcohol misuse, intracranial haemorrhage, and greater severity of injury. Head injuries with amnesia lasting greater than 24 hours are associated with greater severity of injury and are therefore more likely to be associated with epilepsy (Mitchell 2004, p. 131; Yudofsky & Hales 2002, p. 639).

12. HIV disease progression is measured by CD4 counts.

True: CD4 counts are indicators of the stage of HIV infection. It may begin to decline slowly during the asymptomatic phase and decrease more dramatically during the early and late symptomatic phases (Lishman 1997, p. 317; Mitchell 2004, p. 182).

13. HIV infection is a predisposing factor for Alzheimer's disease.

False: Although controversial, HIV-1 Associated Dementia has been described as a subcortical dementia affecting subcortical and frontostriatal brain processes. Cortical symptoms such as aphasia, agnosia, apraxia and other sensory perceptual dysfunctions occur later in the course of the disease, possibly as a result of opportunistic infections or neoplastic invasion of the CNS (Yudofsky & Hales 2002, p. 792).

14. In dementia associated with Huntington's disease, amnesia is similar for all decades of life.

True: Huntington's disease patients do not show gradients of retrograde amnesia (Yudofsky & Hales 2002, p. 929).

15. The globus pallidus is part of the limbic system.

False: The term 'limbic' was coined by Broca (1878) and originally referred to the limbus or rim of cortex adjacent to the corpus callosum and diencephalon. The term limbic system is most often used to describe the areas of the brain involved in emotion, memory or aggression. The precise constituents of the limbic system vary from book to book. Structures considered to be part of the limbic system include the hippocampal formation, septal region, parahippocampal gyrus, cingulate gyrus, insula and amygdala. The globus pallidus is part of the basal ganglia (Fitzgerald 1996, p. 267; Yudofsky & Hales 2002, p. 279).

16. The recency effect is preserved in diencephalic amnesia.

True: Diencephalic amnesia, as exemplified by Korsakoff's syndrome, results in specific memory impairment with other intellectual abilities preserved.

Anterograde memory is most severely affected. Retrograde episodic memory is also affected. Retrograde memory shows a temporal gradient, i.e. more distant memories are spared. Procedural memory and short-term memory (STM, working memory) are not affected. The 'Primacy effect' occurs when the first item on a list is remembered better than later items. The 'Recency effect' occurs when the last item on a list is remembered better than earlier items. In diencephalic amnesia, the recency effect, which is part of the STM, is preserved while the primacy effect, which is part of LTM, is not (Hodges 1994, p. 13).

17. Irritability in multiple sclerosis is often due to a depressive disorder.

True: Major depressive-like disorder due to multiple sclerosis differs from uncomplicated major depression. The typical picture commonly found in uncomplicated major depression, i.e. withdrawn and apathetic, with feelings of guilt and worthlessness, is unusual. Rather, symptoms such as irritability, worry and discouragement predominate (Feinstein 1999, p. 30; Mitchell 2004, p. 144).

18. Paralysis of vertical gaze is characteristically seen in normal pressure hydrocephalus.

False: Classically, normal pressure hydrocephalus presents with gait disturbance, urinary incontinence and dementia. In practice, the clinical picture is more variable (Lindsay & Bone 2004, p. 126; Mitchell 2004, p. 213).

19. Lewy bodies are found in Parkinson's disease.

True: Parkinson's disease is characterized by Lewy bodies and Lewy neurites. They are intracellular aggregates composed of α-synuclein (Gelder et al 2006, p. 341; Mitchell 2004, p. 150; Yudofsky & Hales 2002, p. 337).

20. Hallucinations occur in acute intermittent porphyria.

True: Acute intermittent porphyria is an autosomal dominant disorder resulting in a 50% reduction of porphobilinogen deaminase activity. Attacks are caused by the accumulation of intermediates of haem synthesis. Psychiatric symptoms occur in attacks in 25–75% of cases. They include emotional disturbance, noisy disturbed behaviour, clouding of consciousness, delirium hallucinations and delusions. Coma can develop abruptly (Lishman 1997, p. 567).

21. The serial sevens test can provoke a catastrophic reaction in patients with dementia.

True: Goldstein in 1939 coined the term 'catastrophic reaction' to describe the inability of the organism to cope when faced with physical or cognitive deficits. Catastrophic reaction may involve anxiety, tears, aggressive behaviour, swearing, refusal, renouncement and sometimes compensatory boasting. It occurs in about 20% of stroke patients. It is associated with anterior subcortical lesions, major depression and family or personal history of psychiatric disorders (Yudofsky & Hales 2002, p. 746).

22. Delta waves are maximal in the second half of sleep.

False: After a few minutes of stage 1, sleep progresses through stages 2, 3 and 4 and then enters REM sleep. NREM and REM sleep then alternate in 90–110 minute cycles. In successive cycles the amount of NREM sleep decreases and the amount of REM sleep increases. Stage 3 has 20–50% and stage 4 has >50% slow wave sleep. Stages 3 and 4 are also called slow wave sleep, delta sleep or deep sleep and occur predominantly in the first third of a typical sleep cycle. Delta waves are most prominent in stage 4 sleep (Sadock & Sadock 2005, p. 282; Schneerson 2000, p. 2; Stern & Engel 2004, p. 116).

23. Somnambulism occurs in sleep stages 3 and 4.

True: Somnambulism or sleepwalking is a manifestation of incomplete arousal from stages 3 and 4 NREM sleep in children and young adults. It usually occurs during the first third of the night. Sleepwalking individuals arise from bed and ambulate without awakening. They can engage in a variety of complex behaviours whilst asleep. They often interact with the environment inappropriately, sometimes resulting in injury, rarely committing acts of violence. They are difficult to awaken, and if woken usually appear confused. Sleep deprivation may exacerbate, or even provoke, sleepwalking in susceptible individuals. It has a familial pattern. Up to 17% of people report at least one episode of sleepwalking in childhood with a peak incidence between 4 and 8 years. It usually disappears spontaneously after adolescence. It is rare in adults (Schneerson 2000, p. 143; Wright et al 2005, p. 399; Yudofsky & Hales 2002, pp. 698, 717).

24. Depressive symptoms are less common after breast conserving surgery than radical mastectomy for cancer of the breast.

False: Breast conserving therapy does not reduce the high frequency of depression (Blichert-Toft 1992).

25. Hypothyroidism can cause hirsutism.

False: Hypothyroidism is typically associated with hair loss and thinning (Lishman 1997, p. 512; Sadock & Sadock 2005, p. 2155).

Neuropsychiatry – 7

Rudi Kritzinger and Catherine Corby

	T	F
1. Simultanagnosia is a failure to simultaneously perceive multiple objects.	☐	☐
2. CJD is most common in Libyan Jews.	☐	☐
3. CJD causes spongiform degeneration without plaque formation.	☐	☐
4. EEG has high heritability.	☐	☐
5. The amygdala plays a key role in the genesis of both ictal and inter-ictal anxiety in patients with complex partial seizures.	☐	☐
6. A normal inter-ictal EEG would rule out petit mal epilepsy.	☐	☐
7. Pupillary reaction to light can help differentiate between epileptic and non-epileptic seizures.	☐	☐
8. Akinetic mutism is associated with dysfunction in the orbito-frontal region.	☐	☐
9. The proteasome is the total number of proteins produced by an organism at any point in time.	☐	☐
10. Retrograde amnesia is the best predictor of outcome in head injury.	☐	☐
11. HIV enters the brain through infected macrophages.	☐	☐
12. 60% of those with AIDS develop dementia.	☐	☐
13. Huntington's disease is associated with high amplitude EEG.	☐	☐
14. The dentate gyrus is a part of the limbic system.	☐	☐
15. Insight is retained in diencephalic pathology.	☐	☐
16. The prevalence of depression in multiple sclerosis is comparable to that in the general population.	☐	☐
17. Atypical facial pain characteristically presents as a deep facial pain.	☐	☐
18. Psychosis is a recognized complication in Parkinson's disease.	☐	☐
19. Acute intermittent porphyria is associated with sensitivity to sunlight.	☐	☐
20. In relaxation the skin conductance rises.	☐	☐
21. Most REM sleep occurs in the latter half of the night.	☐	☐
22. Sleepwalking is associated with depression.	☐	☐
23. Tau protein is present in neurofibrillary tangles.	☐	☐
24. Hypothyroidism causes bone pain.	☐	☐

25. Writer's cramp is a dystonia.

T   F
☐   ☐

ANSWERS

1. Simultanagnosia is a failure to simultaneously perceive multiple objects.

True: Simultanagnosia or visual disorientation is the inability to attend to more than a very limited sector of the visual field at any given moment, the rest being in a sort of fog or out of focus. It is detected by asking the subject to describe a complex design (Lishman 1997, p. 61; Yudofsky & Hales 2002, pp. 85, 174).

2. CJD is most common in Libyan Jews.

True: There is a familial form of CJD seen in Libyan and Tunisian Jews which gives them 100 × the risk of the general population. Before the mutation was found, the high incidence of CJD was attributed to eating sheep's eyes. A very high incidence of CJD has been described in Libyan Jewish immigrants to Israel (Lishman 1997, p. 475).

3. CJD causes spongiform degeneration without plaque formation.

True: The neuropathological characteristics of CJD are neuronal loss, spongiform vacuolation and reactive astrogliosis. There are no neurofibrillary tangles, senile plaques, circumscribed atrophy or inflammatory reaction. However, extracellular amyloid plaques are present in 10% of cases, especially in the cerebellum. In contrast, the essential diagnostic pathological feature of nvCJD is the presence of multiple, florid, large, fibrillary amyloid plaques in the cerebral and cerebellar cortices, especially in the occipital cortex (Lishman 1997, p. 478; Sadock & Sadock 2005, p. 471; Wright et al 2005, p. 387).

4. EEG has high heritability.

True: A number of family and twin studies have demonstrated high heritability of EEG alpha power (80%) and alpha peak frequency (80%), P300 amplitude (60%) and P300 latency (50%).

5. The amygdala plays a key role in the genesis of both ictal and inter-ictal anxiety in patients with complex partial seizures.

True: The amygdala is involved in emotion recognition and fear conditioning. The projections of the central nucleus of the amygdala to the locus coeruleus and hypothalamus mediate the arousal and autonomic responses associated with fear and anxiety. Thus, the amygdala plays a key role in the integration of the behavioural and neuroendocrine components of the stress response as well as anxiety symptoms associated with complex partial seizures. MRI studies show smaller amygdala volumes in patients with complex partial seizures who have ictal fear than those who do not (Mitchell 2004, p. 438; Trimble & Schmitz 2002, p. 32).

6. A normal inter-ictal EEG would rule out petit mal epilepsy.

False: A normal inter-ictal EEG does not rule out the possibility of seizure disorders. However, a normal EEG during a seizure would (Mitchell 2004, p. 116; Yudofsky & Hales 2002, p. 678).

7. Pupillary reaction to light can help differentiate between epileptic and non-epileptic seizures.

True: Non-epileptic seizures are notoriously difficult to distinguish from epileptic seizures. During and immediately after generalized tonic-clonic seizures there are usually up-going plantars and wide-fixed pupils. This is not seen in non-epileptic seizures (Lishman 1997, p. 292).

8. Akinetic mutism is associated with dysfunction in the orbito-frontal region.

False: The prefrontal cortex projects to subcortical structures in a series of distinct closed loops. Disruption of any of these produces a pattern of discrete deficits. However, these clinical syndromes seldom present as neatly in clinical practice as pathological lesions seldom respect anatomy. The syndromes are:

1. Dorsolateral prefrontal cortex. Damage here may be caused by trauma, stroke or damage to the subcortical structures, e.g. Parkinson's disease. It presents with damaged executive function manifest as poor problem solving and difficulties with working memory.
2. Dorsomedial prefrontal cortex. Lesions may be due to stroke or tumours. This presents with apathy, poor motivation and problems with initiation of action. Akinetic mutism is the most extreme form.
3. Orbito-frontal cortex. Damage is often secondary to trauma and damage to sense of smell is a related clinical sign. Otherwise, bedside neuropsychological tests may be normal. This syndrome presents with change in personality. Most commonly this involves impulsivity, disinhibition, emotional lability, poor judgement and lack of insight.

The mnemonic 'Don't Let Exam Demons Marr Any Opportunity For Passing' can be used to help remember this. The initial letters spell DLEDMAOFP. DorsoLateral – Executive function. DorsoMedial – Akinetic mutism (also apathy and attention). Orbito-Frontal – Personality change.

Though clinical lesions seldom fall neatly into these categories it is the dorsomedial syndrome which is most closely associated with akinetic mutism (Lindsay & Bone 2004, p. 109; Mitchell 2004, pp. 57, 77; Sadock & Sadock 2005, p. 325).

9. The proteasome is the total number of proteins produced by an organism at any point in time.

False: The proteasome is an intracellular structure involved in the degradation of misfolded proteins. The proteome is the total number of proteins produced by a genome (Alberts et al 2000, p. 358).

10. Retrograde amnesia is the best predictor of outcome in head injury.

False: Post-traumatic amnesia (PTA) is a more valid and useful guide to the severity of head injury and subsequent prognosis than retrograde amnesia, the duration of unconsciousness or overt confusion. PTA is highly variable from case to case and serves as an index of severity. It is a permanent index of severity and is available to the clinician who enquires long after the injury. PTA in closed head injuries is also an indicator of the time lapse before the patient returns to work (Lishman 1997, p. 171; Mitchell 2004, p. 128).

11. HIV enters the brain through infected macrophages.

True: The 'Trojan horse theory' postulates that the HI virus enters the brain through infected macrophages and microglia (Lishman 1997, p. 322).

12. 60% of those with AIDS develop dementia.

False: The cumulative lifetime prevalence of HIV dementia in infected adults is about 15%. Highly active antiretroviral therapy (HAART) reduces the incidence by about 50%. HIV-associated dementia is usually seen in the late stages of HIV illness, CD4 cell count nadir less than 200 per μL, higher HIV RNA viral load, lower educational level, older age, anaemia, illicit drug use and female gender (Lishman 1997, p. 324; Mitchell 2004, p. 186; Sadock & Sadock 2005, p. 433).

13. Huntington's disease is associated with high amplitude EEG.

False: The EEG in Huntington's disease shows loss of alpha rhythm. There may be generalized low voltage fast activity or random slow activity. As the disease progresses the amplitude decreases and the EEG may become completely flat. These changes are not ubiquitous. Normal traces may be seen even in advanced disease (Lishman 1997, p. 470; Yudofsky & Hales 2002, p. 964).

14. The dentate gyrus is a part of the limbic system.

True: The dentate gyrus is part of the hippocampal formation along with the hippocampus and subiculum. Broca in 1878 coined the term 'limbic' for the limbus or rim of cortex adjacent to the corpus callosum and diencephalon. The term limbic system is most often used to describe the areas of the brain involved in emotion, memory or aggression, e.g. the hippocampal formation, septal region, parahippocampal gyrus, cingulate gyrus, insula and amygdala (Fitzgerald 1996, p. 267; Yudofsky & Hales 2002, p. 279).

15. Insight is retained in diencephalic pathology.

False: In diencephalic lesions, e.g. in Korsakoff's syndrome, patients are usually unaware of their illness and may deny they have any impairment (Lishman 1997, pp. 19, 69).

16. The prevalence of depression in multiple sclerosis is comparable to that in the general population.

False: The lifetime prevalence of major depression in multiple sclerosis is 25–50%, i.e. three times the general population rate. Physical disability and fatigue are indirectly associated with depression via their effects on day-to-day functioning (Feinstein 1999, p. 29; Mitchell 2004, p. 143).

17. Atypical facial pain characteristically presents as a deep facial pain.

True: Two facial pain syndromes may respond to antidepressants. In temporomandibular joint dysfunction (Costen's syndrome, facial arthralgia) there is a dull ache around the joint. In contrast, atypical facial pain is a deeper aching or throbbing pain (Gelder et al 2006, p. 212).

18. Psychosis is a recognized complication in Parkinson's disease.

True: Psychosis, particularly affective psychosis, occurs in Parkinson's disease. In most cases medications and overmedication can be implicated. Non-drug related cases are usually transient and often associated with dementia. Schizophrenia-like psychosis is rare (Lishman 1997, p. 657; Mitchell 2004, p. 152).

19. Acute intermittent porphyria is associated with sensitivity to sunlight.

False: Unlike many porphyrias, acute intermittent porphyria is not associated with skin rashes. Symptoms of acute intermittent porphyria are caused when intermediates of haem synthesis accumulate in abnormal and toxic amounts. Symptoms include abdominal pain, vomiting, constipation, muscle weakness, hypertension, tachycardia, peripheral neuropathy and mental state changes (Lishman 1997, p. 116).

20. In relaxation the skin conductance rises.

False: The electrodermal system is under the sole control of the sympathetic nervous system rather than a dynamic balance between sympathetic and parasympathetic. Sympathetic activation may be tonic or phasic. Anxiety increases tonic sympathetic activity and sweating and hence increases conductance. Depression may decrease skin conductance. Relaxation decreases skin conductance (Sadock & Sadock 2005, p. 1729).

21. Most REM sleep occurs in the latter half of the night.

True: NREM sleep predominates at all times in the night though REM gets proportionately greater. In successive sleep cycles the amount of NREM sleep decreases and the amount of REM sleep increases. REM accounts for 25% of the total sleep time. Most REM periods occur during the last third of the night, as opposed to stage 4 sleep, where most occurs in the first third of the night (Gelder et al 2000, p. 996).

22. Sleepwalking is associated with depression.

True: Sleepwalking may be precipitated by traumatic events such as parental death or divorce, change of school or birth of a sibling. There may be a disturbed family background or a difficult relationship with the parents. The majority have a history of acting out behaviours, delinquency and theft. Many show evidence of anxiety, depression and depersonalization. The majority of adult sleepwalkers have no psychiatric disorders (Lishman 1997, p. 736).

23. Tau protein is present in neurofibrillary tangles.

True: Neurofibrillary tangles are largely composed of phosphorylated tau protein (Lishman 1997, p. 441).

24. Hypothyroidism causes bone pain.

False: However, hyperparathyroidism does. Hyperparathyroidism may present with malaise, depression, renal calculi, peptic ulcers and corneal calcification. Hyperparathyroidism leads to absorption of bone which when advanced may lead to cysts or destructive 'brown tumours'.

25. Writer's cramp is a dystonia.

True: Writer's cramp, torticollis, and blepharospasm with jaw and mouth movements (Meige syndrome) are focal dystonias (Yudofsky & Hales 2002, p. 164).

Neurotic disorders – 1

Ben Underwood

	T	F

1. Suffocation false alarm theory explains panic attacks. ☐ ☐

2. There is an increased prevalence of mitral valve prolapse in patients with generalized anxiety disorder. ☐ ☐

3. Compulsive buying is classified under impulse control disorders in DSM-IV. ☐ ☐

4. It is rare for factitious disorder to present with anaemia. ☐ ☐

5. According to the concept of 'Illness behaviour', it is the ill person's responsibility to seek a medical diagnosis. ☐ ☐

6. Psychiatrists are able to detect the majority of malingerers. ☐ ☐

7. In OCD there is decreased blood flow in the prefrontal cortex. ☐ ☐

8. OCD has a poorer prognosis if the ruminations are not accompanied by rituals. ☐ ☐

9. Cognitive restructuring can be used in pain management. ☐ ☐

10. 10–20% of patients with panic disorder relapse when the SSRIs are discontinued. ☐ ☐

11. In borderline personality disorder, analytically orientated day hospital service is effective. ☐ ☐

12. Psychotherapy is not effective in dissocial personality disorder. ☐ ☐

13. Rational emotive behavioural therapy (REBT) is of proven benefit for patients with emotionally unstable personality disorder. ☐ ☐

14. Psychopaths accommodate to the galvanic skin response faster than normal subjects. ☐ ☐

15. Habituation can exacerbate phobic avoidance. ☐ ☐

16. Fear of heights appears in the first year. ☐ ☐

17. Derealization is common in agoraphobia. ☐ ☐

18. Animal phobia is more common in boys. ☐ ☐

19. Failure to remember aspects of the trauma is characteristic of PTSD. ☐ ☐

20. Yohimbine injection in PTSD patients can precipitate panic attacks. ☐ ☐

21. Emotional blunting is a common feature of PTSD. ☐ ☐

22. Panic attacks are a common feature of PTSD. ☐ ☐

T   F

23. Stress can cause aphthous ulcers. ☐ ☐

24. High-pressure jobs are associated with increased risk of ischaemic heart disease irrespective of the level of control. ☐ ☐

25. There is a U-shaped association between medically certified sickness absence and mortality. ☐ ☐

ANSWERS

1. Suffocation false alarm theory explains panic attacks.

True: Klein's (1993) suffocation false alarm theory hypothesizes that panic attacks represent a false triggering of a suffocation alarm. Many spontaneous panic attacks are due to a 'suffocation monitor' in the brain erroneously signalling a lack of useful air, and triggering an evolved 'suffocation alarm system'. He proposed that carbon dioxide acts as a panic stimulus because rising arterial carbon dioxide suggests that suffocation may be imminent (Klein 1993; Sadock & Sadock 2005, p. 1732).

2. There is an increased prevalence of mitral valve prolapse in patients with generalized anxiety disorder.

True: The prevalence of mitral valve prolapse is 5% in the general population and as high as 37% in anxiety disorder (Gelder et al 2000, p. 59).

3. Compulsive buying is classified under impulse control disorders in DSM-IV.

True: In DSM-IV, 'Impulse control disorders not *elsewhere* classified' includes intermittent explosive disorder, kleptomania, pathological gambling, pyromania, trichotillomania and impulse control disorders not *otherwise* specified. The latter includes compulsive buying or oniomania, delicate self-cutting, compulsive skin picking, severe nail biting, internet compulsion, mobile phone compulsion and compulsive sexual behavior (Sadock & Sadock 2002, p. 792).

4. It is rare for factitious disorder to present with anaemia.

False: There are two broad groups of patients with factitious disorders: the less common group present repeatedly to hospital emergency departments with symptoms suggesting medical or surgical emergencies. In the more common group, signs of disease are fabricated in a subtle and deceitful manner. They may produce superficial ulcerating wounds or they may repeatedly bleed themselves to induce the clinical and laboratory picture of iron-deficiency anaemia (Murray et al 1997, p. 549).

5. According to the concept of 'Illness behaviour', it is the ill person's responsibility to seek a medical diagnosis.

False: Mechanic (1962) defined 'illness behaviour' as the ways in which given symptoms may be differentially perceived, evaluated and acted (or not acted) upon by different kinds of persons. This may include consulting doctors, taking medicines, seeking help from relatives and friends and giving up inappropriate activities.

Abnormal illness behaviour (Pilowsky 1969) or dysnosognosia is persistently pathological modes of experiencing, evaluating and responding to one's own health status despite lucid and accurate appraisal and management options provided by health professionals (Gelder et al 2006, p. 165; Johnstone et al 2004, p. 687; Murray et al 1997, pp. 51, 483; Stein & Wilkinson 1998, p. 719).

6. Psychiatrists are able to detect the majority of malingerers.

False: Health professionals can detect subjects simulating illness effectively if they are forewarned that simulation is a possibility. If not forewarned, they wrongly accept symptoms at face value. David Rosenhan's study of malingerers faking psychosis on an inpatient psychiatric ward confirms the inability of psychiatrists to differentiate real from feigned mental illness, at least in certain contexts (Gelder et al 2000, p. 1130; Sadock & Sadock 2005, p. 2252).

7. In OCD there is decreased blood flow in the prefrontal cortex.

False: PET studies in OCD show abnormally increased resting blood flow and glucose metabolism in the orbital cortex and caudate nucleus. On symptom provocation with exposure to relevant stimuli, the flow increases further in the prefrontal cortex and basal ganglia: prefrontal, orbital, anterior cingulate, lateral frontal, anterior temporal, parietal and insular cortices, caudate, putamen and thalamus (Gelder et al 2000, p. 825; Gelder et al 2006, p. 198; Sadock & Sadock 2005, p. 1755).

8. OCD has a poorer prognosis if the ruminations are not accompanied by rituals.

False: In general, the type of symptoms or pre-treatment severity has no prognostic value in OCD.

However, poor prognosis has been associated with early onset and associated personality disorders, especially schizotypal personality disorder. Overvalued or fixed obsessive ideation, hoarding behaviour and avoidance behaviour have been associated with poor response to behavioural treatments. Somatic obsessions and poor insight are also associated with poor prognosis.

Indicators of better prognosis include a precipitating factor, good social and occupational adjustment, episodic course and a positive family history (Gelder et al 2000, p. 825; Gelder et al 2006, p. 199).

9. Cognitive restructuring can be used in pain management.

True: Cognitive restructuring and reconceptualization of the individual's experience of pain are used in pain management. They may increase self-efficacy as well as alter the patient's appraisal of their ability to manage pain (Sadock & Sadock 2005, p. 2192).

10. 10–20% of patients with panic disorder relapse when the SSRIs are discontinued.

False: In panic disorder the optimum duration of treatment with SSRIs is unknown but at least 8–18 months is recommended. The recurrence rate on stopping SSRIs is 30–90% (Sadock & Sadock 2002, p. 608; Taylor et al 2005, p. 186).

11. In borderline personality disorder, analytically orientated day hospital service is effective.

True: In a randomized controlled trial, compared to treatment as usual, psychoanalytically informed day hospital significantly reduced self-harm behaviour, hospitalization and psychiatric symptoms and improved self-reported mood (Gelder et al 2006, p. 149).

12. Psychotherapy is not effective in dissocial personality disorder.

False: There have been reports of improvement in dissocial personality disorder with supportive psychotherapy, problem-solving counselling, Beckian cognitive therapy adapted for personality disorders, individual dynamic psychotherapy in which individuals are confronted repeatedly and directly with evidence of their abnormal behaviour and small-group therapy with groups comprising entirely of patients with dissocial personality disorders. The Henderson Hospital runs a therapeutic community for patients with antisocial and other personality disorders. Follow-up studies have shown improvement in general social functioning, employment and reconviction rates (Bateman & Tyrer 2004; Gelder et al 2006, p. 145; Johnstone et al 2004, p. 517; Sadock & Sadock 2005, p. 2493).

13. Rational emotive behavioural therapy (REBT) is of proven benefit for patients with emotionally unstable personality disorder.

False: REBT was developed by Albert Ellis in 1955 in the USA. He emphasized the importance of thoughts and philosophies in creating and maintaining psychological disturbance. REBT emphasizes the importance of the interaction between cognitive, emotive and behavioural factors in human functioning as well as in dysfunction. There is no evidence for REBT in the treatment of emotionally unstable personality disorder (Bateman & Tyrer 2004).

14. Psychopaths accommodate to the galvanic skin response faster than normal subjects.

True: There are two theories that explain this phenomenon. Lykken's punishment/low-fear theory focuses on sensation-seeking and insensitivity to punishment. Blair's violence inhibition mechanism deficit hypothesis focuses on the specific failure of basic emotions. These include failure of fear to cause autonomic arousal and the inhibition of ongoing behaviour in individuals with psychopathic personality (Dolan 2004).

15. Habituation can exacerbate phobic avoidance.

False: Habituation is a form of counter-conditioning whereby the successive presentation of a stimulus leads to a decrease in the intensity of the response which it elicits. Instinctive and acquired fear responses can be extinguished by habituation in animals and in humans. Systematic desensitization is an example of habituation. The converse of habituation is sensitization where responses are increased. Once sensitized with an electric shock, the previously sub-threshold stimulus causes the animal to withdraw. It is sensitization which may increase phobic avoidance (Munafo 2002, p. 10; Sadock & Sadock 2002, p. 147).

16. Fear of heights appears in the first year.

True: The famous 'cliff experiment' by Gibson & Walk in 1960 demonstrated that babies can perceive depth and the danger associated with heights within the first year of life (Gross 2001, p. 237).

17. Derealization is common in agoraphobia.

True: Derealization and depersonalization are features of panic attacks (in panic disorder with agoraphobia) and 'panic-like symptoms' (in agoraphobia without history of panic disorder) (DSM-IV 1994, pp. 395, 403; Sims 2004, p. 237).

18. Animal phobia is more common in boys.

False: Animal phobias in children occur equally in both sexes. Boys lose their animal phobias around puberty. A few girls maintain theirs. Women comprise 95% of the adult sufferers of animal phobia.

19. Failure to remember aspects of the trauma is characteristic of PTSD.

True: DSM-IV criterion C (3) is 'inability to recall an important aspect of the trauma'.

20. Yohimbine injection in PTSD patients can precipitate panic attacks.

True: Yohimbine is an α_2-adrenergic receptor blocker. It provokes panic attacks in patients with a history of panic attacks. It can worsen the core symptoms including startle responses, intrusive thoughts and emotional numbing in PTSD patients. It can provoke flashbacks and panic attacks in a subgroup of PTSD patients (Gelder et al 2000, p. 764; Sadock & Sadock 2005, p. 2999).

21. Emotional blunting is a common feature of PTSD.

True: Sense of 'numbness' and emotional blunting, detachment from others, unresponsiveness to surroundings and anhedonia are typical symptoms of PTSD (Gelder et al 2000, p. 760).

22. Panic attacks are a common feature of PTSD.

False: Dramatic acute bursts of fear, panic or aggression triggered by reminders are rare symptoms of PTSD. They are neither necessary for a diagnosis, or typical nor common (Gelder et al 2000, p. 759).

23. Stress can cause aphthous ulcers.

True: Aphthous ulcers or canker sores are ulcers on the mucous membranes of the mouth or genitals. The commonest form is recurrent aphthous stomatitis. Aphthous ulcers may be precipitated by emotional stress, lack of sleep or deficiency of vitamins.

24. High-pressure jobs are associated with increased risk of ischaemic heart disease irrespective of the level of control.

False: Low control in the work environment is associated with an increased risk of coronary heart disease. This association could not be explained by employment grade, negative affectivity, or classic coronary risk factors. Job demands and social support at work were not related to the risk of coronary heart disease. Giving employees more variety in tasks and a stronger say in decisions about work may decrease the risk of coronary heart disease (Bosma et al 1997).

25. There is a U-shaped association between medically certified sickness absence and mortality.

True: Kivimaki et al (2003) found that male and female employees taking a medically certified sick leave (>7 days) on average more than once in 2 years had mortality rates 2 to 5 times greater than their colleagues with no such absence. However, compared with no absence, taking a few brief absences decreases rather than increases the risk of mortality. This U-shaped association was statistically significant in men. Short-term absences may represent healthy coping behaviours or may be otherwise affected by factors causing variation in the threshold of taking sick leave.

Neurotic disorders – 2

Judy Chan

37

	T	F
1. Orthopnoea is a common symptom of cardiac neurosis.	☐	☐
2. Sedation threshold is raised in panic disorder.	☐	☐
3. Weight loss can occur in normal bereavement.	☐	☐
4. Imipramine and CBT are equally effective in treating moderately severe depression.	☐	☐
5. The sick role is synonymous with illness behaviour.	☐	☐
6. Life events are more common preceding schizophrenia than depression.	☐	☐
7. Shoplifting is more common in OCD than in the general population.	☐	☐
8. In OCD, ruminations, as opposed to rituals, respond better to CBT.	☐	☐
9. Obsessive ruminations disappear with thought stopping.	☐	☐
10. Panic attacks are usually predictable.	☐	☐
11. People with dissocial personality disorder continue to have interpersonal difficulties later on in life.	☐	☐
12. Sublimation is seen in borderline personality disorder.	☐	☐
13. Psychoanalytically oriented therapy is beneficial in borderline personality disorder.	☐	☐
14. Dialectic behaviour therapy (DBT) is beneficial in borderline personality disorder.	☐	☐
15. Neurotic traits predispose to the development of phobias.	☐	☐
16. Negative reinforcement can exacerbate avoidance in phobia.	☐	☐
17. Fear of open spaces is the central feature of agoraphobia.	☐	☐
18. Agoraphobia is associated with catastrophization.	☐	☐
19. Agoraphobia responds well to exposure in imagination.	☐	☐
20. In PTSD the cortisol levels are raised.	☐	☐
21. The Implied Event Scale is used in the assessment of PTSD.	☐	☐
22. PTSD is more likely after rape than other types of trauma.	☐	☐
23. Victims of childhood sexual abuse have a high incidence of alcohol and drug abuse in later life.	☐	☐

T F

24. Tics respond to habit reversal training. ☐ ☐

25. Women working in the civil service are more likely to call in sick than men. ☐ ☐

ANSWERS

1. Orthopnoea is a common symptom of cardiac neurosis.

False: Cardiac neurosis, Da Costa's syndrome or neurocirculatory asthenia is a 'somatoform autonomic dysfunction' (F45.3) involving the heart and cardiovascular system. The diagnostic features of F45.3 include symptoms of autonomic arousal, subjective symptoms referred to a specific organ or system, preoccupation with and distress about the possibility of a serious disorder and no evidence of a significant disturbance of structure or function of the stated system or organ.

Orthopnoea is discomfort in breathing that is relieved by sitting up or standing. It is not a feature of cardiac neurosis but a sign of cardiac failure (ICD-10 1992).

2. Sedation threshold is raised in panic disorder.

True: Panic disorder patients are less sensitive than controls to the effects of diazepam. This may suggest a decreased functional sensitivity of the GABA–benzodiazepine supramolecular complex (Sadock & Sadock 2005, p. 1744).

3. Weight loss can occur in normal bereavement.

True: The symptoms of normal bereavement may meet the criteria for major depression, including weight loss. However, normal grief is not associated with morbid feelings of guilt and worthlessness, suicidal thoughts, psychomotor retardation or severe functional impairment (DSM-IV 1994).

4. Imipramine and CBT are equally effective in treating moderately severe depression.

True: CBT, interpersonal therapy and imipramine have been found to be equally effective and superior to placebo in moderate depression. Moreover, 1 year after treatment discontinuation, the relapse rate in CBT patients was one-half that of the antidepressant drug group, who were not on maintenance treatment (Sadock & Sadock 2005, p. 2609).

5. The sick role is synonymous with illness behaviour.

False: Sick role (Parsons 1951) involves:

1. Exemption from normal social role responsibilities
2. Right to expect help and care
3. Desire to get well and
4. Obligation to seek and cooperate with treatment.

Mechanic (1962) defined 'illness behaviour' as the ways in which given symptoms may be differentially perceived, evaluated and acted (or not acted) upon by different kinds of persons. This may include consulting doctors, taking medicines, seeking help from relatives and friends and giving up inappropriate activities (Gelder et al 2006, p. 165; Murray et al 1997, p. 51; Stein & Wilkinson 1998, p. 719).

6. Life events are more common preceding schizophrenia than depression.

False: Compared to the general population, independent life events are more likely to occur prior to episodes of both schizophrenia and depression. In schizophrenia, independent life events are more likely to occur prior to relapse rather than prior to first onset. Life events are more likely prior to both the first episode and relapses of depression than those of schizophrenia.

Adverse life events, particularly loss events, increase the risk of an episode of major depression. The increased vulnerability to an episode appears to last for 2 to 3 months following such an event. Some studies show that in the 6–12 months prior to the onset of depression, compared with normal controls, patients have a 3 to 5-fold greater chance of having suffered at least one life event with major negative long-term implications (Puri & Hall 2004, p. 141; Gelder et al 2000, pp. 603, 699).

7. Shoplifting is more common in OCD than in the general population.

False: OCD spectrum disorders have been described on a dimension of compulsivity and impulsivity. Compulsivity reflects harm-avoidance while impulsivity reflects risk-seeking. Thus OCD falls at the compulsive end. Tourette syndrome, trichotillomania and anankastic personality disorder have both compulsive and impulsive features. Kleptomania, pathological gambling, pyromania and uncontrolled buying fall at the impulsive end. Rarely, there are some patients with kleptomania who show compulsive features, e.g. they have to steal exactly three items on each occasion, while others hoard stolen items. Shoplifters, however, do not have true compulsive rituals. They have an impulse to steal as opposed to a compulsion (Bluglass & Bowden 1990, p. 793).

8. In OCD, ruminations, as opposed to rituals, respond better to CBT.

False: About two-thirds of patients with moderately severe obsessional rituals improve substantially with exposure and response prevention. When rituals improve with CBT, the accompanying ruminations usually improve as well. CBT is much less effective for obsessional ruminations without rituals (Gelder et al 2006, p. 200).

9. Obsessive ruminations disappear with thought stopping.

False: There is no evidence of a specific effect (Gelder et al 2006, p. 200).

10. Panic attacks are usually predictable.

False: There are three types of panic attacks with respect to the presence or absence of triggers: unexpected, situationally bound and situationally triggered. Unexpected or uncued panic attacks occur out of the blue. Recurrent unexpected panic attacks are essential for a diagnosis of panic disorder (DSM-IV 1994, p. 395).

11. People with dissocial personality disorder continue to have interpersonal difficulties later on in life.

True: About a third of people with persistent antisocial behaviour in early adult life improve later, as indicated by the number of arrests and contacts with social agencies. However, they still have problems in relationships, as indicated by hostility to partners and neighbours. They also have an increased suicide rate (Gelder et al 2006, p. 144).

12. Sublimation is seen in borderline personality disorder.

False: Sublimation is a mature defence mechanism. It involves satisfying an unacceptable desire indirectly in a socially acceptable manner. Patients with personality disorders use immature and primitive defence mechanisms. Patients with borderline personality disorder often use defence mechanisms such as splitting and projective identification (Gelder et al 2000, p. 341; Johnstone et al 2004, p. 313; Sadock & Sadock 2005, p. 723).

13. Psychoanalytically oriented therapy is beneficial in borderline personality disorder.

True: Psychoanalytically oriented therapies, especially mentalization-based treatment, have been shown to be efficacious and cost effective in borderline personality disorder (Bateman & Tyrer 2004).

14. Dialectic behaviour therapy (DBT) is beneficial in borderline personality disorder.

True: DBT was initially devised for the treatment of patients who repeatedly harm themselves. Later it was developed as a treatment for borderline personality disorder. DBT is based on CBT, dialectical influences and Zen principles. Clinical trials have shown DBT to be of some benefit in treating borderline personality disorder (Bateman & Tyrer 2004; Gelder et al 2006, p. 149).

15. Neurotic traits predispose to the development of phobias.

True: The most common anxiety disorder is specific phobia, followed by social phobia, generalized anxiety disorder and other anxiety disorder subtypes. An early indicator of the vulnerability to develop anxiety disorders is behavioural inhibition, i.e. increased physiological reactivity or behavioural withdrawal in the face of novel or challenging situations. Another indicator is anxiety sensitivity, i.e. the belief that anxiety sensations are indicative of harmful physiological, psychological or social consequence (Gelder et al 2000, p. 811; Sadock & Sadock 2005, p. 1726).

16. Negative reinforcement can exacerbate avoidance in phobia.

True: In negative reinforcement, a response that leads to the removal of an aversive event is increased. Any behaviour that enables a person or animal to avoid or escape a punishing consequence is strengthened. In phobia the subject tries to avoid the feared object or situation and this is rewarded by a reduction in anxiety. This becomes a learned behaviour and negatively reinforces the avoidant behaviour (Sadock & Sadock 2002, p. 146).

17. Fear of open spaces is the central feature of agoraphobia.

False: Anxiety about being in places or situations from which escape may be difficult or help may not be available in case of having a panic attack is the central feature of agoraphobia. These circumstances may include being outside home alone, being in crowds or public places or travelling alone (DSM-IV 1994; ICD-10 1992).

18. Agoraphobia is associated with catastrophization.

True: Aaron Beck suggested that in anxiety states individuals systematically overestimate the danger inherent in a given situation. David Clark elaborated this cognitive concept. He proposed that the external and internal stimuli are perceived as threats and result in a state of apprehension. The wide range of bodily sensation that normally accompanies apprehension is interpreted in a catastrophic fashion and a further increase in apprehension occurs. Further apprehension produces further increase in bodily sensation, resulting in a vicious circle which culminates in a panic attack.

19. Agoraphobia responds well to exposure in imagination.

False: Exposure in vivo with anxiety management produces better long-term results than exposure in imagination or exposure alone. Partner-assisted and therapist-assisted exposure improves the outcome (Gelder et al 2000, p. 818).

20. In PTSD the cortisol levels are raised.

False: The hypothalamic-pituitary-adrenal axis is dysregulated in PTSD. Even though stress usually causes an increase in cortisol levels, patients with PTSD have low circulating cortisol levels. Moreover, they show enhanced response to the dexamethasone suppression test, in contrast to depression. One hypothesis is that an increase in glucocorticoid receptors in the hypothalamus results in supersuppression to cortisol feedback and hence decreased peripheral cortisol. Low cortisol levels immediately after trauma are associated with the development of PTSD, while high levels are associated with depression (Gelder et al 2000, p. 764; Gelder et al 2006, p. 160; Sadock & Sadock 2005, p. 1741).

21. The Implied Event Scale is used in the assessment of PTSD.

False: The Impact of Event Scale (IES) was developed to assess current subjective distress to any specific event. IES used to be the most widely used self-report measure of PTSD. It contained an intrusion scale and an avoidance scale. The revised version (IES-R) included an additional hyperarousal scale. The Post-traumatic Stress Diagnostic Scale (PSDS) is modelled on DSM-IV and is now commonly used in research.

22. PTSD is more likely after rape than other types of trauma.

True: Rape is associated with the highest rates of PTSD. Two-thirds of male and one-half of female victims of rape develop trauma. Other traumatic events associated with high rates of PTSD include combat exposure, childhood neglect and physical abuse, and sexual molestation (Gelder et al 2000, p. 762).

23. Victims of childhood sexual abuse have a high incidence of alcohol and drug abuse in later life.

True: Adult survivors of childhood sexual abuse have high rates of depression, guilt, low self-esteem, alcoholism, sexual problems, eating disorders, agoraphobia, panic disorder, self-harm and further victimization. However, most of them have no significant abuse-related symptoms (Gelder et al 2000, p. 1827; Johnstone et al 2004, p. 716; Sadock & Sadock 2005, p. 3416).

24. Tics respond to habit reversal training.

True: Habit reversal training (HRT) was developed by Azrin and Nunn for the treatment of tics and other habits. HRT includes behaviour monitoring, relaxation and competing-response training. A competing response is a response incompatible with the tic. The patient performs this competing response, e.g. clenching a fist for 3 minutes, when faced with the urge to perform the tic or when catching themselves performing the tic. HRT has been found to be useful in Tourette syndrome. HRT has been shown to be superior to negative practice in trichotillomania. Relaxation and massed practice can also be helpful (Gelder et al 2000, p. 989; Johnstone et al 2004, p. 597; Sadock & Sadock 2005, p. 3234).

25. Women working in the civil service are more likely to call in sick than men.

True: After adjustment for differences in age and grade, women have a 1.5-fold higher risk of medically certified sickness absence and a 1.2-fold higher risk of self-certified sickness absence compared with men (Kivimaki et al 2003).

Old age psychiatry – 1

Alan Murtagh

38

	T	F

1. Compared to verbal skills, digit span is preserved in old age.

2. Depression is more likely to improve spontaneously in older age.

3. A manic episode in an elderly person is usually treated with lithium alone.

4. Late onset schizophrenia is more common in women.

5. Low fecundity is seen in late onset delusional disorder.

6. Self-neglect in the elderly (Diogenes syndrome) is likely to be caused by delusions.

7. People with mild cognitive impairment progress to dementia at a rate of 20% per annum.

8. Mutations in the APP gene account for 10% of cases of Alzheimer's disease.

9. In dementia associated with Alzheimer's disease, the amnesia is similar for all decades of life.

10. Lewy body dementia is characterized by progressive deterioration of cognitive functions.

11. In semantic dementia the ability to list objects from a class is retained.

12. Early onset of apraxia indicates Pick's disease rather than Alzheimer's disease.

13. Personality changes before memory changes suggest Pick's rather than Alzheimer's disease.

14. Plaques occur in the brain in normal ageing.

15. An elderly patient who suffers a first episode of depression is more likely to have larger ventricles than someone of the same age who had not had an episode of depression.

16. The hippocampus is spared in Alzheimer's disease.

17. In early dementia, progressive agnosia is more suggestive of Alzheimer's than vascular dementia.

18. Neurofibrillary tangles are very rare in Lewy body dementia.

19. Leukoaraiosis is associated with gait disturbances.

T   F

20. Carers of the opposite sex are more likely to abuse a patient in a nursing home for the elderly than carers of the same sex. ☐ ☐

21. Hospital admission is essential for elderly patients with delusional disorder. ☐ ☐

22. In the elderly, the proportion of body fat is increased. ☐ ☐

23. Up to 15% of elderly depressed patients develop agitation when prescribed SSRIs. ☐ ☐

24. Because of its long half-life, donepezil is given once daily. ☐ ☐

25. Memantine is useful in Alzheimer's dementia. ☐ ☐

ANSWERS

1. Compared to verbal skills, digit span is preserved in old age.

True: Short-term memory as tested by digit span does not decline with age as much as verbal skills, e.g. verbal fluency, do. Sensory memory or extremely brief sensory record of a stimulus; primary memory, e.g. by the ability to recall a series of digits long enough to repeat them; and tertiary memory or memories of childhood have no significant age effects. Verbal expression and verbal reasoning skills show subtle changes with age and language may become less precise and more repetitive over time. However, performance IQ declines more rapidly than verbal in the elderly (Sadock & Sadock 2005, p. 3628).

2. Depression is more likely to improve spontaneously in older age.

False: Episodes of depression tend to last longer in old age. When depression is untreated one-third remain unwell at 3-year follow-up. However, with treatment the prognosis of late-life depression can be as good as that of depression in younger adults. This emphasizes the need for early detection and adequate treatment of depression in the elderly. However, true comparative studies with depression in younger people are rare (Lawlor 2001, p. 228; Norman & Redfern 1996, p. 154).

3. A manic episode in an elderly person is usually treated with lithium alone.

False: Lithium or another mood stabilizer + an antipsychotic combination is the most common treatment (Gelder et al 2000, p. 1650; Jacoby & Oppenheimer 2002, p. 689; Johnstone et al 2004, p. 648).

4. Late onset schizophrenia is more common in women.

True: Late onset schizophrenia is 3–9 times more common in women than in men (Butler & Pitt 1998, p. 153).

5. Low fecundity is seen in late onset delusional disorder.

True: Fecundity relates to the potential reproductive capacity of an organism. Patients with late onset delusional disorders are less likely to have been married. They have fewer children even if they were married (Johnstone et al 2004, p. 644).

6. Self-neglect in the elderly (Diogenes syndrome) is likely to be caused by delusions.

False: Diogenes syndrome, senile self-neglect or senile squalor is characterized by severe self-neglect unaccompanied by any psychiatric disorder sufficient to account for the squalor in which the patient exists. Although burnt out personality disorder, end-stage personality disorder or personality reaction to stress and loneliness have been suggested, it is currently thought to involve a complex interplay of personality traits, psychosocial stressors and medical/psychiatric conditions. If delusions were causing the presentation, then the patient would receive a diagnosis relating to those delusions, e.g. late onset schizophrenia with secondary extreme self-neglect, and not Diogenes syndrome. The syndrome is named after the Greek philosopher 'Diogenes the cynic' (412–323 BC). He attempted to have as simple a life as possible and allegedly lived in a wooden tub belonging to the temple of Cybele (Jacoby & Oppenheimer 2002, p. 730; Sims 2004, p. 371; Wright et al 2005, p. 487).

7. People with mild cognitive impairment progress to dementia at a rate of 20% per annum.

False: Mild cognitive impairment is usually considered an intermediate state between normal ageing and dementia. It is characterized by subjective complaints of poor memory and objective evidence of impaired memory for age and education but with preserved general cognitive function and intact activities of daily living in the absence of dementia. The progression to dementia is 10–15%/year (Copeland et al 2002, p. 306; Johnstone et al 2004, p. 628; Mitchell 2004, p. 265).

8. Mutations in the APP gene account for 10% of cases of Alzheimer's disease.

False: Mutations in the amyloid precursor protein gene are thought to account for only a proportion of the 5% of cases of familial Alzheimer's disease (Johnstone et al 2004, p. 630).

9. In dementia associated with Alzheimer's disease, the amnesia is similar for all decades of life.

False: In the early stages of Alzheimer's disease, there is failure of new learning. Hence, memory for recent events is impaired while the recall of previously learned information remains good. As the disease progresses the memory impairment broadens to involve retrieval of more and more distant memories. This results in the patient appearing to live in the ever-more-distant past (Jacoby & Oppenheimer 2002, p. 512; Mitchell 2004, p. 280).

10. Lewy body dementia is characterized by progressive deterioration of cognitive functions.

True: The consensus criteria for Lewy body dementia include progressive decline in cognitive functions and two of the following core features: fluctuating cognition, visual hallucinations, motor features of Parkinsonism (Johnstone et al 2004, p. 633; Mitchell 2004, p. 261).

11. In semantic dementia the ability to list objects from a class is retained.

False: Semantic dementia or progressive fluent aphasia is a frontotemporal dementia in which the patient loses their ability to understand and recognize words. The language disorder is characterized by progressive, fluent, empty, spontaneous speech. Loss of word meaning is manifest by impaired naming and comprehension and semantic paraphasias. The ability to list objects from a class is impaired (Lishman 1997, p. 753; Mitchell 2004, p. 289).

12. Early onset of apraxia indicates Pick's disease rather than Alzheimer's disease.

False: Pick's typically begins with changes of character and social behaviour before progressing to deficits in spatial orientation and memory. Praxis is generally preserved until late in the disease (Lishman 1997, p. 461).

13. Personality changes before memory changes suggest Pick's rather than Alzheimer's disease.

True: Pick's is characterized by changes in personality and behaviour, affective symptoms, and a progressive reduction of expressive speech (Gelder et al 2000, p. 398; Mitchell 2004, p. 288).

14. Plaques occur in the brain in normal ageing.

True: Senile plaques and neurofibrillary tangles appear in normal ageing (Esiri et al 2004, p. 113; Sadock & Sadock 2005, p. 3611).

15. An elderly patient who suffers a first episode of depression is more likely to have larger ventricles than someone of the same age who had not had an episode of depression.

True: Elderly patients with a first episode of depression have larger ventricles than age-matched healthy controls. This may be predictive of increased mortality on follow-up (Lishman 1997, p. 140).

16. The hippocampus is spared in Alzheimer's disease.

False: The earliest changes seen on neuroimaging are usually in the hippocampus. This is consistent with the clinical picture where laying down of new memories is often the first deficit noted in dementia (Esiri et al 2004, p. 168; Mitchell 2004, p. 268).

17. In early dementia, progressive agnosia is more suggestive of Alzheimer's than vascular dementia.

True: The term 'agnosia' was introduced by Freud in 1891. Agnosia is a failure of recognition which is not due to a primary sensory defect or to generalized intellectual impairment. Progressive deterioration of cognitive functions such as language (aphasia), motor skills (apraxia) and perception (agnosia) is a NINCDS-ADRDA criterion for the diagnosis of probable Alzheimer's disease. According to NINDS-AIREN criteria, progressive worsening of memory and other cognitive functions in the absence of corresponding focal lesions on brain imaging make the diagnosis of vascular dementia unlikely (Johnstone et al 2004, p. 630; Lishman 1997, p. 58; Mitchell 2004, p. 74).

18. Neurofibrillary tangles are very rare in Lewy body dementia.

True: Neurofibrillary tangles are intraneuronal aggregations of insoluble phosphorylated tau protein. Neurofibrillary tangles are not specific for Alzheimer's disease. They are found in the normal elderly as well as in other neurodegenerative disorders such as dementia pugilistica. In Lewy body dementia, neurofibrillary tangles are typically few or absent (Gelder et al 2006, p. 340; Johnstone et al 2004, p. 71; Lishman 1997, p. 453).

19. Leukoaraiosis is associated with gait disturbances.

True: Leukoaraiosis (Greek for white matter of loose texture) is a diminution of white matter intensity in the periventricular regions on brain imaging. It is thought to be ischaemic in origin. It is associated with limb weakness, extensor plantars and gait disturbances. Both leukoaraiosis and gait disturbance suggest poorer prognosis (Briley et al 2000; Copeland et al 2002, pp. 23, 252; Lishman 1997, p. 460).

20. Carers of the opposite sex are more likely to abuse a patient in a nursing home for the elderly than carers of the same sex.

False: Male carers more commonly abuse male patients and female carers more commonly abuse females (Payne & Cikovic 1995).

21. Hospital admission is essential for elderly patients with delusional disorder.

False: There is no single strategy that suits all patients. Some patients will accept a brief admission to the hospital in order to get to the bottom of the problem. A compulsory admission may reduce the prospect of establishing a trusting relationship. The need for admission depends on such factors as risk, associated distress, response to interventions delivered to their homes and response to attendance at day hospitals and day centres (Jacoby & Oppenheimer 2002, p. 755).

22. In the elderly, the proportion of body fat is increased.

True: The relative proportion of body fat increases and the total body water decreases with age. Consequently, the half-life of lipid soluble drugs is increased. Other changes include reduced hepatic metabolism and renal function (King 2004, p. 449; Norman & Redfern 1996, p. 421).

23. Up to 15% of elderly depressed patients develop agitation when prescribed SSRIs.

True: Common side-effects of SSRIs in the elderly include anxiety/agitation (2–15%), nausea (15%), diarrhoea (10%) and insomnia (5–15%) (Jacoby & Oppenheimer 2002, p. 653).

24. Because of its long half-life, donepezil is given once daily.

True: Donepezil has a half-life of 70 hours, lending itself to once daily administration (Johnstone et al 2004, p. 636).

25. Memantine is useful in Alzheimer's dementia.

True: Memantine is an NMDA channel blocker. It is used in moderate to severe Alzheimer's dementia (BNF 2005, 4.11; Mitchell 2004, p. 370).

Old age psychiatry – 2

Alan Murtagh

	T	F

1. The prevalence of depression in old age is 13%.

2. Visual hallucinations are common in elderly depressed patients.

3. The relapse rate of depression in the elderly is significantly reduced by maintenance medication.

4. One-third of neurotic disorder of the elderly starts before age 65 years.

5. The prevalence of psychotic symptoms in those aged above 70 years is 10%.

6. Visual hallucinations are common in elderly people with paraphrenia.

7. Diogenes syndrome is associated with fronto-temporal dementia.

8. Low IQ is a risk factor for dementia.

9. Determining Apoprotein E genotype is useful for counselling relatives of the risk of Alzheimer's disease.

10. A similarity between impaired cognition in old age and Alzheimer's disease is an impaired visuospatial sketchpad.

11. Antipsychotic drugs can cause lethal side-effects in Lewy body dementia.

12. Spontaneous speech is fluent in semantic dementia.

13. Emotional lability indicates vascular dementia rather than Alzheimer's disease.

14. Urinary incontinence suggests vascular dementia rather than Alzheimer's disease.

15. Shrinkage of cells in the cerebral cortex occurs in normal ageing.

16. The latency of evoked responses is decreased in Alzheimer's disease.

17. A normal MRI is possible in Alzheimer's disease.

18. Neurofibrillary tangles are seen in dementia due to boxing.

19. Multi-infarct dementia may be diagnosed despite a normal CT brain scan.

20. Non-pharmacological interventions can delay institutional care in dementia.

21. Paraphrenia responds well to antipsychotic drug treatment.

22. In co-morbid epilepsy and depression in the elderly, improved control of epilepsy improves depression.

23. SSRIs have proven value in treating non-cognitive features of dementia.

T F

24. Donepezil has a short biological half-life. ☐ ☐

25. Memantine is useful in vascular dementia. ☐ ☐

ANSWERS

1. The prevalence of depression in old age is 13%.

False: Although the prevalence of depressive symptoms is about 15%, the prevalence of depression itself is 3% (1–9%). Both depression and depressive symptoms are higher in nursing home settings (Jacoby & Oppenheimer 2002, p. 630).

2. Visual hallucinations are common in elderly depressed patients.

False: Only a small minority of depressed patients have fleeting auditory or visual hallucinations with extremely unpleasant content in keeping with their delusions e.g. hearing accusatory voices or seeing themselves in graveyards or prisons (Gelder et al 2006, p. 511; Sadock & Sadock 2005, p. 1617).

3. The relapse rate of depression in the elderly is significantly reduced by maintenance medication.

True: Maintenance therapy is thought to reduce rates of relapse by up to a factor of 2.5. Up to 70% of patients on maintenance treatment may remain well at 4 years. Given the detrimental impact and high probability of relapse in patients not on maintenance therapy, it is not surprising that some clinicians recommend indefinite prophylaxis (Copeland et al 2002, p. 440; Johnstone et al 2004, p. 647; King 2004, p. 460).

4. One-third of neurotic disorder of the elderly starts before age 65 years.

False: Although there tends to be a wide range, it is generally accepted that about one-third of neurotic disorders are of late onset, i.e. starting after age 65 years. This makes sense when considering that just under two-thirds of total anxiety disorders are accounted for by agoraphobia and about half of these cases are late onset. Moreover, about 10% of generalized anxiety disorder begins after age 65 years. It is still very rare, however, for panic disorder without agoraphobia and obsessive compulsive disorder to begin after age 65 years (Butler & Pitt 1998, p. 136; Gelder et al 2000, p. 1653; Johnstone et al 2004, p. 648).

5. The prevalence of psychotic symptoms in those aged above 70 years is 10%.

False: The prevalence of paranoid symptoms in the elderly is estimated at 5%. The prevalence of psychotic disorders in the elderly in the community ranges from 0.2% to 4.7%. The prevalence is 10% in a nursing home population and as high as 63% in a study of Alzheimer's disease patients (Copeland et al 2002, p. 521).

6. Visual hallucinations are common in elderly people with paraphrenia.

False: The commonest hallucinations in paraphrenia are auditory. Tactile and olfactory hallucinations are infrequent. Visual hallucinations are rare (Gelder et al 2006, p. 514; Johnstone et al 2004, p. 644).

7. Diogenes syndrome is associated with fronto-temporal dementia.

False: Diogenes syndrome, senile self-neglect or senile squalor is characterized by severe self-neglect unaccompanied by any psychiatric disorder sufficient to account for the squalor in which the patient exists. Diogenes syndrome has been found to be associated with frontal lobe dysfunction, but is not generally associated with fronto-temporal dementia (Lishman 1997, p. 495).

8. Low IQ is a risk factor for dementia.

True: People with lower intelligence, lower educational achievement and lower verbal ability are at increased risk of developing Alzheimer's disease. People with bigger brains may have a reduced risk of developing dementia. Total brain volume has been correlated with IQ scores and hence greater brain reserve (Jacoby & Oppenheimer 2002, p. 494).

9. Determining Apoprotein E genotype is useful for counselling relatives of the risk of Alzheimer's disease.

False: Presence of Apoprotein E4 does not predict progression to Alzheimer's disease but it does increase the likelihood. It seems to operate in conjunction with other genetic factors by decreasing the age of onset of the illness. It is generally held that it is of insufficient predictive power to justify its use in genetic counselling (Copeland et al 2002, p. 219).

10. A similarity between impaired cognition in old age and Alzheimer's disease is an impaired visuospatial sketchpad.

True: Baddeley et al described working memory as consisting of a central executive and two slave systems: a phonological loop concerned with verbal and acoustic information and a visuospatial sketchpad concerned with visuospatial information. The visuospatial sketchpad is a temporary system used in creating and manipulating visual images. Children predominantly use a visuospatial encoding until age 5 years when they switch to a phonological–verbal system. The visuospatial sketchpad and hence the visual short-term memory deteriorates in old age as well as in Alzheimer's disease (Gelder et al 2000, pp. 264, 274).

11. Antipsychotic drugs can cause lethal side-effects in Lewy body dementia.

True: The Newcastle group found that approximately half of all patients with Lewy body dementia show extreme sensitivity to antipsychotic drugs resulting in a two- to three-fold increase in mortality. Severe reactions can precipitate irreversible Parkinsonism, further impair consciousness and induce autonomic disturbances similar to neuroleptic malignant syndrome. The effect of atypical antipsychotics is not yet certain (Johnstone et al 2004, p. 633).

12. Spontaneous speech is fluent in semantic dementia.

True: Semantic dementia is a form of fronto-temporal dementia in which the patient loses their ability to recognize and understand words. The language disorder is characterized by progressive, fluent, empty spontaneous speech. Loss of word meaning is manifest by impaired naming and comprehension, and semantic paraphasias (Lishman 1997, p. 753; Mitchell 2004, p. 289).

13. Emotional lability indicates vascular dementia rather than Alzheimer's disease.

True: Emotional lability and explosive emotional outbursts are common in vascular dementia due to lesions in the basal parts of the brain. In contrast, Alzheimer's disease is associated with blunted affect (Gelder et al 2000, p. 431; Lishman 1997, p. 454).

14. Urinary incontinence suggests vascular dementia rather than Alzheimer's disease.

True: Clinical diagnosis of vascular dementia can be difficult. Efforts have been made to create clinical criteria to make this easier. An example of this was collaboration between the Neuroepidemiology Branch of the National Institute of Neurological Disorders and Stroke (NINDS) and the Association Internationale pour la Recherche et l'Enseignement en Neurosciences (AIREN) to create the NINDS-AIREN criteria. Urinary incontinence suggests probable vascular dementia according to these criteria. They have 80% specificity and 58% sensitivity in detecting vascular dementia (Gelder et al 2000, p. 431).

15. Shrinkage of cells in the cerebral cortex occurs in normal ageing.

True: The main changes in normal ageing are decrease in volume of larger neurons and regression of dendrites, especially in the frontal and temporal lobes, decrease in the number of oligodendrocytes and increase in the number of small neurons, astrocytes and microglia (Jacoby & Oppenheimer 2002, p. 104; Sadock & Sadock 2005, p. 3614).

16. The latency of evoked responses is decreased in Alzheimer's disease.

False: P300 reflects the fundamental cognitive processes involved in stimulus evaluation and immediate memory. The latency of evoked response is increased and, hence, the P300 is delayed in Alzheimer's disease. However, delayed P300 is more apparent in subcortical dementias (Lishman 1997, p. 132).

17. A normal MRI is possible in Alzheimer's disease.

True: However, the majority of cases show some abnormalities such as decreased hippocampal size, decreased volume of the entorhinal cortex, changes in the fusiform gyrus and the amygdala. None of these predict progression better than clinical examination findings (Jacoby & Oppenheimer 2002, p. 510).

18. Neurofibrillary tangles are seen in dementia due to boxing.

True: Neurofibrillary tangles are found in Alzheimer's disease, dementia pugilistica (punch drunk syndrome or dementia due to boxing), post-encephalitic conditions and Down's syndrome.

Other features of dementia due to boxing include cerebral atrophy, ventricular enlargement and a perforated septum pellucidum seen on CT scan or at autopsy. Microscopic findings include neuronal loss, tearing of white matter axons, diffuse axonal swelling and haemorrhages. Senile plaques are not seen (Lishman 1997, p. 442; Mitchell 2004, p. 137).

19. Multi-infarct dementia may be diagnosed despite a normal CT brain scan.

True: Small infarcts in deep white matter are often missed on CT. These may be visible on MRI (Gelder et al 2000, p. 431; Mitchell 2004, p. 46).

20. Non-pharmacological interventions can delay institutional care in dementia.

True: There is some evidence that psychosocial interventions, and especially carer directed support, may be useful in delaying institutionalization in dementia. However, more research is needed in the area (Brodaty et al 2003).

21. Paraphrenia responds well to antipsychotic drug treatment.

True: Contrary to the studies in the 1960s, studies over the past decade suggest that paraphrenia responds well to antipsychotic drugs, with 50–75% showing a full or partial response. Lower doses than those used in a younger population are usually sufficient. However, compliance is often a major problem (Gelder et al 2000, p. 670; Gelder et al 2006, p. 514; Jacoby & Oppenheimer 2002, p. 756; Johnstone et al 2004, p. 644).

22. In co-morbid epilepsy and depression in the elderly, improved control of epilepsy improves depression.

False: Although this would seem intuitive, no such link has been proven (Jacoby & Oppenheimer 2002, p. 303).

23. SSRIs have proven value in treating non-cognitive features of dementia.

True: Depression occurs in 20% of patients with dementia living in the community. SSRIs are also used to treat repetitive behaviours and emotional lability/emotionalism. SSRIs are known to improve functional status, and neurological and cognitive functions (Johnstone et al 2004, p. 639; Mitchell 2004, p. 321).

24. Donepezil has a short biological half-life.

False: The half-life of Donepezil is 70 hours in younger patients. It may be even longer in the elderly. Hence, it can be given once daily (BNF 2005, 4.11; Johnstone et al 2004, p. 636).

25. Memantine is useful in vascular dementia.

True: A number of small studies have demonstrated benefits in patients with vascular dementia (King 2004, p. 474).

Old age psychiatry – 3

Alan Murtagh

T F

1. The female to male ratio for the prevalence of depression increases as people enter old age.

2. The onset of depression in a man aged 65 years without any previous history of depression suggests dementia.

3. The dexamethasone suppression test (DST) is a reliable test for depression in the elderly.

4. Generalized anxiety disorder presenting in old age is likely to have started in adulthood.

5. Sensory deprivation may lead to persecutory delusions in the elderly.

6. Delusional disorder of old age (paraphrenia) usually progresses to dementia.

7. Diogenes syndrome responds well to inpatient treatment.

8. Viral infection is a recognized cause of dementia.

9. Tobacco smoking increases the risk of Alzheimer's disease.

10. Recognition is impaired before recall in Alzheimer's disease.

11. Lewy body spectrum disorder includes Parkinson's disease.

12. The pathology of semantic dementia involves the fronto-temporal region.

13. Dementia involving the frontal lobe is more likely to be due to Pick's disease than Alzheimer's disease.

14. Vascular dementia is more common than Alzheimer's disease in 65–75-year-olds.

15. Old age and Alzheimer's disease both show neuronal degeneration in layer 2 of the entorhinal cortex.

16. Old age depression is not associated with significant structural changes in brain imaging.

17. Leukoaraiosis is strongly associated with cognitive decline.

18. Narrow sulci are a characteristic pathological feature of Alzheimer's disease.

19. In Pick's disease, the atrophy is mostly fronto-temporal.

20. The use of day hospitals in old age psychiatry reduces the number of admissions.

21. Treating hypertension would reduce the risk of Alzheimer's disease.

22. In elderly patients antidepressants are safer than ECT. ☐ ☐

23. Cholinesterase inhibitors improve cognitive function in 65% of cases of mild Alzheimer's disease. ☐ ☐

24. Donepezil is an anticholinergic. ☐ ☐

25. Rivastigmine is a selective inhibitor of butyryl cholinesterase. ☐ ☐

ANSWERS

1. The female to male ratio for the prevalence of depression increases as people enter old age.

False: It is not known exactly why, but the female: male ratio actually decreases with age. It may reflect the increased importance of common risk factors such as chronic illness, changing psychosocial circumstances, hormonal or vascular factors in the aetiology of depression with advancing age (Copeland et al 2002, p. 381; Jacoby & Oppenheimer 2002, p. 636).

2. The onset of depression in a man aged 65 years without any previous history of depression suggests dementia.

False: At this age, the incidence of dementia is less than 0.5%. Hence, the incidence of dementia presenting as depression would be substantially less than this. Although an exact incidence rate of depression at this age is difficult to establish, it would be much higher than that of dementia. Therefore, depression is the more likely diagnosis (Johnstone et al 2004, p. 646; Schweitzer et al 2002).

3. The dexamethasone suppression test (DST) is a reliable test for depression in the elderly.

False: A positive DST differentiates depressed patients from healthy controls in most but not all cases, especially in melancholic or psychotic depressions. The DST does not differentiate between depressed and other patient groups (for example those who abuse alcohol) sufficiently well to be used as a diagnostic test (Gelder et al 2000, p. 715).

4. Generalized anxiety disorder presenting in old age is likely to have started in adulthood.

True: About 10–20% of generalized anxiety disorders in the elderly are new cases. They often follow adverse life events or physical illness (Jacoby & Oppenheimer 2002, p. 698).

5. Sensory deprivation may lead to persecutory delusions in the elderly.

True: Hearing impairment has been experimentally and clinically associated with the development of paranoid symptoms (Copeland et al 2002, p. 505).

6. Delusional disorder of old age (paraphrenia) usually progresses to dementia.

False: Kraepelin's (1909) paraphrenia included patients with chronic delusions and hallucinations without the characteristic personality deterioration of dementia praecox. Roth's (1965) 'late paraphrenia' described paranoid conditions starting after age 60 years in a setting of well preserved personality and affective response. Recent follow-up studies of patients with late paraphrenia show heterogeneous outcomes with only some developing dementia. This may not be significantly more than the number of cases of dementia expected in this age group anyway (Johnstone et al 2004, p. 644).

7. Diogenes syndrome responds well to inpatient treatment.

False: The prognosis of Diogenes syndrome is very poor. Inpatient admission, training, supervision and rehabilitation are almost inevitably followed by relapse into squalid conditions. Indefinite daycare may maintain improvements for longer periods, but often institutional or residential care becomes necessary. Hospital admission is also associated with high mortality (Gelder et al 2006, p. 515; Jacoby & Oppenheimer 2002, p. 730).

8. Viral infection is a recognized cause of dementia.

True: Viruses that can cause dementia include HIV and possibly herpes simplex virus and cytomegalovirus (Jacoby & Oppenheimer 2002, p. 495; Mitchell 2004, p. 199).

9. Tobacco smoking increases the risk of Alzheimer's disease.

True: Although smoking was once believed to reduce the risk of developing Alzheimer's disease, more recent evidence suggests that the opposite may be true (Jacoby & Oppenheimer 2002, p. 827).

10. Recognition is impaired before recall in Alzheimer's disease.

False: Recognition involves being able to recognize but not recall spontaneously an answer to a question. Recall involves actively searching the memory stores and reproducing something that was learnt. Recall is probably more cognitively demanding and hence is affected before recognition in Alzheimer's disease. However, both recall and recognition are severely affected in Alzheimer's disease (Hodges 1994, p. 36; Mitchell 2004, p. 280).

11. Lewy body spectrum disorder includes Parkinson's disease.

True: Parkinson's disease is associated with Lewy bodies in the brainstem region, whereas Lewy body dementia is associated with diffuse Lewy bodies. Parkinson's disease and Lewy body dementia are now considered to be part of a spectrum of disorders (Gelder et al 2000, p. 415; Lishman 1997, p. 450; Mitchell 2004, p. 292).

12. The pathology of semantic dementia involves the fronto-temporal region.

True: Semantic dementia or temporal variant of fronto-temporal dementia is seen with focal cortical atrophy of the dominant lateral temporal neocortex (Gelder et al 2000, p. 274; Lishman 1997, p. 754; Mitchell 2004, p. 289; Sadock & Sadock 2005, p. 3634).

13. Dementia involving the frontal lobe is more likely to be due to Pick's disease than Alzheimer's disease.

False: Pick's disease accounts for about 1–2% of all dementias, fronto-temporal dementia for about 7% and Alzheimer's disease for 50%. Dementia of frontal type refers to the clinical presentation of the dementia. Therefore Alzheimer's disease is much more likely to present with dementia of frontal type than Pick's (Gelder et al 2000, p. 398).

14. Vascular dementia is more common than Alzheimer's disease in 65–75-year-olds.

False: In Western countries, Alzheimer's disease accounts for 50–70% and vascular dementia for 20–30% of all dementias. The prevalence rate for dementia doubles every 5.1 years, Alzheimer's disease every 4.5 years and vascular dementia every 5.3 years. Even though in many non-Western countries vascular dementia is relatively more common, the trend is changing (Jacoby & Oppenheimer 2002, p. 487).

15. Old age and Alzheimer's disease both show neuronal degeneration in layer 2 of the entorhinal cortex.

False: The entorhinal cortex receives afferents from the sensory areas and sends efferents to the hippocampus. Loss of neurons in this area is seen with memory loss and even in very mild Alzheimer's disease, but not in normal ageing (Esiri 2004, p. 116; Mitchell 2004, p. 257).

16. Old age depression is not associated with significant structural changes in brain imaging.

False: Most studies have shown some cortical changes including mild volume reductions in the prefrontal and medial temporal regions (Jacoby & Oppenheimer 2002, p. 279).

17. Leukoaraiosis is strongly associated with cognitive decline.

False: Leukoaraiosis is a diminution of white matter intensity in the periventricular regions on brain imaging. It is thought to be ischaemic in origin. Although it is associated with vascular dementia and although its presence does worsen the prognosis, it is not strongly associated with cognitive decline in itself. It seems that it might act as a marker for 'brain ageing' and might suggest vulnerability to future compromise (Copeland et al 2002, pp. 23, 252).

18. Narrow sulci are a characteristic pathological feature of Alzheimer's disease.

False: The sulci are widened and the gyri narrowed (Johnstone et al 2004, p. 70).

19. In Pick's disease, the atrophy is mostly fronto-temporal.

True: Pick's disease is characterized pathologically by circumscribed, asymmetrical knife-blade fronto-temporal atrophy (Gelder et al 2006, p. 342; Mitchell 2004, p. 44).

20. The use of day hospitals in old age psychiatry reduces the number of admissions.

False: Day hospitals may reduce admissions when compared to no treatment at all. However, compared to other treatments, day hospitals are not definitively proven to reduce admission rates (Copeland et al 2002, p. 682; Johnstone et al 2004, p. 615).

21. Treating hypertension would reduce the risk of Alzheimer's disease.

True: Hypertension is a risk factor for the development of Alzheimer's disease. Treating systolic hypertension in the elderly reduces the rates of dementia including Alzheimer's disease (Jacoby & Oppenheimer 2002, p. 523).

22. In elderly patients antidepressants are safer than ECT.

False: Drug-induced morbidity is a major problem in the elderly, partly because of the changes in pharmacokinetics. ECT is at least as safe as antidepressants (Copeland et al 2002, p. 434).

23. Cholinesterase inhibitors improve cognitive function in 65% of cases of mild Alzheimer's disease.

False: Approximately 40–50% of patients with mild to moderate Alzheimer's disease respond to treatment. A few show a dramatic response, while the majority show a modest benefit of relative stability or slower decline. They enhance not only cognition, but also non-cognitive symptoms, quality of life and ability to perform activities of daily living (Johnstone et al 2004, p. 636; Mitchell 2004, p. 425).

24. Donepezil is an anticholinergic.

False: Donepezil is an acetylcholinesterase inhibitor (Johnstone et al 2004, p. 636).

25. Rivastigmine is a selective inhibitor of butyryl cholinesterase.

False: Rivastigmine inhibits both acetylcholinesterase and butyryl cholinesterase (Johnstone et al 2004, p. 636).

Old age psychiatry – 4

Alan Murtagh

	T	F

1. General practitioners overdiagnose depression in the elderly.

2. Late onset depression is a risk factor for dementia.

3. Mania accounts for one-third of all psychiatric problems in those aged over 65 years.

4. Pseudodementia is associated with later cognitive decline.

5. In the elderly with paranoid disorders there is equal prevalence of visual and hearing impairment.

6. Visual hallucinations are common in Charles Bonnet syndrome.

7. 12% of people aged >75 years have moderate or severe dementia.

8. People with dementia cannot make valid financial decisions.

9. In women on HRT the risk of Alzheimer's disease is lower than in the general population.

10. Cerebrospinal fluid (CSF) corticotropin-releasing factor (CRF) is reduced in Alzheimer's disease.

11. Vascular dementia is associated with gait disturbance.

12. Episodic memory is usually impaired in semantic dementia.

13. Having a seizure is more suggestive of Pick's disease than Alzheimer's disease.

14. Normal ageing is associated with increased numbers of Lewy bodies.

15. In a 70-year-old with suspected depression, a CT scan showing dilated ventricles does not rule out the diagnosis.

16. Most people with Down's syndrome have the neuropathological changes of Alzheimer's disease by age 40 years.

17. Lewy bodies are present in 40% of dementias.

18. In dementia with white matter lesions on CT, there is an increased risk of ataxia.

19. Post-mortem studies conducted on patients with fronto-temporal dementia show that the pathology is mainly due to Pick's disease.

20. Day hospitals manage people with mild to moderate dementia significantly better than day centres.

T F

21. Clomethiazole is a useful hypnotic in elderly patients due to its freedom from 'hangover' effects. ☐ ☐

22. In the elderly, relapse of depression is more likely following ECT than using tricyclic antidepressants. ☐ ☐

23. Cholinesterase inhibitors are useful in the treatment of apathy in Alzheimer's disease. ☐ ☐

24. Galantamine treatment should be reviewed for efficacy every 6 months. ☐ ☐

25. Rivastigmine is a nicotinic receptor agonist. ☐ ☐

ANSWERS

1. General practitioners overdiagnose depression in the elderly.

False: Under-diagnosis is more common. This may be due to presentation with somatic symptoms, masking with alcohol abuse or the complex combination of medical, social and psychiatric problems that can occur in patients of this age group (Norman & Redfern 1996, p. 147; Roose & Sackeim 2004, p. 29).

2. Late onset depression is a risk factor for dementia.

True: Late onset depression is different from early onset depression. Patients with late onset depression have more cognitive impairment and more deep white matter lesions. Schweitzer et al (2002) argue that late onset depression is a prodrome to dementia in a higher than expected number of cases. Depressive symptoms without apparent cognitive decline predict later cognitive decline and development of dementia, especially in those with more severe and persistent symptoms. However the impact of early onset depression on later dementia is controversial (Jacoby & Oppenheimer 2002, p. 637; Johnstone et al 2004, p. 646; Lawlor 2001, p. 229; Schweitzer et al 2002).

3. Mania accounts for one-third of all psychiatric problems in those aged over 65 years.

False: Mania is rare in the elderly. The incidence is 1:1000 in those aged over 65 years. Mania accounts for 9% of admissions to psychogeriatric wards for treatment of affective disorders (Gelder et al 2000, p. 1650; Jacoby & Oppenheimer 2002, p. 684; Norman & Redfern 1996, p. 154).

4. Pseudodementia is associated with later cognitive decline.

True: This is a reasonably consistent finding (Butler & Pitt 1998, p. 117; Jacoby & Oppenheimer 2002, p. 637; Lawlor 2001, p. 227).

5. In the elderly with paranoid disorders there is equal prevalence of visual and hearing impairment.

False: Deafness is present in 25–40% of cases. Visual impairment is less common (Johnstone et al 2004, p. 644).

6. Visual hallucinations are common in Charles Bonnet syndrome.

True: In Charles Bonnet syndrome the patient experiences complex, persistent, repetitive and stereotyped visual hallucinations. The patient recognizes them as not real. There are no associated hallucinations in other modalities, delusions or altered consciousness. Most cases are reported in the elderly. The syndrome occurs in the context of visual impairment. It is named after a Swiss philosopher who first described the condition in 1760. He noticed that his grandfather, who suffered from cataracts, was complaining of seeing birds (Johnstone et al 2004, p. 805; Mitchell 2004, p. 23).

7. 12% of people aged >75 years have moderate or severe dementia.

False: About 12% of people aged over 75 years suffer from dementia. Only a proportion of these will have moderate or severe dementia (Butler & Pitt 1998, p. 50).

8. People with dementia cannot make valid financial decisions.

False: The ability to make financial decisions must be assessed formally. Inability cannot be assumed on the basis of a diagnosis of dementia (Johnstone et al 2004, p. 640).

9. In women on HRT the risk of Alzheimer's disease is lower than in the general population.

False: It was once thought that HRT might be protective. Subsequent studies suggest that HRT may increase the risk. This is an ongoing area of contention (Bluming 2004; Jacoby & Oppenheimer 2002, p. 495).

10. Cerebrospinal fluid (CSF) corticotropin-releasing factor (CRF) is reduced in Alzheimer's disease.

False: CSF CRF is reduced in fronto-temporal dementia, but not in Alzheimer's disease. CSF somatostatin level is reduced both in fronto-temporal dementia and Alzheimer's disease. Delta-sleep-inducing peptide is significantly reduced in Alzheimer's disease, but not in fronto-temporal dementia (Gelder et al 2000, p. 402).

11. Vascular dementia is associated with gait disturbance.

True: Gait disturbances occur in up to 25% of patients with vascular dementia. They are included in the DSM-IV criteria for vascular dementia and the NINDS-AIREN criteria for probable vascular dementia. Gait may be hemiplegic, apraxic-ataxic or short-stepped (Gelder et al 2000, p. 431; Mitchell 2004, p. 38).

12. Episodic memory is usually impaired in semantic dementia.

False: Semantic dementia is fairly specific for language difficulties (Lishman 1997, p. 753; Mitchell 2004, p. 290).

13. Having a seizure is more suggestive of Pick's disease than Alzheimer's disease.

False: Seizures are uncommon in Pick's disease (Lishman 1997, p. 461).

14. Normal ageing is associated with increased numbers of Lewy bodies.

False: Lewy bodies are abnormal intracellular bodies. They occur in the brains of only 0–5% of the 'normal' elderly. They are common in patients with Parkinson's disease (Jacoby & Oppenheimer 2002, p. 106).

15. In a 70-year-old with suspected depression, a CT scan showing dilated ventricles does not rule out the diagnosis.

True: In normal people, from about the age of 50 years, the brain weight and volume fall and ventricular and subarachnoid volumes rise (Lishman 1997, p. 140).

16. Most people with Down's syndrome have the neuropathological changes of Alzheimer's disease by age 40 years.

True: Almost all have the neuropathological changes but only 10% develop dementia by age 40 years (Johnstone et al 2004, p. 544).

17. Lewy bodies are present in 40% of dementias.

False: Lewy bodies are rounded eosinophilic inclusions within neurons. They are seen in 0–5% of the normal elderly population and 10–25% of patients with dementia (Lishman 1997, p. 450; Mitchell 2004, p. 292; Sadock & Sadock 2005, p. 1084).

18. In dementia with white matter lesions on CT, there is an increased risk of ataxia.

True: White matter lesions are thought to reflect underlying cerebral vascular pathology and have been associated with increased rates of ataxia and a poorer general prognosis (Briley et al 2000; Lishman 1997, p. 460).

19. Post-mortem studies conducted on patients with fronto-temporal dementia show that the pathology is mainly due to Pick's disease.

False: Pure Pick's disease is rare. There is a much larger group of frontal-lobe dementias clinically similar to Pick's but lacking the pathological characteristics of Pick's or Alzheimer's diseases (Gelder et al 2000, p. 397).

20. Day hospitals manage people with mild to moderate dementia significantly better than day centres.

False: This has not been proven to be the case (Copeland et al 2002, p. 682).

21. Clomethiazole is a useful hypnotic in elderly patients due to its freedom from 'hangover' effects.

True: Clomethiazole has a short half-life. Therefore it is relatively free of the hangover effects associated with other drugs. Hepatic disease can slow down the rate of its metabolism. It is used for the short-term treatment of severe anxiety in the elderly and also for alcohol withdrawal (BNF 2005, 4.1.2).

22. In the elderly, relapse of depression is more likely following ECT than using tricyclic antidepressants.

True: ECT is a more effective and faster treatment than tricyclics. 50–70% of patients have a good response. Patients relapse more quickly following ECT. An extended period of, or indefinite, antidepressant maintenance treatment following ECT is necessary. There are conflicting reports on the efficacy of maintenance treatment. Even with continued antidepressants, up to 50% of patients may relapse within 6–12 months (Johnstone et al 2004, p. 647).

23. Cholinesterase inhibitors are useful in the treatment of apathy in Alzheimer's disease.

True: Apathy is present in one-third of patients with Alzheimer's disease. The severity of apathy correlates with age, cognitive decline and loss of insight. Apathy is more common in patients with Alzheimer's disease who are depressed. Apathy also correlates with prefrontal and anterior temporal perfusion deficits. Cholinesterase inhibitors have been shown to improve apathy in Alzheimer's disease (Copeland et al 2002, p. 231; Mitchell 2004, pp. 278, 441, 370).

24. Galantamine treatment should be reviewed for efficacy every 6 months.

True: The NICE guidelines recommend that patients should be assessed between 2 and 4 months after reaching the maintenance dose of cholinesterase inhibitors. Treatment should be continued beyond this time only if there is an improvement or no deterioration in the MMSE score and evidence of global improvement from behavioural and functional assessment. Subsequently, patients should be assessed every 6 months and the treatment should be continued only if the MMSE score remains above 12 and the patient's global, functional and behavioural condition supports continuation of treatment (NICE).

25. Rivastigmine is a nicotinic receptor agonist.

False: Rivastigmine inhibits both acetylcholinesterase and butyryl cholinesterase. Galantamine is a reversible inhibitor of acetylcholinesterase and also a nicotinic receptor agonist (Johnstone et al 2004, p. 636).

42 Old age psychiatry – 5

Ben Underwood

		T	F
1.	Depression in the elderly is a risk factor for dementia.	☐	☐
2.	Prognosis for depression in the elderly is better if depression also occurred earlier in life.	☐	☐
3.	98% of elderly patients who have an episode of mania also develop depressive episodes.	☐	☐
4.	Cognitive testing may help differentiate depressive pseudodementia from dementia.	☐	☐
5.	Late onset schizophrenia is not associated with paranoid premorbid personality.	☐	☐
6.	Self-neglect in the elderly (Diogenes syndrome) is generally thought to be burnt out personality disorder.	☐	☐
7.	The prevalence of dementia doubles every 5 years after age 65 years, until age 85 years.	☐	☐
8.	There is an increased incidence of Alzheimer's disease in cerebral palsy.	☐	☐
9.	Oestrogen HRT is proven to delay the onset of Alzheimer's dementia.	☐	☐
10.	Stepwise cognitive decline is a recognized feature of Lewy body dementia.	☐	☐
11.	Disorders of praxis are associated with Pick's disease.	☐	☐
12.	Hachinski Ischaemia Score can differentiate Alzheimer's disease from vascular dementia.	☐	☐
13.	Gait disturbance suggests vascular dementia rather than Alzheimer's disease.	☐	☐
14.	Normal ageing is associated with a decrease in astrocytes.	☐	☐
15.	An elderly patient who suffers the first episode of depression is more likely to have large ventricles than someone of the same age who had several previous episodes.	☐	☐
16.	Hyperphosphorylated tau leads to the formation of tangles in Alzheimer's disease.	☐	☐
17.	Neurofibrillary tangles are composed of tau protein.	☐	☐
18.	White matter lesions on CT indicate better prognosis in dementia.	☐	☐
19.	The Barthel index is used to monitor behavioural disturbance in the elderly.	☐	☐

T   F

20. The Royal College of Psychiatrists recommends one Consultant in Old Age Psychiatry per 100 000 people aged over 65 years. ☐ ☐

21. Gastric pH is decreased in the elderly. ☐ ☐

22. Relapse of depression in the elderly is significantly reduced by maintenance medication. ☐ ☐

23. Cholinesterase inhibitors should be discontinued in patients with MMSE scores of less than 5/30. ☐ ☐

24. Memantine blocks NMDA receptors. ☐ ☐

25. Antioxidants have been tried in Alzheimer's disease. ☐ ☐

ANSWERS

1. Depression in the elderly is a risk factor for dementia.

True: There is a particularly strong risk for depression associated with 'pseudodementia', i.e. depression with cognitive impairment that resolves on remission of depression. There may be many reasons for the association between depression and dementia. Dementia may lead to depression as a result of increased subjective awareness of cognitive decline. Alternatively, a common factor may cause both depression and dementia (an example of this might be atherosclerosis). Depression may increase the risk of dementia via behaviours that increase the risk of vascular dementia such as smoking. These risks may also apply to depression occurring in midlife (Jacoby & Oppenheimer 2002, p. 637; Mitchell 2004, p. 277).

2. Prognosis for depression in the elderly is better if depression also occurred earlier in life.

False: Factors associated with poor outcomes include a slower initial improvement, incomplete recovery, more severe initial depression, duration of illness more than 2 years, three or more previous episodes of depression, previous episodes of dysthymia, psychotic symptoms and certain types of brain disease (Gelder et al 2000, p. 1647; Jacoby & Oppenheimer 2002, p. 663).

3. 98% of elderly patients who have an episode of mania also develop depressive episodes.

False: Up to 12% of elderly patients with mania do not develop depressive episodes. They have unipolar mania. Unipolar mania is more likely to be secondary mania due to an organic cause (Johnstone et al 2004, p. 648; Mitchell 2004, p. 439).

4. Cognitive testing may help differentiate depressive pseudodementia from dementia.

True: Higher cortical functions such as praxis are preserved in depressive pseudodementia but lost in true dementia, though not necessarily in the early stages. Verbal fluency and delayed recall is usually more severely affected in true dementias even in the early stages (Lishman 1997, p. 488; Mitchell 2004, p. 277).

5. Late onset schizophrenia is not associated with paranoid premorbid personality.

False: Paranoid or schizoid personality traits have been found in up to 45% of patients with late onset schizophrenia. These include jealousy, suspiciousness, emotional coldness, arrogance, egocentricity, explosiveness, oversensitivity and extreme solitariness. They also have lower rates of marriage and lower fecundity (Jacoby & Oppenheimer 2002, p. 754).

6. Self-neglect in the elderly (Diogenes syndrome) is generally thought to be burnt out personality disorder.

False: Diogenes syndrome, senile self-neglect or senile squalor, is characterized by severe self-neglect unaccompanied by any psychiatric disorder sufficient to account for the squalor in which the patient exists. Although burnt out personality disorder, end-stage personality disorder, personality reaction to stress and loneliness have been suggested, it is generally thought to involve a complex interplay of personality traits, psychosocial stressors and medical/psychiatric conditions (Jacoby & Oppenheimer 2002, p. 730).

7. The prevalence of dementia doubles every 5 years after age 65 years, until age 85 years.

True: The doubling of prevalence for every 5 years is a generally accepted 'rule of thumb'. The prevalence of dementia is c. 1% in 65–69-year-olds and c. 12% in 80–84-year-olds. The prevalence increases even more steeply after age 85 years (Butler & Pitt 1998, p. 50; Mitchell 2004, p. 258).

8. There is an increased incidence of Alzheimer's disease in cerebral palsy.

False: Cerebral palsy is not considered an independent risk factor.

9. Oestrogen HRT is proven to delay the onset of Alzheimer's dementia.

False: The role of HRT in preventing Alzheimer's disease is currently a source of much debate. It appears that the neuroprotection offered by oestrogen may depend on individual patient factors (Bluming 2004; Jacoby & Oppenheimer 2002, p. 495).

10. Stepwise cognitive decline is a recognized feature of Lewy body dementia.

False: Stepwise cognitive decline is a feature of multi-infarct dementia. The key features of Lewy body dementia include fluctuating cognition with pronounced disturbances in attention and concentration, visual hallucinations and spontaneous Parkinsonism (Johnstone et al 2004, p. 633; Mitchell 2004, p. 292).

11. Disorders of praxis are associated with Pick's disease.

False: Praxis relates to 'putting ideas into action'. Praxis is usually spared in Pick's disease (Lishman 1997, p. 461).

12. Hachinski Ischaemia Score can differentiate Alzheimer's disease from vascular dementia.

True: Hachinski Ischaemia Score incorporates the cardinal features of vascular dementia. It can differentiate Alzheimer's disease from vascular dementia. However, it cannot differentiate between vascular dementia and Alzheimer's disease with cerebrovascular disease (Gelder et al 2000, p. 432; Lishman 1997, p. 456).

13. Gait disturbance suggests vascular dementia rather than Alzheimer's disease.

True: Gait disturbances occur in up to 25% of patients with vascular dementia. They are included in the DSM-IV criteria for vascular dementia and the NINDS-AIREN criteria for probable vascular dementia. Gait may be hemiplegic, apraxic-ataxic, short-stepped or Parkinsonian. Gait disorders are more common in vascular dementia than in Alzheimer's disease (Gelder et al 2000, p. 431).

14. Normal ageing is associated with a decrease in astrocytes.

False: Glial cells are 10 times more numerous than neurons. The oligodendrocytes and Schwann cells form the myelin sheaths. The astrocytes participate in the blood–brain barrier, remove certain neurotransmitters from the synaptic cleft, buffer the extracellular potassium concentration and possibly have a nutritive role. The microglia serve as scavengers. With ageing, oligodendrocytes are decreased, consistent with disproportionate white matter loss on MRI, but astrocytes and microglia are increased (Lawlor 2001, p. 224; Sadock & Sadock 2005, pp. 4, 3613).

15. An elderly patient who suffers the first episode of depression is more likely to have large ventricles than someone of the same age who had several previous episodes.

False: Dolan and colleagues in 1985 studied CT brain scans of 101 patients with depression. Although their ventricles were enlarged relative to healthy controls, the degree of enlargement did not relate to illness duration or treatment parameters, suggesting that ventricular enlargement antedated the onset of the illness (Lishman 1997, p. 140).

16. Hyperphosphorylated tau leads to the formation of tangles in Alzheimer's disease.

True: Tau protein is important in stabilizing the microtubules in the neuronal cytoplasm. Hyperphosphorylation is seen in Alzheimer's disease (Johnstone et al 2004, p. 68; Lishman 1997, p. 442; Mitchell 2004, p. 272).

17. Neurofibrillary tangles are composed of tau protein.

True: Tau protein normally plays a role in the cytoskeleton, linking neurofilaments and microtubules. Paired helices of tau form neurofibrillary tangles (Lishman 1997, p. 442).

18. White matter lesions on CT indicate better prognosis in dementia.

False: White matter lesions are associated with a worse prognosis. This may be because they are reflective of underlying generalized vascular pathology (Briley et al 2000).

19. The Barthel index is used to monitor behavioural disturbance in the elderly.

False: The Barthel index is a standardized assessment scale for activities of daily living (Jacoby & Oppenheimer 2002, p. 229).

20. The Royal College of Psychiatrists recommends one Consultant in Old Age Psychiatry per 100 000 people aged over 65 years.

False: The correct figure is 1 per 10 000. Of 10 000 people over 65 years, there will be on average 500 with dementia, 1400 with depression, 160 with psychosis and 160 with other conditions (Jacoby & Oppenheimer 2002, p. 430).

21. Gastric pH is decreased in the elderly.

False: Ageing decreases gastric acid secretion. The prevalence of gastric achlorhydria increases with age. The elderly have reduced gastric acid production, gastric emptying, gastrointestinal motility, absorptive gut surface area and intestinal blood flow, all of which may reduce the absorption of some drugs (Jacoby & Oppenheimer 2002, p. 286; King 2004, p. 449; Sadock & Sadock 2005, p. 3717).

22. Relapse of depression in the elderly is significantly reduced by maintenance medication.

True: Maintenance therapy is thought to reduce rates of relapse by a factor of up to 2.5. Up to 70% of patients on maintenance treatment may remain well at 4 years (Copeland et al 2002, p. 440; Johnstone et al 2004, p. 647; King 2004, p. 460).

23. Cholinesterase inhibitors should be discontinued in patients with MMSE scores of less than 5/30.

True: This area is controversial. Cholinesterase inhibitors are considered to be most effective in mild to moderate dementia. Hence, the NICE guidelines suggest discontinuing them if the MMSE scores drop below 12/30 (BNF 2005, 4.11; Jacoby & Oppenheimer 2002, p. 572; NICE).

24. Memantine blocks NMDA receptors.

True: Memantine is an NMDA (N-Methyl-D-Aspartate) receptor antagonist. It has been used in moderate to severe Alzheimer's dementia (BNF 2005, 4.11).

25. Antioxidants have been tried in Alzheimer's disease.

True: Antioxidant therapy has been tried in Alzheimer's disease. This is based on the hypothesis that cellular respiration produces oxygen derivatives and other free radicals that may be harmful to intracellular structures. Vitamin E and vitamin C have been tried in Alzheimer's disease. The results have been conflicting, though predominantly negative (Jacoby & Oppenheimer 2002, pp. 496, 574).

Pharmacology – 1

Graham Murray

	T	F
1. Chronic administration of agonists results in both receptor desensitization and down-regulation.	☐	☐
2. Antagonists bind with agonists and prevent them reaching the receptors.	☐	☐
3. The area under the curve is greater if the drug elimination is faster.	☐	☐
4. In zero-order kinetics the rate of elimination is directly proportional to the amount of drug remaining.	☐	☐
5. Second messengers are characteristic of ion-channel receptors.	☐	☐
6. Therapeutic index is the ratio of the maximum tolerated concentration and the minimum effective concentration.	☐	☐
7. The binding of two acetylcholine molecules at the two beta subunits of a nicotinic receptor-channel results in the opening of that channel.	☐	☐
8. Albumin has a low affinity for acidic drugs.	☐	☐
9. D-Cycloserine enhances the extinction of fear.	☐	☐
10. Dopamine neurons that innervate the nucleus accumbens have their cell bodies in the ventral tegmental area of the midbrain.	☐	☐
11. Lithium decreases dopaminergic effects in the CNS.	☐	☐
12. Bromocriptine decreases dopaminergic effects in the CNS.	☐	☐
13. D_1 and D_2 receptors belong to the same family.	☐	☐
14. Endorphins are implicated in the gate theory of pain.	☐	☐
15. Glutamate is an NMDA antagonist.	☐	☐
16. Melatonin has a narrow therapeutic index.	☐	☐
17. Nicotinic receptors control cation channels.	☐	☐
18. Nicotine improves cognitive performance in non-smokers.	☐	☐
19. Nicotinic receptors are ligand-gated.	☐	☐
20. Noradrenaline reuptake inhibitors increase the sensitivity of presynaptic α_2-receptors.	☐	☐
21. The QT interval is dependent on heart rate.	☐	☐
22. 5-HT_{1A} receptors are called 5-HT_B receptors.	☐	☐

T F

23. Some serotonin receptors are metabotropic while others are ionotropic. ☐ ☐

24. 5-HT$_3$ receptor is ionotropic. ☐ ☐

25. Substance P antagonists reduce pain. ☐ ☐

ANSWERS

1. Chronic administration of agonists results in both receptor desensitization and down-regulation.

True: Prolonged exposure to agonists causes receptors to both desensitize and down-regulate.

Desensitization occurs first (within minutes) and may be related to receptor phosphorylation.

Down-regulation occurs later (a timeframe of hours) and is due to receptor internalization and degradation, though decreased levels of receptor mRNA are also seen.

The opposite is true in that chronic administration of antagonists results in receptor up-regulation (Cooper et al 2003, p. 81).

2. Antagonists bind with agonists and prevent them reaching the receptors.

False: The binding of antagonists to agonists and the prevention thereby of them reaching receptors is known as chemical antagonism. For example, a chelating agent may be used to counter the effect of heavy metals. It is a rare form of antagonism. Most antagonists bind with the receptor, thus preventing the agonist reaching the receptor (Rang et al 2003, p. 18).

3. The area under the curve is greater if the drug elimination is faster.

False: The area under the curve (AUC) refers to the area under the plasma concentration–time curve. AUC is lesser if the drug elimination is faster (Anderson & Reid 2002, p. 28; Rang et al 2003, p. 116).

4. In zero-order kinetics the rate of elimination is directly proportional to the amount of drug remaining.

False: In first-order kinetics the rate of absorption or elimination is directly proportional to the amount of drug remaining.

In zero-order kinetics a fixed amount of drug is absorbed or eliminated per minute, independent of the drug concentrations. This is because of rate limiting factors, e.g. in the metabolism of alcohol (Anderson & Reid 2002, p. 27).

5. Second messengers are characteristic of ion-channel receptors.

False: Second messengers are characteristic of G-protein coupled receptors (Rang et al 2003, p. 33).

6. Therapeutic index is the ratio of the maximum tolerated concentration and the minimum effective concentration.

True: Therapeutic range is the range of plasma concentrations that yield therapeutic success. The size of therapeutic window, i.e. the therapeutic index (TI), is the ratio of the maximum tolerated concentration to the minimum effective concentration. In practice, we compare the dose at which 50% of the people have the desired outcome (effective dose 50 or ED_{50}) with the dose at which 50% have side-effects (toxic dose 50 or TD_{50}). TI is the ratio of the TD_{50} to the ED_{50}. The closer TD_{50} is to ED_{50}, the narrower the margin of safety and the greater the risk of side-effects (Bennett & Brown 2003, p. 94; King 2004, p. 72).

7. The binding of two acetylcholine molecules at the two beta subunits of a nicotinic receptor-channel results in the opening of that channel.

False: The binding of two acetylcholine molecules at the two *alpha* subunits of a nicotinic receptor-channel results in the opening of that channel (Kandel et al 2000, p. 200).

8. Albumin has a low affinity for acidic drugs.

False: Albumin has a high affinity for acidic drugs, although a low capacity for binding acidic drugs. Acidic drugs bind in small quantities, but they do bind strongly and are hard to displace. This is particularly relevant in renal failure, when the concentration of acidic drugs such as phenytoin may be affected. The unbound percentage of phenytoin may increase from the usual 9% to 19% in renal disease (Bennett & Brown 2003, p. 111).

9. D-Cycloserine enhances the extinction of fear.

True: D-Cycloserine is a partial agonist at the NMDA glutamate receptor. It enhances the extinction of conditioned fear in rodents. It is being investigated in the treatment of phobias.

10. Dopamine neurons that innervate the nucleus accumbens have their cell bodies in the ventral tegmental area of the midbrain.

True: There are three main dopamine pathways:

- Nigrostriatal: from substantia nigra to basal ganglia
- Mesocortical and mesolimbic: from ventral tegmental area to nucleus accumbens, amygdala and prefrontal cortex
- Tuberoinfundibular: from median eminence to the pituitary (Anderson & Reid 2002, p. 11).

11. Lithium decreases dopaminergic effects in the CNS.

False: Although often used in concert with dopamine antagonists in the treatment of acute mania, lithium does not have any effect on dopamine levels, dopamine turnover or dopamine receptor mediated behaviour (Anderson & Reid 2002, p. 80).

12. Bromocriptine decreases dopaminergic effects in the CNS.

False: Bromocriptine is a dopamine agonist. It is used to treat Parkinsonism, extrapyramidal syndromes, hyperprolactinaemia, galactorrhoea and neuroleptic malignant syndrome (Sadock & Sadock 2005, p. 2999).

13. D_1 and D_2 receptors belong to the same family.

False: The dopamine receptors belong to two families. The 'D$_1$ like' include the D_1 and D_5 receptors, which are positively coupled to cAMP. The 'D$_2$ like' include the D_2, D_3 and D_4 receptors, which inhibit cAMP (Anderson & Reid 2002, p. 12).

14. Endorphins are implicated in the gate theory of pain.

True: The gate theory of pain suggests that pain results from the balance of activity in nociceptive and non-nociceptive afferents. Morphine produces analgesia partly by activating descending inhibitory pathways. Such pathways may also be activated by endogenous opioid peptides such as endorphins (Kandel et al 2000, p. 483).

15. Glutamate is an NMDA antagonist.

False: Glutamate is an NMDA agonist. Glutamate is the major excitatory transmitter in the brain and spinal cord. The glutamate receptors include: the ionotropic receptors that directly gate channels and the metabotropic receptors that indirectly gate channels through second messengers. The subtypes of ionotropic glutamate receptors are AMPA, kainate and NMDA, named according to the agonists that activate them. The action of glutamate on the ionotropic receptors is always excitatory. The activation of metabotropic receptors can produce either excitation or inhibition (Kandel et al 2000, p. 212).

16. Melatonin has a narrow therapeutic index.

False: Melatonin is a hormone secreted by the pineal gland during darkness. It is thought to play a role in the sleep–wake cycle, and hence, used to treat insomnia and jet-lag. Prolonged use may lead to dependence. It is generally considered to have minimal side-effects (Bennett & Brown 2003, p. 404; King 2004, p. 438).

17. Nicotinic receptors control cation channels.

True: The cholinergic receptors are subdivided into nicotinic and muscarinic. The nicotinic receptors are directly coupled to cation channels and are involved in fast excitatory transmission (Anderson & Reid 2002, p. 22).

18. Nicotine improves cognitive performance in non-smokers.

True: Clinical and pre-clinical evidence show the cognitive enhancing properties of nicotine (Rang et al 2003, p. 599).

19. Nicotinic receptors are ligand-gated.

True: Nicotinic receptors are ligand-gated ionotropic channels. Their activation leads to a rapid transient increase in membrane permeability to either cations (especially sodium and calcium) or anions (mainly chloride). They are excitatory. They are blocked by curare. In contrast, muscarinic receptors are G-protein linked, can be excitatory or inhibitory and are blocked by atropine, scopolamine and other anticholinergics (Cookson et al 2002, p. 66; Kandel et al 2000, p. 185; Stahl 2000, p. 468).

20. Noradrenaline reuptake inhibitors increase the sensitivity of presynaptic α_2-receptors.

False: Administration of noradrenaline reuptake inhibitors leads to increased levels of noradrenaline, and, as a consequence, increased stimulation of presynaptic α_2-receptors. However, this increased stimulation then leads to down-regulation of presynaptic α_2-receptors, leading to reduced sensitivity (Cookson et al 2002, p. 267).

21. The QT interval is dependent on heart rate.

True: The QT interval represents the time between the onset of electrical depolarization and the end of depolarization of the ventricles. Prolongation of the QT interval increases the vulnerability of the myocardium during which ventricular arrhythmias may be precipitated. The length of the QT interval is influenced by the heart rate. Hence, a rate correction is required to interpret its length. QTc is calculated using Bazett's formula (QT/√RR interval) (King 2004, p. 581).

22. $5\text{-}HT_{1A}$ receptors are called $5\text{-}HT_B$ receptors.

False: There are seven distinct types of 5-HT receptors: $5\text{-}HT_1$, $5\text{-}HT_2$, $5\text{-}HT_3$, $5\text{-}HT_4$, $5\text{-}HT_5$, $5\text{-}HT_6$, and $5\text{-}HT_7$. The $5\text{-}HT_1$ family contains receptors that are negatively coupled to adenylate cyclase ($5\text{-}HT_{1A}$, $5\text{-}HT_{1B}$, $5\text{-}HT_{1D}$, $5\text{-}HT_{1E}$, $5\text{-}HT_{1F}$). $5\text{-}HT_{1C}$ receptors have been reclassified as $5\text{-}HT_{2C}$ (King 2004, p. 26).

23. Some serotonin receptors are metabotropic while others are ionotropic.

True: There are 14 different serotonin receptors, belonging to 7 groups.

The $5\text{-}HT_1$ group of receptors ($5\text{-}HT_{1A}$, $5\text{-}HT_{1B}$, $5\text{-}HT_{1D}$, $5\text{-}HT_{1E}$, $5\text{-}HT_{1F}$) are inhibitory and are negatively coupled to cAMP. The $5\text{-}HT_{1C}$ receptor has been reclassified as $5\text{-}HT_{2C}$.

$5\text{-}HT_2$ receptors ($5\text{-}HT_{2A}$, $5\text{-}HT_{2B}$, $5\text{-}HT_{2C}$) are excitatory. They act through the phospholipase C/inositol phosphate pathway.

The $5\text{-}HT_3$ receptor is a non-selective cation channel receptor which is permeable to both sodium and potassium ions. Because both calcium and magnesium ions can modulate its activity, it resembles the glutamate NMDA receptor.

$5\text{-}HT_4$, $5\text{-}HT_5$, $5\text{-}HT_6$, and $5\text{-}HT_7$ are excitatory. They act through the phospholipase C/inositol phosphate pathway.

Thus, all serotonin receptors are G-protein coupled (metabotropic), except $5\text{-}HT_3$ which is a ligand-gated ion channel (ionotropic) (Anderson & Reid 2002, p. 18; Cooper et al 2003, p. 295; King 2004, p. 26; Rang et al 2003, p. 481).

24. 5-HT$_3$ receptor is ionotropic.

True: The 5-HT$_3$ receptor is a ligand-gated ion channel receptor (ionotropic receptor). It is a non-selective cation channel receptor permeable to both sodium and potassium ions. Both calcium and magnesium ions can modulate its activity, and thus it resembles the glutamate NMDA receptor (Cooper et al 2003, p. 295; King 2004, p. 26).

25. Substance P antagonists reduce pain.

False: Substance P is a pain neurotransmitter. Administration of substance P in animals elicits behavioural and cardiovascular effects resembling stress response. Plasma levels of substance P are elevated in depression. Substance P receptor antagonists improve depression, anxiety and emesis, but surprisingly not pain (Sadock & Sadock 2005, pp. 83, 135).

Pharmacology – 2

Konstantinos Stagias

	T	F

1. The use of ethanol in methanol poisoning is an example of competitive agonism. ☐ ☐

2. Compliance therapy has been shown to improve the outcome in patients prescribed neuroleptic medication. ☐ ☐

3. Zero-order kinetics can be correctly described in terms of half-life. ☐ ☐

4. Heteroceptors regulate neurotransmitter release. ☐ ☐

5. Heteroceptors can be ionotropic or metabotropic. ☐ ☐

6. Acetylcholine is a transmitter at some postganglionic sympathetic neuroeffector junctions. ☐ ☐

7. Muscarinic receptors are coupled to ion channels. ☐ ☐

8. Pregabalin binds to the alpha 2 delta subunit of voltage-sensitive calcium channels. ☐ ☐

9. DHEA has an effect opposite to that of cortisol. ☐ ☐

10. Benzhexol inhibits dopamine secretion. ☐ ☐

11. The firing rate of neurons in the mesolimbic pathway changes in anticipation of pleasurable stimuli. ☐ ☐

12. Dopamine receptors are postsynaptic but not presynaptic. ☐ ☐

13. Raclopride is used to study dopamine receptor binding. ☐ ☐

14. Opiates regulate dopamine activity. ☐ ☐

15. Glutamate concentration is increased in post-mortems of schizophrenic brains. ☐ ☐

16. Magnesium ions block NMDA receptors. ☐ ☐

17. Nicotine reaches the brain within 5–6 seconds after inhalation. ☐ ☐

18. Nicotine increases the brain dopamine in the mesolimbic region. ☐ ☐

19. The NMDA receptor is a voltage gated channel. ☐ ☐

20. β-adrenergic receptors are stimulatory. ☐ ☐

21. The upper limit for a normal QT interval is approximately 400 ms. ☐ ☐

22. Increased 5-HT in the periaqueductal grey matter increases the fright/flight response. ☐ ☐

T F

23. Serotonin transporter gene polymorphisms are associated with violence. ☐ ☐

24. In neuroimaging, iodobenzamide may be used as a ligand for 5-HT$_{2A}$ ☐ ☐
receptors.

25. Yohimbine is an α_2-noradrenergic receptor antagonist. ☐ ☐

ANSWERS

1. The use of ethanol in methanol poisoning is an example of competitive agonism.

False: Ethanol competes for occupancy of the enzyme alcohol dehydrogenase, and thus prevents the metabolism of methanol to its toxic metabolite formic acid. This is an example of competitive antagonism (Bennett & Brown 2003, p. 92; King 2004, p. 76).

2. Compliance therapy has been shown to improve the outcome in patients prescribed neuroleptic medication.

True: Compliance therapy, i.e. the use of a cognitive strategy that helps the patient weigh advantages and disadvantages of drug treatment, has been shown to improve the outcome in patients with schizophrenia.

3. Zero-order kinetics can be correctly described in terms of half-life.

False: In zero-order kinetics the rate of the metabolism or elimination is not related to the concentration of the drug, but occurs at a constant rate, e.g. the metabolism of alcohol. First-order kinetics can be described in terms of half-life (Anderson & Reid 2002, p. 28; Bennett & Brown 2003, p. 99).

4. Heteroceptors regulate neurotransmitter release.

True: Neurotransmitter receptors are usually located on a membrane on the far side of the synapse to the point of release. When these postsynaptic receptors are located on the dendrites or the soma of a neuron they regulate cell firing. When located on a nerve terminal and regulating neurotransmitter release they are called presynaptic heteroceptors. Presynaptic heteroceptors regulate neurotransmitter release by the axon terminal on which they are located. For example, mirtazapine blocks α_2-heteroceptors on serotonergic neurons, resulting in increased serotonin release (Anderson & Reid 2002, p. 10).

5. Heteroceptors can be ionotropic or metabotropic.

True: Ionotropic receptors are ligand-gated ion channels that respond to neurotransmitters by allowing ion flux across cell membranes. Metabotropic receptors, however, mediate neurotransmission less directly by activating second messenger molecules which subsequently modulate cellular communication (Rang et al 2003, p. 22).

6. Acetylcholine is a transmitter at some postganglionic sympathetic neuroeffector junctions.

True: The sympathetic transmitter at the postganglionic synapse is usually noradrenaline, but in sweat glands and in some blood vessels it is acetylcholine. The postganglionic parasympathetic neurotransmitter is acetylcholine (Rang et al 2003, p. 123).

7. Muscarinic receptors are coupled to ion channels.

False: Muscarinic receptors are G-protein coupled (Anderson & Reid 2002, p. 22).

8. Pregabalin binds to the alpha 2 delta subunit of voltage-sensitive calcium channels.

True: Pregabalin is a leucine analogue. It binds to the alpha 2 delta subunit of voltage-sensitive calcium channels. This diminishes neuronal activity and neurotransmitter release. Pregabalin is used in peripheral neuropathic pain and as adjunctive therapy for partial seizures. Its efficacy in anxiety, social phobia and pain is under investigation.

9. DHEA has an effect opposite to that of cortisol.

True: DHEA can act as an anti-glucocorticoid (Goodyer et al 2003).

10. Benzhexol inhibits dopamine secretion.

True: Anticholinergic drugs exert an excitatory effect, opposite to that of dopamine, on striatal neurons. They also exert a presynaptic inhibitory effect on dopaminergic nerve terminals and hence inhibit dopamine secretion (Rang et al 2003, p. 500).

11. The firing rate of neurons in the mesolimbic pathway changes in anticipation of pleasurable stimuli.

True: The dopamine firing rate changes during the anticipation and possibly also during the experience of pleasurable or dreaded stimuli. This pathway is strongly associated with motivation, reward behaviour and dependence on drugs of abuse (Anderson & Reid 2002, p. 12; Sadock & Sadock 2005, p. 1393).

12. Dopamine receptors are postsynaptic but not presynaptic.

False: Dopamine receptors can be pre- or postsynaptic. Postsynaptic dopamine receptors are located on the far side of the synapse to the point of release. The presynaptic receptors are located on the dopamine neurons and are called autoreceptors. Stimulation of these autoreceptors inhibits the release of dopamine by the neuron. The D_2 receptors are located post- as well as presynaptically (Anderson & Reid 2002, p. 10; Cooper et al 2003, p. 240).

13. Raclopride is used to study dopamine receptor binding.

True: Raclopride is a D_2 receptor antagonist. Other compounds used to image dopamine receptors include other benzamides such as iodobenzamide and fallypride, and butyrophenones such as spiperone/spiroperidol derivatives (King 2004, p. 24).

14. Opiates regulate dopamine activity.

True: β-endorphin neurons, via μ receptors, inhibit GABA neurons that inhibit dopaminergic neurons. This results in increased mesolimbic dopaminergic activity. Dynorphin, via κ receptors, tonically inhibits mesolimbic dopamine release. Basal dopamine release is determined by the balance between these two opioid systems.

15. Glutamate concentration is increased in post-mortems of schizophrenic brains.

False: Post-mortem studies in schizophrenic brains show reduced concentrations of glutamate in the hippocampus and the prefrontal cortex. This suggests that there is decreased glutaminergic transmission in schizophrenia (Sadock & Sadock 2005, p. 70).

16. Magnesium ions block NMDA receptors.

True: Magnesium readily blocks NMDA receptors. This block shows marked voltage dependence, occurring at physiological magnesium concentrations when the cell is normally polarized, but is overcome if the cell is depolarized (Kandel et al 2000, p. 212; Rang et al 2003, p. 466).

17. Nicotine reaches the brain within 5–6 seconds after inhalation.

True: Nicotine is absorbed through the skin, mucous membranes and lungs. With smoking, nicotine is rapidly absorbed across the lung mucosa and produces effects on the brain within about 7 seconds (King 2004, p. 507).

18. Nicotine increases the brain dopamine in the mesolimbic region.

True: The mesolimbic dopaminergic pathway that projects from the ventral tegmental area to the nucleus accumbens is strongly associated with motivation, reward behaviour and dependence on drugs of abuse. The stimulant and rewarding effects of nicotine are mediated via the nicotinic cholinergic receptors that indirectly increase the release of dopamine from the nucleus accumbens (Anderson & Reid 2002, p. 12; King 2004, p. 506; Sadock & Sadock 2005, p. 1393).

19. The NMDA receptor is a voltage-gated channel.

False: The NMDA receptor is a ligand-gated ion channel, activated by glutamate. The NMDA receptor is unique among transmitter-gated channels because its opening also depends on membrane voltage (which will expel Mg^{2+} from the channel by electrostatic repulsion, allowing Ca^{2+} and Na^+ to enter). Thus it is sensitive to voltage. It controls a cation channel that is permeable to Ca^{2+} as well as to Na^+ and K^+ (Cooper et al 2003, p. 139; Kandel et al 2000, p. 212).

20. β-adrenergic receptors are stimulatory.

True: β-adrenoceptors are stimulatory. Their stimulation increases cAMP (Anderson & Reid 2002, p. 16).

21. The upper limit for a normal QT interval is approximately 400 ms.

False: The QT interval is the time in milliseconds between the beginning of the QRS complex and the end of the T wave. Prolongation is associated with ventricular arrhythmias and sudden death. QT is dependent on heart rate. The Bazett's formula (QT/√RR interval) is applied to give a QT corrected for rate (QTc). Normal QTc is <450 ms in women and <430 ms in men. Prolonged values are >470 ms in women and >450 ms in men (King 2004, p. 581).

22. Increased 5-HT in the periaqueductal grey matter increases the fright/flight response.

False: The serotonergic pathway that connects the dorsal raphe nuclei to the dorsal periaqueductal grey matter is implicated in the regulation of escape behaviour and panic. A number of animal studies have shown that increased 5-HT in the periaqueductal grey matter inhibits the fright/flight response. This may be mediated via 5-HT$_{1A}$ and 5-HT$_{2A}$ receptors. This may explain why SSRIs are effective in the treatment of anxiety disorders.

23. Serotonin transporter gene polymorphisms are associated with violence.

True: Transporters or monoamine plasma membrane transported proteins mediate the reuptake of monoamines released into the synaptic cleft back into the presynaptic terminal. There is an inverse association between 5-HT and impulsivity, aggression and violence (Johnstone et al 2004, p. 509; Sadock & Sadock 2005, p. 54).

24. In neuroimaging, iodobenzamide may be used as a ligand for 5-HT$_{2A}$ receptors.

False: [^{123}I]-iodobenzamide ([^{123}I]IBZM) is a radioligand that is widely used for SPECT imaging of dopamine receptors D$_2$ and D$_3$.

25. Yohimbine is an α_2-noradrenergic receptor antagonist.

True: Yohimbine is an α_2 antagonist which increases noradrenaline release. It precipitates panic attacks in patients with panic disorder, but not in healthy volunteers. It was considered an aphrodisiac. It sometimes helps in psychogenic impotence (Anderson & Reid 2002, p. 96; King 2004, p. 560).

Psychology – 1

Salbu Krishnan

		T	F
1.	Acting out is a means of ventilating inner feelings without restriction.	☐	☐
2.	In looking through telephone book numbers, looking for letters next to numbers is a test of divided attention.	☐	☐
3.	The fundamental attribution error explains why we attribute other people's mistakes to situational reasons.	☐	☐
4.	The fundamental attribution error is less likely to occur in collectivist societies.	☐	☐
5.	Social role valorization is the new aim of mental health services.	☐	☐
6.	The semantic content is completely contained in the word.	☐	☐
7.	Telephone conversations are longer than face-to-face conversations.	☐	☐
8.	The congruity theory holds that if a person does not agree with a message from a person they like, they will change both the attitude towards the person and to the message.	☐	☐
9.	Deviancy amplification spiral leads to secondary deviance.	☐	☐
10.	In a stable community of wild baboons, the dominant male is the most aggressive.	☐	☐
11.	In baboons, female dominance comes from the mother.	☐	☐
12.	According to Eysenck, introverts condition quicker than extroverts.	☐	☐
13.	Eysenck's personality theory is idiographic.	☐	☐
14.	Disorders in the children of parents with depression are secondary to the core symptoms in the parents.	☐	☐
15.	Friendships in teenagers are based on standards that are opposed to parental standards.	☐	☐
16.	The parents of a child with learning disabilities would show bereavement response.	☐	☐
17.	Groups tend to make more extreme decisions than individuals.	☐	☐
18.	Social iatrogenesis includes side-effects of mass vaccination.	☐	☐
19.	Labelling theory implies the understanding by the labelled individual of the specific behaviour expected to be associated with the particular label.	☐	☐
20.	Charismatic leaders have referent power.	☐	☐

	T	F
21. Leadership ability depends on task orientation.	☐	☐
22. Norms is synonymous with values.	☐	☐
23. Social cohesion promotes racial prejudice.	☐	☐
24. In the UK, the Registrar General determines social class based on occupation.	☐	☐
25. Acute stress causes cutaneous vasodilation.	☐	☐

ANSWERS

1. Acting out is a means of ventilating inner feelings without restriction.

False: Engaging in activities which can be interpreted as a substitute for remembering past events is termed acting out. In essence thoughts are replaced by actions, implying that such memories lack verbal representation or the impulse is too intense to be discharged in verbal form. Acts within the session such as pacing up and down, throwing things, etc. are referred to as acting in. Both acting out and acting in are examples of enactment. Acting out implies regression to a pre-reflective preverbal level (Bateman & Holmes 1995, p. 195).

2. In looking through telephone book numbers, looking for letters next to numbers is a test of divided attention.

True: Attention tests are of two types – focused and divided. Focused attention tests require subjects to attend only to one stimulus whilst being distracted by others. Divided attention tests require subjects to attend to multiple stimuli simultaneously (Munafo 2002, p. 20).

3. The fundamental attribution error explains why we attribute other people's mistakes to situational reasons.

False: The fundamental attribution error occurs when we explain the bad behaviour of others by referring to the individual's personal or dispositional factors. When analysing our own behaviour we are more likely to blame bad behaviour on situational factors (Gross 2001, p. 345; Wright et al 2005, p. 80).

4. The fundamental attribution error is less likely to occur in collectivist societies.

True: The fundamental attribution error may be limited to Western societies. It may be more pronounced when people are required to attribute behaviour to a single cause (Fear 2004, p. 32; Gross 2001, p. 345; Wright et al 2005, p. 80).

5. Social role valorization is the new aim of mental health services.

True: Mental health care traditionally followed the deviancy approach with labelling, segregation and institutional care of the mentally ill. The normalization approach or social role valorization approach was initially developed in learning disabilities. It aims to reverse the devaluation of the disabled person and the group while accepting that disability exists. It capitalizes on the strengths and ambitions of the person to improve the person's quality of life. It uses person-centred planning to identify what it would take to offer 'normal' opportunities for living, work, friendships and relationships (Fear 2004, p. 497; Gelder et al 2000, p. 1503).

6. The semantic content is completely contained in the word.

False: Semantics is the study of the meaning of language, i.e. the meaning underlying words and sentences. It is divided into morphemes and sentences. Morphemes include words as well as prefixes and suffixes which may alter the meaning of a word. Meaning is also influenced by context and thus the sentence in which the word is contained is also important (Fear 2004, p. 48; Gross 2001, p. 279).

7. Telephone conversations are longer than face-to-face conversations.

True: In telephone conversations all the information has to be conveyed solely via the audible component. In face-to-face communication the additional visual component involving facial expression, gestures, proximity, etc. carries a lot of information. This necessitates telephone conversations to be longer and more articulate than face-to-face conversations in order to convey the same amount of information.

8. The congruity theory holds that if a person does not agree with a message from a person they like, they will change both the attitude towards the person and to the message.

True: According to Osgood and Tannenbaum's congruity theory (1955), incongruity makes people feel uncomfortable and motivates them to change their attitudes to make them congruent. Both attitudes change. The weaker attitude changes more and the stronger attitude changes less. Attitudes do not change direction (Osgood & Tannenbaum 1955).

9. Deviancy amplification spiral leads to secondary deviance.

False: Primary deviance is a deviant act. Secondary deviance refers to the change in behaviour as a result of being labelled a deviant due to the primary act. Cohen in 1972 coined the term deviancy amplification spiral. It is the modern mass media phenomenon of an increasing cycle of reporting on a category of antisocial behaviour or other undesirable events resulting in a moral panic which causes change out of proportion to the real threat (Cohen 1992; Puri & Tyrer 1998, p. 333).

10. In a stable community of wild baboons, the dominant male is the most aggressive.

True: Aggression is a spontaneously generated force which helps maintain dominance hierarchies and aids the process of natural selection. Animals that live in groups often develop a social order based on dominance hierarchies.

In baboons the dominant male usually achieves his status through victory in several aggressive threat displays and encounters. After this, his status is settled for a while and lower ranking baboons generally step aside for his convenience (Gleitman 1996, p. 302).

11. In baboons female dominance comes from the mother.

True: In many primate societies, females compete as much as the males do. The females develop hierarchies that are often more stable than those of males. The female rank has more important long-term consequences than the male rank. The mothers tend to bequeath their social rank to their offspring, especially to their daughters (Gleitman 1996, p. 302).

12. According to Eysenck, introverts condition quicker than extroverts.

True: Eysenck hypothesized that the ascending reticular activating system of introverts is sensitive and chronically over-aroused. Strong stimuli facilitate stimulus–response associations. As introverts are more easily stimulated than extroverts, they should, in theory, be more prone to conditioning. Experimental evidence does not strongly support this (Gelder et al 2000, p. 707; Gross 2001, p. 617).

13. Eysenck's personality theory is idiographic.

False: Personality theories may be nomothetic or idiographic. The nomothetic approach describes personality in terms of shared attributes, i.e. there are a limited number of variables on which people differ. The idiographic approach considers each individual as unique. The nomothetic approach has two variants – type and trait approaches. Type theories are categorical or non-continuous, e.g. the use of diagnostic categories for various personality disorders. In the trait approach there are a limited number of personality variables, but they are continuous in nature. Eysenck's three dimensions of personality, i.e. neuroticism, extraversion and psychoticism, belong to the nomothetic and trait type (Johnstone et al 2004, p.111; Wright et al 2005, p. 75).

14. Disorders in the children of parents with depression are secondary to the core symptoms in the parents.

False: Parental depression is associated with a greatly increased risk of psychopathology and developmental difficulties in children. This is due to a complex bi-directional interaction between genetic vulnerability, influence of depression on parenting behaviour, parent–child relationships and social disadvantage, not just the core symptoms (Gelder et al 2000, p. 1848).

15. Friendships in teenagers are based on standards that are opposed to parental standards.

False: Teenagers' standards are remarkably in tune with those of their parents. Peer and friendship groups work in concert with, rather than in opposition to, adult values, attitudes, goals and achievements (Gross 2001, p. 540; Sadock & Sadock 2005, p. 3040).

16. The parents of a child with learning disabilities would show bereavement response.

True: The parents respond with grief, similar to that which occurs with a sudden loss. Every expectant parent daydreams about the child. The arrival of a sick or damaged baby destroys many of those dreams. The phases of the response are also similar to normal grief, involving shock, denial and anger followed by constructive active adaptation, which might involve learning about the condition or joining a parents' association, leading on to resolution (Gelder et al 2000, p. 2001).

17. Groups tend to make more extreme decisions than individuals.

True: Group discussions tend to lead to decisions that are more extreme than individual decisions. If the group members were initially inclined to take risks with regard to a particular issue, the group would make even riskier decisions. Similarly, if the group members were cautious to start with, the group decision would be even more cautious. This is called the group polarization effect (Wright et al 2005, p. 81).

18. Social iatrogenesis includes side-effects of mass vaccination.

False: (Clinical) iatrogenesis is the state of ill health, adverse effect or complication resulting from medical treatment. The word literally means 'brought forth by a doctor' (*iatros* means physician in Greek). From a sociological point of view there are three types of iatrogenesis: clinical, social and cultural.

Social iatrogenesis results from the medicalization of life. More and more problems are seen as amenable to medical intervention. Normal phenomena such as relationships, sex, pregnancy, menstruation, and especially childbirth are medicalized. Pharmaceutical companies develop expensive treatments for non-diseases. Social problems such as homelessness, child abuse, violence and alcohol intoxication have become redefined as medical areas. Medicalization of such areas is a more effective way of controlling such deviance than legal punishment (Illich 2001).

19. Labelling theory implies the understanding by the labelled individual of the specific behaviour expected to be associated with the particular label.

True: Howard Becker proposed labelling theory to explain the role of society in creating deviance. Many people commit criminal acts but not all are prosecuted. The society picks on those it decides are 'deviant', labels them 'whore', 'thief', 'abuser', 'junkie', etc. and segregates them from the rest of society. This creates 'outsiders' who are outcast from society. They are thus forced to associate with others who have also been cast out. When society treats them as deviants, they respond as such. Thus the deviant reacts to such a response by continuing to engage in the behaviour society now expects from them (Fear 2004, p. 82; Giddens 1997, p. 178).

20. Charismatic leaders have referent power.

True: Charismatic leaders show referent power, i.e. they are liked by others. French & Raven (1960) described referent power (being charismatic and liked by others) as a type of social power. The other four types of power are authority (power derived from role), reward (power comes from ability to reward), coercive (power derived from ability to punish) and expert (power derived from skill) (Puri & Hall 2004, p. 53).

21. Leadership ability depends on task orientation.

True: Leadership ability may depend on task orientation but the nature of the task is also important. Task orientated leaders are better for structured tasks and emotion orientated leaders for unstructured tasks (Munafo 2002, p. 79).

22. Norms is synonymous with values.

False: Every culture has a number of unwritten laws or guidelines that direct conduct in particular situations and tell us what is right to do and what is wrong. They are called norms. Norms are specific guides to action, which define acceptable and appropriate behaviour in particular situations. Norms are enforced by positive and negative sanctions, i.e. rewards and punishments. Some norms vary from person to person, but others are collective within a society or even across cultures. For example, all societies have norms governing dress. A 70-year-old grandmother dressed as a teenager would contravene the norms for her age group.

Unlike norms, which provide specific directives for conduct, values provide more general guidelines. A value is a belief that something is good and desirable. It is an abstract concept. It defines what is ideal, important, worthwhile and worth striving for. Generally, norms reflect values (Giddens 1997, p. 172).

23. Social cohesion promotes racial prejudice.

False: Social cohesion is where the following exist:

- There is a common vision and a sense of belonging for all communities
- The diversity of people's different backgrounds and circumstances are appreciated and positively valued
- Those from different backgrounds have similar life opportunities
- Strong and positive relationships are being developed between people from different backgrounds in the workplace, in schools and within neighbourhoods. Therefore social cohesion protects against racial prejudice (The Home Office).

24. In the UK, the Registrar General determines social class based on occupation.

True: In the UK, the Office of Population Censuses and Surveys has traditionally divided the population into six groups depending on an individual's occupation or the occupation of the head of the household. This was expanded in 2001 to reflect some of the social change which has occurred since the original scale was designed in 1911. There are now eight social classes:

1. higher managerial and professional
2. lower managerial and professional
3. intermediate occupations
4. small employers and own account workers
5. lower supervisory, craft and related
6. semi-routine
7. routine
8. long-term unemployed (Fear 2004, p. 86; Puri & Hall 2004, p. 129).

25. Acute stress causes cutaneous vasodilation.

False: Acute stress reaction or the fight or flight reaction results from increased sympathetic activation. The sympathetic activation increases heart rate, blood pressure, blood sugar level, blood flow in heart muscle, lungs and skeletal muscle, and causes vasoconstriction and decreased blood flow in smooth muscle, skin and the digestive tract. People turn pale as a result of decreased blood flow to the skin (Sadock & Sadock 2005, p. 1729; Wright et al 2005, p. 74).

Psychology – 2

Ben Underwood

	T	F
1. Modern social anthropology is concerned with ontogeny.	☐	☐
2. A person's perceived tallness creates a positive attitude towards them.	☐	☐
3. In Western societies we attribute others' behaviour to the context.	☐	☐
4. Attribution error involves an unstable/stable component.	☐	☐
5. The non-verbal communication gaze theory suggests that long glances occur before the speech ends.	☐	☐
6. The physical attractiveness of the speaker does not affect the reception of the message.	☐	☐
7. Cognitive consistency promotes problem solving.	☐	☐
8. Projective identification is a defence against unconscious anxiety.	☐	☐
9. Aggression is expressed in hierarchies in wild baboons.	☐	☐
10. The alpha male monkey performs ritualistic appeasement before mating.	☐	☐
11. According to Eysenck, extroverts have a more reactive reticular system.	☐	☐
12. Introversion is thought to be associated with autonomic lability.	☐	☐
13. Family size predicts delinquency.	☐	☐
14. Coercive power is rarely used in families.	☐	☐
15. Gestalt determinants of grouping include closure.	☐	☐
16. Open debate promotes group think phenomenon.	☐	☐
17. Decision-making in groups is influenced by majority opinion.	☐	☐
18. Cultural iatrogenesis refers to the side-effects of herbal remedies.	☐	☐
19. In autocratic leadership, productivity increases when the leader is away.	☐	☐
20. Leadership skills are independent of specific situations.	☐	☐
21. The theory of mind refers to the ability to understand the false beliefs of others.	☐	☐
22. Risk-taking behaviour is one of the 'big five' dimensions of personality.	☐	☐
23. Stigma is associated with actual, not perceived, status.	☐	☐
24. Japanese Americans migrating to the USA but maintaining their traditions are at increased risk of cardiovascular disease than those adapting to the local norms.	☐	☐

T F

25. Having an appendicectomy is a significant life event.

☐ ☐

ANSWERS

1. Modern social anthropology is concerned with ontogeny.

False: *Social anthropology* is the study of ethnological, ethnographic, linguistic, social and psychological development of human cultures.

Modern social anthropology is the comparative study of societies, and cultural and social variety. It focuses on small-scale social groups. Data is collected usually through participant observation.

Ontogeny or ontogenesis is the origin and development of an individual organism from embryo to adult.

2. A person's perceived tallness creates a positive attitude towards them.

True: Attitude change may be incentive based or argument based. The status, expertise, personality, attractiveness, enthusiasm, motivation and non-verbal cues of the person presenting the information can modify the effectiveness of argument based persuasion (Fear 2004, p. 32; Munafo 2002, p. 66; Puri & Hall 2004, p. 50).

3. In Western societies we attribute others' behaviour to the context.

False: The fundamental attribution error occurs when we explain the behaviour of others by attributing it to that individual's personal or dispositional factors. When analysing our own behaviour we are more likely to blame behaviour on situational factors. This phenomenon may be more likely to happen in Western societies (Fear 2004, p. 32; Wright et al 2005, p. 80).

4. Attribution error involves an unstable/stable component.

False: The fundamental attribution error occurs when we explain the behaviour of others by attributing it to personal/dispositional rather than situational/environmental factors. This tends to make others' behaviour seem more predictable which in turn enhances our sense of control over the environment. It does not involve a 'stable/unstable' component (Fear 2004, p. 32; Wright et al 2005, p. 80).

5. The non-verbal communication gaze theory suggests that long glances occur before the speech ends.

True: Speakers tend not to look at the person they are talking to unless they are attempting to impose their authority. When they come to the end of what they are saying they glance at the listener to signal that it is the listener's turn to speak. Listeners tend to look at speakers (Hayes 1994, p. 516).

6. The physical attractiveness of the speaker does not affect the reception of the message.

False: Important aspects in communication include the speaker, the listener, the message and the context. Physically attractive speakers are more persuasive communicators. Other features of the speaker that influence communication include ability of the audience to identify with the speaker, credibility, expertise, motivation, non-verbal communication and being an opinion leader (Fear 2004, p. 32; Munafo 2002, p. 66; Puri & Hall 2004, p. 50).

7. Cognitive consistency promotes problem solving.

False: Cognitive dissonance refers to the discomfort caused by inconsistent cognitions, i.e. those which appear to conflict with one another. Cognitive consistency theory suggests that we strive to be consistent in our cognitions, attitudes, beliefs and behaviours in order to minimize this discomfort and that inconsistency or dissonance acts as an irritant or stimulus that motivates us to modify them until they become consistent. Thus, cognitive dissonance may promote problem solving (Atkinson et al 2000, pp. 621, 626; Wright et al 2005, p. 79).

8. Projective identification is a defence against unconscious anxiety.

True: According to Klein, in the first few months of life, the early ego experiences anxiety resulting from a fear of annihilation, which is a manifestation of the death instinct. The early ego deals with the anxiety by using defence mechanisms of splitting, projection, introjection and projective identification. In projective identification the infant in fantasy projects the bad aspects of the self onto the mother in an attempt not only to injure but also to control (Gelder et al 2000, p. 1885; Wright et al 2005, p. 544).

9. Aggression is expressed in hierarchies in wild baboons.

True: Aggression is a spontaneously generated force which helps maintain dominance hierarchies and aids the process of natural selection. Animals that live in groups often develop a social order based on dominance hierarchies. In baboons the dominant male usually achieves his status through victory in several threat displays and aggressive encounters. After this, his status is settled for a while and lower ranking baboons generally step aside for his convenience (Gleitman 1996, p. 302).

10. The alpha male monkey performs ritualistic appeasement before mating.

False: The alpha male chooses whom he mates with and when, and where he sleeps. He eats first. Everyone else steps aside for his convenience. He does not need to appease anyone (Gleitman 1996, p. 302).

11. According to Eysenck, extroverts have a more reactive reticular system.

False: According to Eysenck, introverts have a more reactive reticular system. They attain optimal levels of cortical arousal with low levels of stimulation. Extroverts have a less active reticular system and therefore they have to seek stimuli from outside in order to maintain an optimal level of arousal (Gelder et al 2000, p. 707; Wright et al 2005, p. 75).

12. Introversion is thought to be associated with autonomic lability.

False: According to Eysenck, neuroticism is related to a reactive limbic system and autonomic lability. Introverts have a more reactive reticular activating system (Gelder et al 2000, p. 707).

13. Family size predicts delinquency.

True: In the Cambridge Study, boys having four or more siblings by their 10th birthday had double the risk of being convicted as a juvenile. Large family size predicts self-reported delinquency as well as juvenile and adult convictions (Farrington 1995; Gelder et al 2000, p. 2032).

14. Coercive power is rarely used in families.

False: French & Raven (1960) described five types of power: coercive, reward, legitimate, referent and expert. Coercive power is the power to force someone to do something against his or her will. It involves using threats, punishments and withdrawal of rewards. Parents and governments use coercive power on children and citizens who know no better, in order to maintain peace and order (Munafo 2002, p. 76).

15. Gestalt determinants of grouping include closure.

True: Gestalt determinants of grouping include proximity, similarity, continuity and closure (Fear 2004, p. 8; Wright et al 2005, p. 67).

16. Open debate promotes group think phenomenon.

False: Group think, a term introduced by Irving Janice, refers to the phenomenon in which members of a group are led to suppress their own dissent in the interest of group consensus. Group think is facilitated by pressure on dissenters and self-censorship of dissent. Group think can be prevented by fostering open debate (Wright et al 2005, p. 81).

17. Decision-making in groups is influenced by majority opinion.

True: Even when the opinion of the majority of the group is obviously wrong, group members tend to conform to the majority consensus, especially when the majority of the group is unanimous in their (wrong) opinion. The tendency to agree with others is called conformity (Fear 2004, p. 35; Puri & Tyrer 1998, p. 321; Wright et al 2005, p. 80).

18. Cultural iatrogenesis refers to the side-effects of herbal remedies.

False: Illich considers cultural iatrogenesis to be the worst form of iatrogenesis. Jones (1994) described it as 'the destruction of traditional ways of dealing with and making sense of death, pain and sickness and their replacement by a sanitized technological medical intervention against which individuals and society are unable to fight back' (Fear 2004, p. 90; Illich 2001).

19. In autocratic leadership, productivity increases when the leader is away.

False: Lewin, in 1939, studied the effects of leadership styles adopted by their teacher on three groups of boys making models:

- Democratic: the boys got on well, were productive and worked alone
- Autocratic: the boys were aggressive and stopped working when the leader left, but were productive
- Laissez-faire: the boys were aggressive and did little work under any circumstances (Munafo 2002, p. 76).

20. Leadership skills are independent of specific situations.

False: Lewin described three leadership styles – autocratic (best in urgent situations), democratic (best overall unless highly original product required) and laissez-faire (best for creative, person orientated tasks). Thus, the qualities demanded of a leader depend on the situation (Puri & Hall 2004, p. 53; Puri & Tyrer 1998, p. 321).

21. The theory of mind refers to the ability to understand the false beliefs of others.

True: Theory of mind refers to the ability to know that self and others have mental states, and that these mental states may influence the way we think, feel and behave. Theory of mind typically develops between ages 3 and 4 years. Most children pass first order theory of mind tasks by age 4 years.

In the Sally–Anne test, a child watches two puppets, Sally and Anne. Sally puts a marble in a basket and goes out. While Sally is out, Anne moves the marble from the basket to a box and leaves the room. The child is asked where Sally will look for the marble when she re-enters the room. Most normal 3-year-olds fail the task, and say the box, as they know the marble is in the box. Most normal 4-year-olds will pass the task, saying Sally will act on her false belief and look in the basket. They can be said to have a first order 'theory of mind' – knowing how a person's beliefs will make them act. Most normal children pass a second order theory of mind task (about what Mary thinks John thinks) at age 5–7 years. Most autistic children fail the Sally–Anne test; however, it is important to check that their mental age is at least 4 years. Those who lack theory of mind are unable to infer thoughts and motivations of others and therefore fail to predict others' behaviour and adjust their own actions. This results in a lack of reciprocity in communication and social contact (Gelder et al 2000, p. 1726; Rutter & Taylor 2002, p. 647).

22. Risk-taking behaviour is one of the 'big five' dimensions of personality.

False: Goldberg and McCrae's 'big five' personality dimensions include openness to experience, conscientiousness, extroversion, agreeableness and neuroticism. This gives the acronym OCEAN. They are stable, heritable, adaptive and universal dimensions. The outcome of therapy is better when the patient is aware of their position on these dimensions (Fear 2004, p. 17; Johnstone et al 2004, p. 112; Wright et al 2005, p. 76).

23. Stigma is associated with actual, not perceived, status.

False: Stigma is a label applied to individuals that implies association with undesirable characteristics and avoidance of that individual by others. It is therefore closely linked with how an individual is perceived rather than their actual status (Gelder et al 2000, p. 5; Johnstone et al 2004, p. 123).

24. Japanese Americans migrating to the USA but maintaining their traditions are at increased risk of cardiovascular disease than those adapting to the local norms.

False: The inverse is true (Egusa et al 2002).

25. Having an appendicectomy is a significant life event.

True: Holmes & Rahe's (1967) Social Readjustment Rating Scale rates personal injury or illness at number 6, between death of a close family member and marriage.

Psychometry – 1

Deborah McCartney

	T	F
1. Adaptive Behaviour Scales are used to assess people with learning disabilities.	☐	☐
2. The Beck Depression Inventory was designed to be administered by a trained psychologist.	☐	☐
3. The BPRS is used to screen for psychiatric disorders in the general population.	☐	☐
4. The Clifton Assessment Procedures for the Elderly (CAPE) can identify intellectual deterioration.	☐	☐
5. In a selective attention task the target stimulus is presented amongst a series of random stimuli on a computer screen.	☐	☐
6. The GHQ is used to rule out physical health problems.	☐	☐
7. Goldstein's Object Sorting Test distinguishes between depression and depressive pseudodementia.	☐	☐
8. The Hawthorne effect includes a visual percept.	☐	☐
9. The Hayling Sentence Completion test assesses dorsolateral prefrontal cortical function.	☐	☐
10. Standardized intelligence tests can be modified to suit the individual.	☐	☐
11. The Manchester scale is a self-rated questionnaire.	☐	☐
12. MMPI is used to assess new antidepressants.	☐	☐
13. The Mill Hill Vocabulary Scale (MHVS) can identify intellectual deterioration.	☐	☐
14. 'Pathways to Independence' is used to assess people with mental handicap.	☐	☐
15. Formal psychological testing is essential for the assessment of premorbid personality.	☐	☐
16. The proverb interpretation test distinguishes between dementia and depressive pseudodementia.	☐	☐
17. In subcortical dementia, recall is more disturbed than recognition.	☐	☐
18. The Rey-Osterrieth test is used to assess personality.	☐	☐
19. Spearman's work on intelligence used factor analysis.	☐	☐
20. Reasoning is a component of intelligence as defined by Sternberg.	☐	☐

T   F

21. Patients with Parkinson's disease perform poorly on set-shifting tasks. ☐ ☐

22. The Stroop test is used to assess selective attention. ☐ ☐

23. The Trail Making Test is a test for memory. ☐ ☐

24. In WAIS, digit span is relatively preserved in old age as compared to vocabulary. ☐ ☐

25. The Wisconsin Card Sorting Test is sensitive to frontal damage. ☐ ☐

ANSWERS

1. Adaptive Behaviour Scales are used to assess people with learning disabilities.

True: The Vineland Adaptive Behaviour Scales and the Adaptive Behaviour Scales of the American Association for Mental Retardation are standardized instruments used to evaluate daily living, socialization and motor skills in people with learning disabilities (Gelder et al 2000, p. 1936; Lezak 1995, p. 587).

2. The Beck Depression Inventory was designed to be administered by a trained psychologist.

True: The Beck Depression Inventory was designed to be administered by a trained psychologist who read each statement in the inventory and asked the respondent to select the statement that best fits. In practice, it is usually completed by the patient as a self-report measure.

3. The BPRS is used to screen for psychiatric disorders in the general population.

False: The Brief Psychiatric Rating Scale is used for assessing severity and changes in severity of symptoms in severe mental illness. It is not a screening instrument (Gelder et al 2006, p. 66).

4. The Clifton Assessment Procedures for the Elderly (CAPE) can identify intellectual deterioration.

True: The CAPE was devised as a brief measure of psychological functioning including the level of disability and the need for care in psychogeriatric patients. CAPE has two scales, the cognitive scale with 12 questions on information/orientation and the behaviour rating scale with four subscales. It was designed to be used by nurses. It has been validated against outcome in day hospital and day centre care. It helps distinguish between organic and non-organic conditions in the elderly (Butler & Pitt 1998, p. 10; Lishman 1997, p. 125).

5. In a selective attention task the target stimulus is presented amongst a series of random stimuli on a computer screen.

False: In a selective attention task the target appears on the screen *along with* randomly distributed non-target stimuli.

In a continuous performance test of sustained attention, *a series of* stimuli appear one after another with occasional target stimuli and many distractors preceding and following it (Fear 2004, p. 12; Halligan et al 2003, p. 83).

6. The GHQ is used to rule out physical health problems.

False: The General Health Questionnaire (GHQ) is a self-rated questionnaire for identifying psychiatric 'caseness' in community, general medical and primary care settings. The GHQ was originally designed to assess the psychiatric distress associated with general medical illness. It is not used to rule out physical health problems (Gelder et al 2006, p. 66; Wright et al 2005, p. 127).

7. Goldstein's Object Sorting Test distinguishes between depression and depressive pseudodementia.

False: Goldstein's Object Sorting Test was designed to assess abstract thinking and categorization. It explores the ability to abstract common properties of objects and to shift from one frame of reference to another. These executive functions are particularly vulnerable to frontal lobe lesions. Goldstein's Object Sorting Test would not distinguish between depression and pseudodementia (Lishman 1997, p. 120).

8. The Hawthorne effect includes a visual percept.

False: The 'Hawthorne effect' is a non-specific effect caused by a subject's awareness that they are participating in research. The term originates from the Hawthorne plant in Chicago where in a study the mere presence of observers affected in the way in which the subjects behaved. It does not necessarily include a visual percept (Lawrie et al 2000, p. 254).

9. The Hayling Sentence Completion test assesses dorsolateral prefrontal cortical function.

True: The Hayling Sentence Completion test is designed to assess executive functions such as response initiation and response inhibition. The subject is given 30 sentences from which the last word is omitted. In part 1, the initiation condition, they complete the sentences with a word that makes sense. In part 2, the inhibition condition, they have to supply a word that makes no sense in the context of the sentence, e.g. 'Banana is a yellow *delusion.*' Scoring is based on response latencies and error scores (Halligan et al 2003, p. 315).

10. Standardized intelligence tests can be modified to suit the individual.

False: Standardized intelligence tests cannot be modified, because they are objective, structured, standardized measures. They must be administered in a prescribed manner as laid down in the manuals. They have a normal distribution of scores. They are not culture free, however, and the scores will vary from the expected norms depending on whether the test is standardized and used in the subject's first language, and the language abilities and educational background of the subject.

11. The Manchester scale is a self-rated questionnaire.

False: The Manchester scale or Krawiecka-Manchester scale (K-MS) is a standardized scale for rating positive and negative symptoms in chronic psychosis. It rates four symptoms and four signs on a scale of 0–4. There is no interview schedule. The rating is completed by the clinician.

There are many different Manchester scales including those to assess GP trainees; a self-rated questionnaire assessing quality of clinical supervision; and a scale for grading of hallux valgus (Johnstone et al 2004, p. 182).

12. MMPI is used to assess new antidepressants.

False: The Minnesota Multiphasic Personality Inventory is an objective measure of personality. It was developed as a pencil and paper version of a psychiatric interview. It has 10 clinical scales and 4 correction scales including a lie scale. The original 1943 version has 550 statements concerning attitudes, emotional reactions, physical and psychological symptoms and experiences. The subject has to answer 'true', 'false' or 'cannot say' to each statement. The 1980 revised version, MMPI-2, has 567 questions. There is also an adolescent version, the MMPI-A (Aiken 2000, p. 314; Fear 2004, p. 18; Wright et al 2005, p. 183).

13. The Mill Hill Vocabulary Scale (MHVS) can identify intellectual deterioration.

True: The MHVS is an 80-word multiple-choice vocabulary test. The raw scores are converted to percentiles. It is standardized for ages 20 to 65 years. Vocabulary level is an excellent guide to intellectual performance. MHVS is sensitive to verbal intellectual decline, particularly where there is a lesion in the dominant hemisphere (Lezak 1995, p. 306).

14. 'Pathways to Independence' is used to assess people with mental handicap.

True: These are checklists of daily living skills completed by the rater to assess basic independence skills, strengths and weaknesses, and to highlight areas where training or support may be required.

15. Formal psychological testing is essential for the assessment of premorbid personality.

False: Aspects of personality can be assessed from a patient's and collateral descriptions of their history, relationships, leisure, predominant mood and emotions, attitudes, standards and other character traits, e.g. perfectionist, impulsive, sensitive, controlling, etc. It is important to ask others who know the individual well and to observe the individual's manner and behaviour at the interview (Gelder et al 2006, p. 42).

16. The proverb interpretation test distinguishes between dementia and depressive pseudodementia.

False: Some degree of abstract thinking is necessary to interpret proverbs. For example, 'too many cooks spoil the broth' is not literally a piece of advice for running a kitchen with specific regard to soup preparation but might be taken to be so by patients with concrete thinking. Frontal lobe damage, low educational background and schizophrenia are all potential causes. The proverb interpretation test would not differentiate dementia and depressive pseudodementia (Hodges 1994, p. 119).

17. In subcortical dementia, recall is more disturbed than recognition.

True: Patients with subcortical dementia have difficulty with free recall of information from memory. However, if given cues, as in a recognition test, they perform better. This suggests that the retrieval rather than the encoding process may be impaired in subcortical dementia. Recall and recognition are both severely affected in Alzheimer's disease (Hodges 1994, p. 36).

18. The Rey-Osterrieth test is used to assess personality.

False: The Rey-Osterrieth Complex Figure test requires the subject to copy a complex two-dimensional drawing and then reproduce it later without being warned that they will be asked to do so. It is used to evaluate constructional ability and visual memory, not personality (Hodges 1994, p. 211).

19. Spearman's work on intelligence used factor analysis.

True: Charles Spearman was the originator of factor analysis. He proposed a 2-factor theory of intelligence, i.e. a general factor (g) and a group of specific (s) factors. He believed that 'g' played a part in all intellectual activities, but any given activity was also affected by one of the 's' factors specific to particular abilities. According to him, 'g' factor is the major determinant of performance on intelligence tests.

20. Reasoning is a component of intelligence as defined by Sternberg.

False: Sternberg's Triarchic theory of intelligence has three subtheories:
1. Componential (analytical)
2. Experiential (creative) and
3. Contextual (practical).

Within componential intelligence, there are:

• A1: meta-components that control, monitor and evaluate cognitive processing
• A2: performance components that execute strategies and carry out actions and
• A3: knowledge acquisition components that gain and store new knowledge.

Inductive reasoning, i.e. the ability to generate a rule or relationship that describes a set of observations is one of the primary mental abilities identified by Thurstone.

21. Patients with Parkinson's disease perform poorly on set-shifting tasks.

True: Executive function difficulties in Parkinson's disease include impaired sequencing of voluntary motor activities, difficulty maintaining and switching set, and abnormalities in selective attention (Mitchell 2004, p. 153; Yudofsky & Hales 2002, p. 933).

22. The Stroop test is used to assess selective attention.

True: The Stroop Colour Word Tests are a group of tests based on Stroop's (1935) observation that it takes longer to read printed colour names when they are printed in coloured ink different from the name of the colour word. They are used to assess selective attention maintained in the face of interference. In the Stroop tests, the same task is presented twice, first without and then with distraction or interference by irrelevant stimuli. The subject is asked to read words presented in different colours. In the first presentation, the words are printed in the colour they describe, e.g. the word 'red' is printed in red colour. In the second presentation, the word 'red' is printed in green colour. The subject is asked to read the words as quickly as possible. In the second presentation, the colour of the written word acts as a distracter or interference. This leads to slowing down of performance and mistakes. Thus, it is a test of attention maintained in the face of interference. It detects prefrontal lobe dysfunctions such as response conflict, impaired selective attention and impaired response inhibition (Halligan et al 2003, p. 74; Lishman 1997, p. 118).

23. The Trail Making Test is a test for memory.

False: The Trail Making Test is a quick and simple test of visuomotor skill, tracking, conceptualization, set-shifting and response inhibition. Motor slowing, incoordination, visual scanning difficulties, poor motivation and frontal executive problems result in impaired performance. The Trail Making Test has two parts, A and B. Patients with frontal lobe dysfunction perform disproportionately poorly on part B. It is not a memory test (Hodges 1994, p. 219; Lishman 1997, p. 120).

24. In WAIS, digit span is relatively preserved in old age as compared to vocabulary.

False: 'Hold' tests, e.g. vocabulary, information, object assembly and picture completion are thought to reflect the use of old knowledge and are relatively resistant to the effects of brain damage.

'Don't hold' tests, e.g. digit symbol, digit span, similarities and block design which require speed of response, working memory or the creation of new relations between unrelated items are more likely to show early decline (Lishman 1997, p. 111).

25. The Wisconsin Card Sorting Test is sensitive to frontal damage.

True: It is particularly sensitive to frontal lobe damage, especially lesions of the dorso-lateral convexities of the frontal lobe, and particularly of the left side, rather than inferior and orbital lesions. However, performance can be impaired in subjects with lesions elsewhere (Fear 2004, p. 69; Hodges 1994, p. 226; Lishman 1997, p. 118).

Psychometry – 2

Salbu Krishnan and Deborah McCartney

48

T F

1. The Bannister-Fransella Grid is a personality test.

2. The Beck Depression Inventory (BDI) and the Hamilton Rating Scale for Depression (Ham-D) are used differently.

3. The Camberwell Assessment of Need (CAN) is used in the general population.

4. The likelihood of Alzheimer's disease over vascular dementia can be confirmed by a defective clock face drawing.

5. The 'draw a person' test is used to distinguish between dementia and depressive pseudodementia.

6. The GHQ is frequently used for psychiatric diagnosis.

7. Hare's Psychopathy Checklist is validated for use in the general population.

8. The Halstead–Reitan Battery is used for bedside cognitive function assessment.

9. The Ham-D has more cognitive items than the MADRS.

10. Hayling's test assesses spatial accommodation.

11. Kendrick Assessment Scales help to distinguish between dementia and depressive pseudodementia.

12. The McCollough effect always includes a visual percept.

13. A Mini Mental State Examination (MMSE) score of below 24 is 60% specific for dementia in the over-65 age group.

14. The reverse calendar test is a semi-quantitative test of cognitive function.

15. Compared to patients with dementia, patients with depressive pseudodementia do less well on the Paired Associated Learning Test.

16. The General Health Questionnaire (GHQ) is used to assess premorbid personality.

17. The Raven's Progressive Matrices test gives a percentile score.

18. In assessment of cognitive function, registration is tested by asking the patient to give their telephone number.

19. The Rorschach test is used to measure attitudes.

20. The Stanford–Binet scale is used to assess people with learning disabilities.

T   F

21. Sternberg defined the meta-components of intelligence. ☐ ☐

22. The Thematic Apperception Test is used to assess personality. ☐ ☐

23. The Wechsler Adult Intelligence Scale (WAIS-III) has five verbal and six performance components. ☐ ☐

24. In dementia there is a differential drop in verbal and performance IQ. ☐ ☐

25. The Wisconsin Card Sorting Test (WCST) is a test for planning. ☐ ☐

ANSWERS

1. The Bannister-Fransella Grid is a personality test.

False: The Bannister-Fransella Grid is a test of schizophrenic thought disorder, not personality.

2. The Beck Depression Inventory (BDI) and the Hamilton Rating Scale for Depression (Ham-D) are used differently.

True: The interviewer completes the Ham-D based on an unstructured interview, using his own observations and information from the patient. It measures the severity of the depressive syndrome. The BDI has 21 items, with 4 statements each. The patients complete them themselves by choosing the statements that best apply to their feelings in the previous week (Gelder et al 2006, p. 66).

3. The Camberwell Assessment of Need (CAN) is used in the general population.

False: CAN is used to assess the health and social needs of people with severe mental health problems. It is not for use in the general population. CANE is the version for the elderly mentally ill (Gelder et al 2006, p. 625).

4. The likelihood of Alzheimer's disease over vascular dementia can be confirmed by a defective clock face drawing.

False: In the clock drawing test the patient is asked to draw a clock face, marking the hours, and then to draw the hands to indicate a particular time, e.g. 10 minutes past 11. It tests comprehension, motor function, visuospatial integrity, numerical knowledge and executive function. It is simple to administer, requires no special equipment, is non-threatening and takes only 2 minutes to administer. Common errors in Alzheimer's disease include perseveration, counter-clockwise numbering, absence of numbers and irrelevant spatial arrangement. Errors in vascular dementia may reflect spatial neglect, hemianopsia, sensory loss and cognitive dysfunction. Patients with Alzheimer's disease may do better on copying compared to those with vascular dementia. As a screening test for dementia, it has a sensitivity and specificity of 85%. It cannot differentiate between dementias, and it may be affected by delirium, dysphasia and neglect (Mitchell 2004, p. 86; Sadock & Sadock 2005, p. 872).

5. The 'draw a person' test is used to distinguish between dementia and depressive pseudodementia.

False: The 'draw a person' test is a projective personality measure. Normative data for ages 4–89 years is available. The subject is asked to draw people of both genders. The picture is then analysed to gain insight into the subject's personality and emotional state. Egodystonic unacceptable impulses are often drawn in association with the opposite sex figure whilst the converse is true of acceptable impulses. Some features are held to be more specific, e.g. large eyelashes may be a feature of hysteria. Some features have been correlated with non-verbal intelligence and visuomotor and cognitive functions. Some clinicians use the drawings primarily as a screening technique, particularly to detect brain damage. It is not used to distinguish dementia from depressive pseudodementia (Aiken 2000, p. 334; Sadock & Sadock 2002, p. 185; Sadock & Sadock 2005, p. 3068).

6. The GHQ is frequently used for psychiatric diagnosis.

False: The General Health Questionnaire is a non-specific screening tool for identifying 'caseness' in the community, general medical and primary care settings. It is a screening instrument and not a diagnostic instrument. It is a self-rated questionnaire. The original version has 60 items that can be completed in 10 minutes. Shorter versions with 30, 28 and 20 items are available (Gelder et al 2000, p. 1527; Wright et al 2005, p. 127).

7. Hare's Psychopathy Checklist is validated for use in the general population.

False: The 22-item Hare's Psychopathy Check List (PCL) and its 20-item revised version (PCL-R) are used to measure traits of psychopathic personality disorder in forensic populations. It has not been validated for use in the general population. It is completed based on a semi-structured interview lasting 90–120 minutes. The items are rated on a 3-point scale: 1= item does not apply, 2 = item applies somewhat, 3 = item definitely applies (Wright et al 2005, p. 476).

8. The Halstead–Reitan Battery is used for bedside cognitive function assessment.

False: The Halstead–Reitan Neuropsychological Test Battery is an extensive battery of tests designed for a comprehensive assessment of brain damage, i.e. to detect brain damage, to indicate whether it is focal, diffuse or lateralized, and whether it is acute and progressive or relatively static. Some of the principal tests are Trail making test, Halstead's category test, Critical flicker frequency test, Tactual performance test, Rhythm test, Speech sounds perception test, Finger trapping test, Time sense test and H-A aphasia screening test (Hodges 1994, p. 217; Lishman 1997, p. 121).

9. The Ham-D has more cognitive items than the MADRS.

False: The Montgomery-Åsberg Depression Rating Scale (MADRS) has 10 items concerned with psychological aspects of depression. The Ham-D is concerned with somatic and behavioural features, rather than cognitive features, of depression.

10. Hayling's test assesses spatial accommodation.

False: Hayling's sentence completion test is designed to assess executive functions such as response initiation and response inhibition (Halligan et al 2003, p. 315).

11. Kendrick Assessment Scales help to distinguish between dementia and depressive pseudodementia.

False: Kendrick Assessment Scales of Cognitive Ageing are intended to test cognitive abilities in people without known neuropsychiatric disturbance. They can act as an early warning signal of dementia, indicating a possible need for further assessment or treatment and to provide a baseline for further assessments. They measure the four areas of cognitive function affected in normal ageing, i.e. short-term memory, speed of information processing, reasoning and visuospatial ability. They take about 15 minutes to complete. They do not help distinguish between dementia and depressive pseudodementia.

12. The McCollough effect always includes a visual percept.

True: The McCollough effect occurs when, following exposure to a grid of lines of different colours, a grid of black lines may subsequently be seen as edged with the previously seen colours. It is a contingent after-effect visual adaptation being created by a combination of colour and orientation.

13. A Mini Mental State Examination (MMSE) score of below 24 is 60% specific for dementia in the over-65 age group.

False: Using a cut-off score of 24 the MMSE has a specificity of greater than 60%. Initial values quoted were a specificity of 82% and a sensitivity of 87%. These figures have been questioned as they were obtained in a group of hospitalized and possibly delirious elderly. Despite this, subsequent series have still shown specificity of better than 60% (Hodges 1994, p. 184; Jacoby & Oppenheimer 2002, p. 621; Lishman 1997, p. 123).

14. The reverse calendar test is a semi-quantitative test of cognitive function.

True: The ability to recite familiar sequences backwards is a test of concentration. This is often disrupted in delirium. If the patient is unable to manage months of the year, days of the week may be attempted. It is in a sense semi-quantitative because the number of errors can be counted (Hodges 1994, p. 111).

15. Compared to patients with dementia, patients with depressive pseudodementia do less well on the Paired Associated Learning Test.

False: The Paired Associated Learning Test is a new word learning task. It gives a quantitative estimate of memory impairment. It is not used to differentiate between dementia and pseudodementia (Lishman 1997, p. 114).

16. The General Health Questionnaire (GHQ) is used to assess premorbid personality.

False: The GHQ is a self-rated questionnaire used to screen for potential psychiatric cases. It gives a measure of current psychiatric health. It does not provide information about premorbid personality (Gelder et al 2006, p. 66).

17. The Raven's Progressive Matrices test gives a percentile score.

True: The Raven's Progressive Matrices test was developed as a test of Spearman's general intelligence factor. It is considered as a 'culture fair' test of general intellectual ability. It consists of 60 visually based problem-solving tests arranged in 5 sets of 12 problems of increasing complexity. Each test is a pattern set with a missing piece that the subject must choose from a multiple choice. It initially tests simple pattern matching and moves on to more abstract, complex visuospatial reasoning. The test is simple to administer and takes 20–45 minutes to complete. The raw scores are converted to a percentile. Normative data with percentile scores are available for ages 8 to 65 (Aiken 2000, p. 156; Hodges 1994, p. 207).

18. In assessment of cognitive function, registration is tested by asking the patient to give their telephone number.

False: Registration, used in the context of whether facts are being encoded for recall, is usually assessed as part of the MMSE. The examiner names three objects. The patient is asked to repeat the three words. One point is given for each correct answer.

If a patient can recall an already known telephone number, this would suggest that long-term memory may be unaffected, but this does not tell us whether the patient can register new information.

19. The Rorschach test is used to measure attitudes.

True: The Rorschach Ink Blot test is a projective personality test. The subject is shown a series of 10 standard inkblots, one at a time, and asked to describe what they can see. Initially free association is used. Then the clinician may ask questions. Responses are analysed according to the part of the blot talked about, elements of the blots discussed (colour, shape, etc.) and what the blot is held to represent. Though attempts have been made at standardizing interpretations, the validity of these is questionable.

Attitudes are likes and dislikes, i.e. favourable and unfavourable evaluations of and reactions to objects, people, situations or other aspects of the world.

Even though questionnaires are most commonly used to measure attitudes, personality tests such as the Rorschach test, Thematic Apperception Test and Kelly's Repertory Grid can be used to measure attitudes (Atkinson et al 2000, pp. 466, 658; Fear 2004, p. 18; Wright et al 2005, p. 78).

20. The Stanford–Binet scale is used to assess people with learning disabilities.

True: The Stanford–Binet Intelligence scale consists of pictures, drawings and objects. It gives a mental age score. It provides useful information about people functioning below the standard cut-off score on the Wechsler Intelligence Scales (Gelder et al 2006, p. 659).

21. Sternberg defined the meta-components of intelligence.

True: Sternberg's Triarchic theory of intelligence has three subtheories:

1. Componential (analytical)
2. Experiential (creative)
3. Contextual (practical).

Within componential intelligence, there are

- A1: Meta-components that control, monitor and evaluate cognitive processing
- A2: Performance components that execute the strategies and carry out the action and
- A3: Knowledge acquisition components that gain and store new knowledge.

22. The Thematic Apperception Test is used to assess personality.

True: The Thematic Apperception Test is a widely used projective test of personality for adults. The subject is shown up to 20 ambiguous pictures of persons and themes and asked to make up a story about what is going on in each picture. The stories are analysed for recurrent themes that may reveal the subject's ideas, attitudes, needs, motives and characteristic ways of handling interpersonal relationships (Aiken 2000, p. 337; Fear 2004, p. 18).

23. The Wechsler Adult Intelligence Scale (WAIS-III) has five verbal and six performance components.

False: The Wechsler Adult Intelligence Scale (WAIS-III) has a verbal scale with six compulsory and one optional subtests and a performance scale with five compulsory and two optional subtests. Note that this is different from the older WAIS-R.

The six compulsory subtests of the verbal scale include Arithmetic, Comprehension, Digit span, Information, Similarities and Vocabulary. Letter–number sequencing is optional.

The performance scale includes Block design, Digit symbol-coding, Matrix reasoning, Picture arrangement and Picture completion. Symbol search and Object assembly are optional.

By summating the subset scores and adjusting for age, Verbal, Performance and full IQ, scores can be derived. An average person should score 100 with a standard deviation of 15.

It is a quantitative test battery, with careful timing on some subtests. It is designed to measure intelligence. If repeated after a delay of some months or years, it can identify intellectual deterioration.

There is a deterioration index (DI) to compare scores on the WAIS that tend to be preserved in old age (those that 'hold') compared to those that are likely to decrease (don't hold) in the normal population.

A discrepancy of at least 15 IQ points between the Verbal score and the Performance score is considered significant (Hodges 1994, p. 222; Johnstone et al 2004, p. 142; Lishman 1997, p. 110).

24. In dementia there is a differential drop in verbal and performance IQ.

True: Diffuse brain damage tends to disproportionately lower performance IQ.

However, the opposite might occur in 5% of cases. The performance scale is more sensitive to normal ageing than the verbal scale and the verbal scale is more sensitive to education (Lishman 1997, p. 111; Mitchell 2004, p. 58; Sadock & Sadock 2002, p. 180).

25. The Wisconsin Card Sorting Test (WCST) is a test for planning.

False: The WCST was designed to study abstract thinking and set-shifting ability. It may also test non-verbal reasoning. It is not a test of planning.

The test involves cards with different symbols, e.g. stars, circles or triangles. The number of symbols on each card and their colours vary. The first card is placed down and the examiner creates a rule for which further cards should be matched, e.g. shape, number or colour. When the subject puts a subsequent card down the examiner simply says 'yes' or 'no' until the subject has calculated the rule for matching. Then, the examiner changes the rule. Deficits in motivation, abstract thinking and the verbal regulation of behaviour may contribute to poor performance on WCST (Hodges 1994, p. 226; Lishman 1997, p. 118; Mitchell 2004, p. 78).

49 Psychometry – 3

Ben Underwood and Deborah McCartney

	T	F

1. The Beck Depression Inventory (BDI) cannot be used to measure depression in schizophrenia. ☐ ☐

2. The difference in scores between the Hamilton Rating Scale for Depression (Ham-D) and the Beck Depression Inventory (BDI) relates to the method of administration. ☐ ☐

3. Cattell's 16-personality factor questionnaire includes a factor for intelligence. ☐ ☐

4. In the continuous performance test the target stimulus is presented amongst a series of random stimuli on a computer screen. ☐ ☐

5. Eysenck Personality Questionnaire (EPQ) is an ideographic test. ☐ ☐

6. GHQ is commonly used in defining caseness. ☐ ☐

7. Hachinski Ischaemia Score differentiates between Alzheimer's disease with cerebrovascular disease and vascular dementia. ☐ ☐

8. The Hamilton Depression Rating Scale (Ham-D) is more sensitive to change than the Montgomery and Asberg Depression Rating Scale (MADRS). ☐ ☐

9. The Hospital Anxiety and Depression Scale focuses more on the somatic symptoms of depression than the Ham-D. ☐ ☐

10. Intelligence shows regression towards the mean in generations. ☐ ☐

11. The Flynn effect refers to an increase in IQ test scores. ☐ ☐

12. Likert scales allow for a 5-point response. ☐ ☐

13. MAKATON is used to assess people with learning disabilities. ☐ ☐

14. The Mini Mental State Examination (MMSE) is highly sensitive in detecting delirium and dementia. ☐ ☐

15. Correct awareness of passage of time is a good test of orientation. ☐ ☐

16. Premorbid IQ can be estimated from the WAIS. ☐ ☐

17. Concrete thinking is tested by interpretation of proverbs. ☐ ☐

18. Reasoning is one of the primary mental abilities identified by Thurstone. ☐ ☐

19. Kelly's Repertory Grid (KRG) is usually used to measure attitudes. ☐ ☐

20. Semantic-differential is used to measure attitudes. ☐ ☐

21. The Stanford–Binet Intelligence Scale measures verbal reasoning. ☐ ☐

	T	F

22. Acquisition components of intelligence were defined by Sternberg.

23. Block design is more stable than vocabulary subtest in organic lesions.

24. In selective dominant hemisphere damage the performance scale on the WAIS is more impaired than the verbal scale.

25. The Yale–Brown Obsessive Compulsive Scale (YBOCS) rates obsessive personality traits as well as obsessive compulsive symptoms.

ANSWERS

1. The Beck Depression Inventory (BDI) cannot be used to measure depression in schizophrenia.

False: The BDI is a 21-item inventory. It is usually completed by the patient. Each item has 4–6 statements, one of which is chosen as best describing the current symptoms. BDI can be used to measure the severity of depression in schizophrenia. However, in some patients with schizophrenia, the negative symptoms and cognitive deficits may reduce its reliability. Moreover, in certain neuropsychiatric disorders, the patient may be unaware not only of their physical problems, but also of their cognitive or emotional difficulties. Consequently, assessments based on self-report scales may be less reliable (Gelder et al 2006, p. 66; Halligan et al 2003, p. 382).

2. The difference in scores between the Hamilton Rating Scale for Depression (Ham-D) and the Beck Depression Inventory (BDI) relates to the method of administration.

False: Ham-D and BDI differ in terms of the content, form of administration and scoring. Ham-D is a clinician-administered depression rating scale while BDI is a self-report inventory. Ham-D focuses on somatic and behavioural symptoms of depression while BDI rates the subjective symptoms experienced by the patient. The highest score possible with Ham-D is 52 and with BDI is 60 (Gelder et al 2006, p. 66).

3. Cattell's 16-personality factor questionnaire includes a factor for intelligence.

False: Cattell factor analysed 18 000 adjectives used to describe personality and derived 16 factors. They are reserved vs. warm, concrete vs. abstract, reactive vs. stable, deferential vs. dominant, serious vs. lively, expedient vs. rule-conscious, shy vs. bold, utilitarian vs. sensitive, trusting vs. vigilant, grounded vs. abstract, forthright vs. private, self-assured vs. apprehensive, traditional vs. open to change, group-orientated vs. self-reliant, tolerates disorder vs. perfectionist and relaxed vs. tense. They are further grouped into global factors: self-control, anxiety, extroversion, independence, and tough-mindedness. Even though some of these may indirectly measure some aspects of intelligence (e.g. concrete vs.

abstract), there is no specific factor for intelligence (Aiken 2000, p. 311; Wright et al 2005, p. 76).

4. In the continuous performance test the target stimulus is presented amongst a series of random stimuli on a computer screen.

True: The classical test of sustained attention is the continuous performance test devised by Rosvold in 1956. In the continuous performance test, the subject has to react only to the target stimulus, e.g. letter 'A', which appears occasionally in a long series of letters which are non-target stimuli or distractors (Halligan et al 2003, p. 83).

5. Eysenck Personality Questionnaire (EPQ) is an ideographic test.

False: Personality theories are of two types: *nomothetic* and *ideographic*.

Ideographic approaches consider each individual as unique. EPQ is based on the nomothetic or named category approach, implying that different people have broad personality traits/types/dimensions in common with each other. It scores individuals on neuroticism, extroversion and psychoticism. There is also a lie scale. Normative data exist for children as young as 7 years. EPQ is relatively quick to complete (Aiken 2000, p. 312; Johnstone et al 2004, p. 111; Wright et al 2005, p. 75).

6. GHQ is commonly used in defining caseness.

True: The General Health Questionnaire is a screening tool originally developed for use in primary care. 'Caseness' is a term used in epidemiology to distinguish cases from non-cases. A score on GHQ above a certain level suggests the presence of a 'case', which would require further investigation before a diagnosis could be made (Gelder et al 2000, p. 1527).

7. Hachinski Ischaemia Score differentiates between Alzheimer's disease with cerebrovascular disease and vascular dementia.

False: Hachinski Ischaemia Score differentiates patients with definite Alzheimer's disease from those with definite vascular dementia.

However, it does not differentiate between Alzheimer's disease with cerebrovascular disease and vascular dementia (Gelder et al 2000, p. 432).

8. The Hamilton Depression Rating Scale (Ham-D) is more sensitive to change than the Montgomery and Asberg Depression Rating Scale (MADRS).

False: MADRS was designed to measure treatment-sensitive changes in the severity of depression. MADRS has a higher correlation (0.70) to changes in global ratings than Ham-D (0.59). Hence, MADRS is considered to be more sensitive to change.

9. The Hospital Anxiety and Depression Scale focuses more on the somatic symptoms of depression than the Ham-D.

False: The Ham-D focuses on the somatic and behavioural features of depression. Hence, it tends to overrate depression in the elderly and the medically ill. The Hospital Anxiety and Depression Scale was designed to screen for anxiety and depression in medically ill patients. In order to distinguish between the physical and the psychiatric symptoms, it focuses on the psychological and subjective features of anxiety and depression rather than on the physical signs.

10. Intelligence shows regression towards the mean in generations.

True: Galton investigated geniuses in various fields and their children. He found that their children, though typically gifted, were almost invariably closer to the average than their exceptional parents. He later described the same effect more numerically by comparing fathers' heights to their sons' heights. Galton termed this phenomenon 'regression towards mediocrity' and it is now called 'regression towards the mean'. For example, if a couple's IQ scores are 145 and 150, both higher than 99% of the population, it is likely that the IQ of their children would be closer to the mean IQ of the population, i.e. 100, and less than that of the parents. Similarly, if the parents' IQs were 70 and 80, the children's IQs are likely to be higher than those of the parents and closer to 100.

11. The Flynn effect refers to an increase in IQ test scores.

False: The Flynn effect refers to the large documented worldwide increases in IQ test scores. Suggested explanations include improved nutrition, a trend towards smaller families, better education and greater environmental complexity.

12. Likert scales allow for a 5-point response.

True: Likert scales present a statement and five alternative expressions of level of agreement with that statement, e.g. strongly agree, agree, neither agree nor disagree, disagree and strongly disagree. It is a technique used to measure attitudes. Alternative methods include Thurstone's scales, Geltman's methods and Osgood's semantic-differential scales (Wright et al 2005, p. 78).

13. MAKATON is used to assess people with learning disabilities.

False: MAKATON started as a project to find an effective method of communication between deaf adults who also had learning difficulties. The name arises from the names of the three people who devised it: Margaret Walker, a speech therapist, Kathy Johnson and Tony Cornforth, both psychiatric hospital visitors from the Royal Association in aid of the Deaf and Dumb. Currently MAKATON is the main communication training programme in the UK for those with communication and learning disabilities. It uses speech, signs and written symbols. It is not an assessment tool (www.makaton.org).

14. The Mini Mental State Examination (MMSE) is highly sensitive in detecting delirium and dementia.

False: A score of 24 was initially suggested for distinguishing between impaired and normal subjects with a high degree of specificity (82%) and sensitivity (87%). However, these values were derived from screening elderly hospitalized patients with delirium or fairly advanced dementia. The normative values and 'cut-off' levels generally applied in this test veer towards specificity rather than sensitivity. A score below 24 is a good indicator of dementia in the absence of delirium. However, many patients with early Alzheimer's disease score above this cut-off point. MMSE is insensitive to minor or restricted impairments that occur in early, mild or resolving delirium. Age, education and socio-economic status also affect the performance (Hodges 1994, p. 184; Jacoby & Oppenheimer 2002, p. 621; Lishman 1997, p. 123).

15. Correct awareness of passage of time is a good test of orientation.

True: Orientation is divided into orientation for time, place and person. Of these, orientation to time is often the first to become disturbed and, hence, considered most sensitive. Patients with even mild disorientation misjudge the passage of time. Disorientation is common in patients with delirium (Hodges 1994, p. 110).

16. Premorbid IQ can be estimated from the WAIS.

True: Verbal IQ assessed from the WAIS is often used as an estimate of premorbid IQ because it is an overlearned skill that is rather resistant to deterioration. However, the National Adult Reading Test (NART) gives a more accurate estimate of premorbid IQ (Mitchell 2004, p. 59).

17. Concrete thinking is tested by interpretation of proverbs.

True: Proverbs by their very nature require some elements of abstract thought to interpret them. For example 'too many cooks spoil the broth' is not literally a piece of advice for running a kitchen with specific regard to soup preparation but might be taken to be so by patients with concrete thinking. Frontal lobe damage, low educational background and schizophrenia are all potential causes (Hodges 1994, p. 119).

18. Reasoning is one of the primary mental abilities identified by Thurstone.

True: Thurstone proposed that intelligence can be defined only in terms of essential or primary mental abilities. They are the cognitive skills that enable a person to learn, think and reason. Thurstone's seven primary mental abilities include spatial, perceptual speed, numerical reasoning, verbal meaning, word fluency, memory and inductive reasoning, i.e. the ability to generate a rule or relationship that describes a set of observations. He believed that together these make up intelligence.

19. Kelly's Repertory Grid (KRG) is usually used to measure attitudes.

False: KRG is a personality test. It assesses the subject's personal constructs. Personal constructs are dimensions that individuals use to interpret themselves and their social worlds and to predict events. These constructs tend to take an either/or form.

Usually, Likert scales, Thurstone scales and Semantic-differential scales are used to measure attitudes. Personality tests including KRG, Rorschach test and the Thematic Apperception Test can be used to study constructs.

20. Semantic-differential is used to measure attitudes.

True: Osgood's semantic differential instrument was developed from the Likert scale. The subject is given a word and asked to rate the word with a variety of opposing adjectives on a 7-point scale. It is used to measure attitudes (Fear 2004, p. 28; Wright et al 2005, p. 78).

21. The Stanford–Binet Intelligence Scale measures verbal reasoning.

True: The Stanford–Binet Intelligence Scale contains subtests designed to measure Verbal reasoning, Abstract/visual reasoning, Quantitative reasoning, and Short-term memory. Verbal reasoning includes vocabulary, comprehension, absurdities and verbal relations tests (Aiken 2000, p. 138; Atkinson et al 2000, p. 430; Wright et al 2005, p. 72).

22. Acquisition components of intelligence were defined by Sternberg.

True: Sternberg's Triarchic theory of intelligence has three subtheories:

1. Componential (analytical)
2. Experiential (creative)
3. Contextual (practical).

Within componential intelligence, there are:

- A1: Meta-components that control, monitor and evaluate cognitive processing
- A2: Performance components that execute the strategies and carry out the action and
- A3: Knowledge acquisition components that gain and store new knowledge.

23. Block design is more stable than vocabulary subtest in organic lesions.

False: 'Hold' tests, e.g. vocabulary, information, object assembly and picture completion, reflect the use of old knowledge and are relatively resistant to the effects of brain damage. 'Don't hold' tests, e.g. digit symbol, digit span, similarities and block design, which require speed of response, working memory and the perception of new relations in verbal or spatial content show early decline (Lishman 1997, p. 111).

24. In selective dominant hemisphere damage the performance scale on the WAIS is more impaired than the verbal scale.

False: The dominant hemisphere is specialized for language and for logical, sequential analysis of information. Selective dominant hemisphere damage may severely affect comprehension, arithmetic and vocabulary subtests of the verbal scale, whilst the performance scale is unaffected (Lishman 1997, p. 111).

25. The Yale–Brown Obsessive Compulsive Scale (YBOCS) rates obsessive personality traits as well as obsessive compulsive symptoms.

False: YBOCS rates obsessive compulsive symptoms in those diagnosed to have obsessive compulsive disorder. The clinician rates 10 symptoms using a 4-point scale. It does not rate obsessive personality traits or anxiety or depressive symptoms (Gelder et al 2006, p. 66).

50 | Psychopathology

Claire Dibben and Bipin Ravindran

T   F

1. Passivity phenomena occur in persistent delusional disorder.

2. Dreams are abnormal perceptions.

3. Sensitiver Beziehungswahn is typically associated with hallucinations.

4. Depersonalization is common in agoraphobia.

5. Paraphasias include substitution of words.

6. Weight loss is seen in uncomplicated grief.

7. Repeated suggestion can induce false memories.

8. Waxy flexibility includes resisting passive movements.

9. Morbid jealousy differs from normal jealousy in the quality of evidence for infidelity.

10. Double orientation generally causes little distress to the patient.

11. Grandiose delusions occur in hypomania.

12. Hallucinations are always perceived as emanating from the surrounding environment.

13. Lilliputian hallucinations are often pleasurable.

14. Perceptual disturbances occur in derealization.

15. Pseudohallucinations are sensory deceptions.

16. Pseudohallucinations in the bereaved are indicative of morbid grief.

17. Schneider's first rank symptoms have their emphasis on form rather than content.

18. Intermetamorphosis is a misidentification syndrome.

19. Dereistic thinking is usually goal directed.

20. Circumstantiality is a disorder of reasoning.

21. Overinclusive thinking can be assessed by object sorting tests.

22. Hypochondriacal delusions are found in most patients with dysmorphophobia.

23. Paranoid literally means 'beside the mind'.

24. Out of body experiences may occur in normal people.

T   F

25. Thought broadcasting involves the patient believing that his thoughts are being read by others.

☐ ☐

ANSWERS

1. Passivity phenomena occur in persistent delusional disorder.

False: Non-bizarre delusions constitute the most conspicuous or the only clinical characteristic in persistent delusional disorder. Passivity phenomena are sensations, feelings, impulses or volitional acts that are experienced by the patient as made or influenced by others in some way. They are bizarre delusions suggesting a diagnosis of schizophrenia. ICD-10 specifically excludes 'delusion of control' which is synonymous with passivity experiences from the description of persistent delusional disorder (DSM-IV 1994, 297.1; ICD-10 1992, F22.0; Wright et al 2005, p. 264).

2. Dreams are abnormal perceptions.

False: Dreams are highly complex experiences that occur during REM sleep. They are described by the patient in the way they remember them when they are awake. Daydreams are different and involve fantasy (Johnstone et al 2004, p. 773; Sims 2004, p. 59).

3. Sensitiver Beziehungswahn is typically associated with hallucinations.

False: These are sensitive delusions of reference first described by Kretschmer in 1927. He described a sensitive premorbid personality characterized by shyness and distrust. Such a person would be predisposed to form sensitive ideas of reference, which, following a key experience, would develop into a delusion that is understandable in this context (McKenna 2006, p. 270; Sims 2004, p. 129).

4. Depersonalization is common in agoraphobia.

True: Depersonalization is common in agoraphobia. Roth, in 1959, suggested that depersonalization signified a special subgroup of agoraphobia, the phobic-anxiety-depersonalization syndrome that typically occurs in young married women (DSM-IV 1994; Gelder et al 2006, p. 189; ICD-10 1992, F40.0; Sims 2004, p. 334).

5. Paraphasias include substitution of words.

True: Paraphasia is defined as 'substitutions within a language'.

Paraphasia is a dysphasia that involves substituting correct words with wrong ones, using the right words in wrong combinations, or distortion of syllables or sounds.

Semantic paraphasias involve the use of related words though with a different meaning, e.g. sister for brother.

Literal paraphasia is the misuse of the meanings of words so that the sentence does not make sense.

Phonemic paraphasias involve similar sounding words, e.g. murder for merger.

Verbal paraphasias involve the loss of a word but the substitute still makes sense, e.g. 'four-legged sit-up' for chair (Hodges 1994, p. 95; Lishman 1997, p. 102; Sims 2004, p. 183).

6. Weight loss is seen in uncomplicated grief.

True: Sadness, tearfulness, irritability, anhedonia, early morning wakening, and loss of appetite, weight and libido may all occur in normal grief. One-third of the bereaved meet the criteria for a depressive episode at some point during their grieving. Morbid guilt, suicidal ideation, functional impairment, psychomotor retardation, global loss of self-esteem, worthlessness and persistent hallucinations are more indicative of depression (Gelder et al 2006, p. 169; Puri & Hall 2004, p. 82; Sadock & Sadock 2002, p. 61).

7. Repeated suggestion can induce false memories.

True: Loftus in 1979 showed that people can be misled into remembering things that have never occurred by asking leading questions. In further studies experimenters have falsely suggested to an individual that they experienced a traumatic event as a child. Some of these individuals have subsequently gone on to recall the event in great detail. For example, by repeated suggestion, childhood memories of having been lost in a crowd can be induced in up to 30% of those who had no such memory. However, some think that in order to be 'misled' the false event must in some way be compatible with their personal history (Gross 2001, p. 616).

8. Waxy flexibility includes resisting passive movements.

False: Waxy flexibility or flexibilitas cerea is when the patient allows himself to be moulded into an awkward posture which he will then hold for several minutes. This is a catatonic symptom. The phenomenon of resisting passive movements is called opposition (McKenna 2006, p. 19; Sims 2004, p. 364).

9. Morbid jealousy differs from normal jealousy in the quality of evidence for infidelity.

True: The essential feature of morbid or pathological jealousy is an abnormal belief that the marital partner is being unfaithful. The term should be used only when the jealousy is based on unsound evidence and reasoning (Gelder et al 2006, p. 314; Sims 2004, p. 132).

10. Double orientation generally causes little distress to the patient.

True: Double orientation occurs when patients with chronic schizophrenia behave in a manner incompatible with their firmly held delusions. This delusional belief is thus separate from and therefore does not influence their feelings and behaviour. For example, the patient may believe he is a member of the Royal Family but at the same time lives happily in a hostel (Gelder et al 2006, p. 9; Sims 2004, p. 215).

11. Grandiose delusions occur in hypomania.

False: According to ICD-10, delusions and hallucinations do not occur in hypomania. The presence of grandiose delusions would change the diagnosis to mania with psychotic symptoms (ICD-10 1992, F30.0; Johnstone et al 2004, p. 427).

12. Hallucinations are always perceived as emanating from the surrounding environment.

False: Hallucinations are usually perceived as emanating from the surrounding environment or the outer objective space. However, they can be perceived as arising from within the body or from remote locations as in extracampine hallucinations (Sims 2004, pp. 98, 112).

13. Lilliputian hallucinations are often pleasurable.

True: Lilliputian hallucinations are abnormal perceptions often of little creatures or humans. Here micropsia affects the visual hallucinations. They are accompanied by strong affect, usually a strange mixture of terror and humour. Many patients do enjoy them and are able to watch them with interest and delight. They occur in organic states such as delirium tremens (Lishman 1997, p. 12; Sims 2004, p. 105).

14. Perceptual disturbances occur in derealization.

True: Derealization is an unpleasant feeling of unreality relating to the environment. There can be distortion of time sense, emotional numbing and perceptual changes whilst insight is preserved. The outside world may be experienced as flat, dull and unreal. People can appear as lifeless, two-dimensional 'cardboard' figures. It is often accompanied by depersonalization. It can occur as a transient phenomenon in healthy adults and children, especially when tired (Gelder et al 2006, p. 16; Sims 2004, p. 231).

15. Pseudohallucinations are sensory deceptions.

True: Pseudohallucinations are sensory deceptions. They are false perceptions that are experienced in full consciousness. They are different from normal perception, imagery, illusions, dreams and hallucinations. They are clear, vivid and involuntary but are figurative and occur in inner subjective space (McKenna 2006, p. 10; Sims 2004, p. 108).

16. Pseudohallucinations in the bereaved are indicative of morbid grief.

False: Pseudohallucinations can occur in people free of mental illness at times of crisis, e.g. bereavement. Pseudohallucinations in the bereaved are called hallucinations of widowhood. They occur in up to 50% of the widowed. They do not indicate pathological grief (Gelder et al 2006, p. 169; Sims 2004, p. 111).

17. Schneider's first rank symptoms have their emphasis on form rather than content.

True: Schneider suggested that the presence of any one of the first rank symptoms, in the absence of organic disease, was positive evidence for schizophrenia. It is now recognized that first rank symptoms, whilst highly suggestive of schizophrenia, are not pathognomonic (McKenna 2006, pp. 26, 89; Sims 2004, p. 166).

18. Intermetamorphosis is a misidentification syndrome.

True: Capgras, Fregoli, subjective doubles and intermetamorphosis are the four misidentification syndromes. In intermetamorphosis the patient believes to a delusional level that a familiar person and a misidentified stranger share physical and psychological similarities (Gelder et al 2000, p. 668; Sims 2004, p. 134).

19. Dereistic thinking is usually goal directed.

False: Bleuler coined the term dereistic thinking. It is also known as autistic or undirected fantasy thinking. It refers to preference for an inner personalized idiosyncratic reality rather than external reality (Sims 2004, p. 149).

20. Circumstantiality is a disorder of reasoning.

False: Circumstantiality is a disorder of thinking. It is a pattern of speech which is indirect, delayed at reaching the end goal and frequently includes unnecessary detail. It occurs in schizophrenia, learning disability and epilepsy. It is not uncommon in normal subjects (McKenna 2006, p. 16; Sims 2004, p. 154).

21. Overinclusive thinking can be assessed by object sorting tests.

True: Overinclusive thinking can be demonstrated by sorting tests, e.g. Goldstein-Sheerer Object-Sorting Test. When asked to sort words or pictures into conceptual categories, patients with overinclusive thinking are unable to preserve boundaries.

22. Hypochondriacal delusions are found in most patients with dysmorphophobia.

False: Overvalued ideas are usually found in dysmorphophobia. Delusions do not occur in dysmorphophobia. Hypochondriacal delusions are found in depression, schizophrenia and are most commonly in persistent delusional disorder (Sims 2004, pp. 138, 258).

23. Paranoid literally means 'beside the mind'.

True: In Greek, paranoia means beside the mind. Paranoid is a derivative of this term and translates as 'like paranoia'. The actual meaning and usage of these words in practice is still debated (McKenna 2006, p. 238).

24. Out of body experiences may occur in normal people.

True: Out of body experience is the illusion of being separated from one's own body. Out of body experiences are often accompanied by autoscopy where one sees and feels the presence of one's double. This experience can occur in normal people when deprived of sensory stimuli and also in near death experiences, e.g. after a myocardial infarction (Gelder et al 2006, p. 7; Lishman 1997, p. 73; Sims 2004, p. 215).

25. Thought broadcasting involves the patient believing that his thoughts are being read by others.

False: In thought broadcasting the patient experiences his thoughts as leaving his head and being projected over a wide area and hence others are aware of them. It is a first rank symptom of schizophrenia. It differs from delusions of thoughts being read (McKenna 2006, p. 29; Sims 2004, p. 165).

51 Psychotherapy – 1

Furhan Iqbal

	T	F
1. According to Bion pairing is a therapeutic factor in groups.	☐	☐
2. Interpersonal psychotherapy is beneficial in the treatment of eating disorders.	☐	☐
3. CBT is more effective than waiting list for patients with HIV and depression.	☐	☐
4. CBT is effective in the treatment of delusions.	☐	☐
5. In the treatment of back pain, CBT reduces the intensity of pain, but not the associated physical disability.	☐	☐
6. Cognitive therapy is collaborative in nature.	☐	☐
7. Cognitive therapy uses empirical reasoning.	☐	☐
8. Socratic questioning is used in CBT.	☐	☐
9. Managing enmeshment is part of contingency therapy.	☐	☐
10. Dialectic behavioural therapy includes social skills training.	☐	☐
11. Paradoxical injunction is used in behavioural family therapy.	☐	☐
12. Therapists use introjection in family therapy.	☐	☐
13. In strategic family therapy, direct interventions are used to interrupt unproductive sequences.	☐	☐
14. 'Group analysis' means analysis of the behaviour of the group.	☐	☐
15. Group therapy reduces the chances of intense transference reactions towards the therapist.	☐	☐
16. In dynamic group therapy, the therapist encourages vicarious learning.	☐	☐
17. Large group therapy represents less of a threat to the individual than small group therapy.	☐	☐
18. In psychoanalysis, interpretations are given tentatively.	☐	☐
19. The term 'negative therapeutic reaction' refers to a worsening of symptoms after some progress in psychotherapy.	☐	☐
20. A good response to a trial interpretation would indicate that a patient is likely to respond to psychotherapy.	☐	☐
21. Transference is irrelevant in supportive psychotherapy.	☐	☐

T F

22. Therapeutic communities are characterized by lack of democratic rules. ☐ ☐

23. Therapeutic communities allocate different roles to patients and staff. ☐ ☐

24. Transference phenomena do not affect the therapist. ☐ ☐

25. If a patient becomes upset and distressed in a session, an appropriate intervention is to extend the length of the session. ☐ ☐

ANSWERS

1. According to Bion pairing is a therapeutic factor in groups.

False: Bion developed the idea of basic assumptions as primitive states of mind automatically generated when people combine in a group. The basic assumptions include pairing (the hope that coupling of individuals could lead to the birth of an individual or idea providing salvation), dependence (expecting the leader to provide solutions) and fight/flight (fleeing or engaging in a battle with others). He suggested that fantasies and emotional drives associated with the basic assumptions interfere with the explicit work task, preventing change and development (Brown & Pedder 1991, p. 122).

2. Interpersonal psychotherapy is beneficial in the treatment of eating disorders.

True: Interpersonal psychotherapy reduces psychiatric symptoms by improving the quality of the patient's current interpersonal relations and social functioning. It is indicated in the treatment of depressive disorders, bulimia, binge eating disorder and for individuals facing conflict with significant others or having difficulty adjusting to life transitions. Interpersonal therapy assumes that the social and interpersonal context plays a role in the development and maintenance of some psychiatric disorders. Moreover, the patient's relationships with others influence the response to treatment as well as the overall outcome (Sadock & Sadock 2005, p. 2617).

3. CBT is more effective than waiting list for patients with HIV and depression.

True: Compared to waiting list or routine treatment, interpersonal, supportive, cognitive behavioural and experiential therapies in both individual and group settings are more effective in the treatment of depression, anxiety, anger and distress and in improving quality of life in the context of HIV infection. Moreover, medication plus psychotherapy is more effective than either treatment alone (Sadock & Sadock 2005, p. 435).

4. CBT is effective in the treatment of delusions.

True: The use of CBT techniques in the context of a collaborative therapeutic relationship can reduce the intensity with which delusions are held. Patients are encouraged to test the plausibility of their beliefs through guided discovery, thus

281

enabling them to arrive at their own conclusion regarding the need to revise delusional beliefs (Sadock & Sadock 2005, p. 2603).

5. In the treatment of back pain, CBT reduces the intensity of pain, but not the associated physical disability.

False: In a randomized controlled study comparing operant behavioural treatment and cognitive behavioural treatment with a waiting list control for the treatment of chronic low back pain, Turner & Clancy (1988) showed that both active treatments reduced physical and psychosocial disability as well as self reports of pain.

6. Cognitive therapy is collaborative in nature.

True: In cognitive therapy the therapist actively interacts with the patient, making it a collaborative venture in contrast to some other forms of psychotherapy. The therapy is structured in order to engage the participation of the patient in the empirical investigation of their thoughts, inferences, conclusions and assumptions (Beck et al 1979; Gelder et al 2006, p. 589; Johnstone et al 2004, p. 315).

7. Cognitive therapy uses empirical reasoning.

True: In cognitive therapy, empirical investigation of the patient's automatic thoughts, inferences, conclusions and assumptions is emphasized. The therapist does not accept the patient's conclusions and inferences at face value and instead seeks to determine their validity by looking with the patient at the available evidence (Beck et al 1979; Johnstone et al 2004, p. 315; Sadock & Sadock 2005, p. 2599).

8. Socratic questioning is used in CBT.

True: In cognitive therapy the therapist asks questions in order to elicit the idiosyncratic meanings that cause distress and to look for evidence in favour of or against such thoughts and beliefs. The use of questions to reveal the self-defeating nature of the client's negative automatic thoughts has been termed 'Socratic questioning' (Johnstone et al 2004, p. 315).

9. Managing enmeshment is part of contingency therapy.

False: Enmeshment is a term used in family therapy. In structural family therapy the family is viewed as a system with interacting subsystems. Clarity of boundaries between interacting subsystems is thought to be a good indicator of family functioning and should allow individuals to function without undue interference and also allow contact with other subsystems or individuals within the family. In some families there is a lack of contact (disengaged), whereas in others there is an extreme form of proximity and intensity referred to as 'enmeshment'. In enmeshed families the individual gets lost in the system and the capacity to function independently is impaired (Minuchin 1974, p. 54; Sadock & Sadock 2005, p. 2586).

10. Dialectic behavioural therapy includes social skills training.

True: Linehan developed dialectic behavioural therapy for patients who repeatedly harm themselves, and who have borderline personality disorder.

Patients learn problem-solving techniques for dealing with stressful events, including ways of improving social skills and controlling anger and other emotions (Bateman & Tyrer 2004; Gelder et al 2006, p. 599).

11. Paradoxical injunction is used in behavioural family therapy.

True: The therapist encourages symptomatic behaviours or other undesirable behaviours in an attempt to lessen such behaviours or bring them under control. Such tasks may result in the individual discovering that they do have some control or influence over things which they may have deemed beyond their influence resulting in a sense of helplessness (Dallos & Draper 2000, p. 50; Gelder et al 2006, p. 610).

12. Therapists use introjection in family therapy.

False: Freud originally described introjection as a process of narcissistic identification in which the lost object is introjected and retained as part of the internal psyche. Freud later described it as the primary internalizing mechanism by which parental values are internalized at the resolution of the oedipal phase leading to the origin of the superego (Sadock & Sadock 2005, p. 720).

13. In strategic family therapy, direct interventions are used to interrupt unproductive sequences.

True: Strategic therapy uses interventions to reduce the power of symptoms over the family and to bring about change. It does not use a normative model of healthy family functioning but aims to enable the family to move towards a healthier way of relating. The therapist uses reframing, direct interventions and paradoxical injunctions to interrupt repetitive unproductive patterns (Stein et al 1999, p. 279).

14. 'Group analysis' means analysis of the behaviour of the group.

False: 'Group analysis' refers to the theory and practice of group psychotherapy based on the work of S. H. Foulkes. In group analysis, man is viewed as a social animal born and brought up in a social situation in the context of which the individual's personality develops. The individual is considered as a nodal point in a network of relationships in the group – the matrix. Group analysis attends to the individual's current life situation more directly than in individual analytical therapy, emphasizing the 'here and now' and focusing less on the individual's developmental history. Communication within the group is considered to be central and the group focuses not only on what is said but also on when, how and why. This allows for a deeper and richer understanding of the hidden communication (Aveline & Dryden 1988, p. 19).

15. Group therapy reduces the chances of intense transference reactions towards the therapist.

True: In group psychotherapy the intensity of the transference towards the therapist is less as the group tends to absorb some of the transference feelings. Some of the roles of the therapist, e.g. providing support to struggling members, are taken on by group members, which reduces the intensity of the transference towards the therapist. The diluted transference is worked through in the interactions between group members (Aveline & Dryden 1988, p. 21).

16. In dynamic group therapy, the therapist encourages vicarious learning.

False: In dynamic group psychotherapy, the therapist generally avoids giving direct instructions to the group or group members. Even though vicarious learning inevitably occurs in dynamic group psychotherapy, the therapist does not explicitly encourage this process (Aveline & Dryden 1988, p. 297).

17. Large group therapy represents less of a threat to the individual than small group therapy.

False: The individual in the large group faces a particular dilemma between the wish to lose oneself in the group and maintaining one's identity. This is partly due to the size of the large group, which means that the individual cannot have a relationship with all group members at an individual level, as is perhaps possible in a small group. It is the sense of individual identity acquired in relation to other people (through a process of recognizing one's separateness from others and the separateness of others from oneself) that is under threat in the context of the large group (Kreeger 1975, p. 53).

18. In psychoanalysis, interpretations are given tentatively.

True: An interpretation is a tentative hypothesis, a suggestion rather than a dogmatic assertion. According to psychodynamic therapists, the tentative hypothesis is offered as an invitation to a mutual exploration as opposed to a statement of fact (Brown & Pedder 1991, p. 78).

19. The term 'negative therapeutic reaction' refers to a worsening of symptoms after some progress in psychotherapy.

True: The term 'negative therapeutic reaction' refers to the worsening or reappearance of symptoms following some progress in analysis. Initially, it was thought of as an act of defiance but was later conceptualized as a paradoxical reaction to the accuracy of the interpretation. The negative therapeutic reaction is thought to be determined by aggressive and destructive instincts (Bateman & Holmes 1995, p. 165).

20. A good response to a trial interpretation would indicate that a patient is likely to respond to psychotherapy.

True: Patients with a reasonable level of personality integration (having the capacity to face emotions and continue to function independently), motivation for change, psychological mindedness, average intelligence, realistic expectations of therapy and the absence of psychosis, substance misuse and irresolvable life crisis have favourable outcomes in long-term insight-oriented psychotherapy. A good response to a trial interpretation is helpful in assessing the psychological mindedness of the individual (Mace 1995, pp. 18, 165; Sadock & Sadock 2005, p. 2486).

21. Transference is irrelevant in supportive psychotherapy.

False: Supportive therapy is a long-term psychotherapy aimed at maximizing the patient's strengths, restoring and maintaining psychological equilibrium and acknowledging but attempting to minimize dependence on the therapist. This is achieved by supporting their defences without attempting to restructure their personality, enlarging their behavioural repertoire, alleviating anxiety, and providing a secure and trusting relationship with the therapist. Supportive psychotherapy focuses on fostering and maintaining a positive transference at all times and minimizing the effects of negative transference, should it arise. The therapists need supervision to manage transference and countertransference issues (Sadock & Sadock 2005, p. 2494).

22. Therapeutic communities are characterized by lack of democratic rules.

False: The four themes that characterize therapeutic communities include:

1. Democratization: equal sharing of power of decision-making in the community
2. Permissiveness: the tolerance among community members of behaviours that outside the setting may be viewed as deviant according to 'norms'
3. Reality confrontation: the belief that patients should be continuously presented with how their behaviour is viewed by others, and
4. Communalism: the informality, relationships and sharing of amenities.

Other features of therapeutic communities include: Informality, Mutual help, Directness and honesty, Shared decisions, Shared activities, and Group meetings (Aveline & Dryden 1988, p. 163; Gelder et al 2006, p. 607).

23. Therapeutic communities allocate different roles to patients and staff.

False: In a therapeutic community, staff members are also members of the therapeutic community. They participate in informal social activities and relationships, e.g. preparing meals, etc. This helps break down the patient–staff barriers. However, such democratization has its limits and it is important to remember that the staff are there for the therapeutic benefit of patients and not for the gratification of their own personal needs (Aveline & Dryden 1988, p. 168).

24. Transference phenomena do not affect the therapist.

False: Transference is an unconscious process in which the individual transfers onto the therapist and others experiences, attitudes and feelings experienced in the past in relation to significant others in early life. Inevitably, it affects the therapist and provides important information regarding the patient's internal world.

25. If a patient becomes upset and distressed in a session, an appropriate intervention is to extend the length of the session.

False: If a patient becomes distressed in a session, the therapist should attend to the individual's distress sensitively. It is important to allow the patient to be upset and express their distress. The therapist should also try to establish why the person became upset; cognitive therapists may choose to focus on the thoughts (hot cognitions) whereas a dynamic therapist may focus on the feelings. Generally speaking, the therapist should not extend the length of the session and should attempt to contain the distress within the boundary of the session. On occasions, patients may become extremely distressed and if there is a concern regarding their own safety or the safety of others then the assessment and management of risk should be the priority.

Psychotherapy – 2

Furhan Iqbal

T   F

1. Transference is not discussed in brief dynamic psychotherapy.

2. Brief psychodynamic therapy is useful in adjustment disorder.

3. In CBT for relationship difficulties, homework may be included.

4. In the treatment of generalized anxiety disorder (GAD), CBT is significantly more effective than relaxation training.

5. In pain disorders in children, CBT reduces the intensity of pain as well as improving the non-pain outcomes.

6. In cognitive therapy for depression, cognitive changes generally precede behavioural changes.

7. Collaborative empiricism is used in CBT.

8. Contingency management includes consideration of internal motives.

9. An experienced psychotherapist can avoid countertransference.

10. Circular questioning is used in family therapy.

11. Triangulation is a concept used in family therapy.

12. In structural family therapy, the therapist uses a directive approach.

13. Systems theory of family therapy assumes that the symptom in one member enables homeostasis.

14. Foulkes is associated with the development of group analysis.

15. Imparting of information by the therapist is a therapeutic factor in group psychotherapy.

16. Advice is an important therapeutic factor in group therapy.

17. Resistance in group therapy may be expressed as scapegoating.

18. Contract marital therapy requires the cooperation of both partners.

19. In psychotherapy the term negative therapeutic reaction means that the patient idolizes the therapist.

20. A diagnosis understandable in psychological terms is an indicator of likely response to psychotherapy.

21. In supportive psychotherapy, it is not necessary to do a psychodynamic formulation.

T F

22. The ethos of therapeutic community includes normalization. ☐ ☐

23. The therapist's account of the strength of a therapeutic relationship is related to the outcome. ☐ ☐

24. Underlying assumptions are processes that belong to the dynamic unconsciousness. ☐ ☐

25. In psychoanalysis, working alliance is the same as transference relationship. ☐ ☐

ANSWERS

1. Transference is not discussed in brief dynamic psychotherapy.

False: In transference, the patient relates to the therapist as though he/she was a significant object from the past. In brief psychodynamic psychotherapy, transference is discussed and analysed (Gelder et al 2000, p. 1423; Sadock & Sadock 2005, p. 2641).

2. Brief psychodynamic therapy is useful in adjustment disorder.

True: Brief psychodynamic psychotherapy is a time-limited therapy based on psychodynamic principles. It is useful in patients who present with a circumscribed set of problems with a focus that can be understood in dynamic terms; in individuals with transitional crises, e.g. parenthood, leaving home, abnormal grief reaction; PTSD; adolescents with emotional or conduct problems; and in issues of illness, treatment and decline in the elderly (Stein et al 1999, pp. 155–173).

3. In CBT for relationship difficulties, homework may be included.

True: Homework is not absolutely necessary for improvement in CBT. However, patients who engage in homework make quicker, longer lasting and more generalized progress. CBT for relationship difficulties involves helping the couple reformulate their problems and develop new rules in a spirit of collaboration and shared goals. Homework assignments often involve putting the new revised rules into practice, so that the couple can appreciate the level of functionality that is possible and make further adjustments as necessary (Sadock & Sadock 2005, pp. 2601, 2604).

4. In the treatment of generalized anxiety disorder (GAD), CBT is significantly more effective than relaxation training.

True: Relaxation training is useful as a basic treatment for anxiety. The training consists of instructions that aid progressive muscle relaxation. CBT specifically targets cognitive, e.g. worry, and behavioural, e.g. avoidance, features. Combined cognitive and behavioural treatments are more effective than either treatment alone. CBT is the most effective psychological treatment for GAD. It reduces the severity of anxiety by about 50%. It is as effective as treatment with benzodiazepines in GAD (Gelder et al 2000, p. 791; Gelder et al 2006, p. 182; Johnstone et al 2004, p. 468).

5. In pain disorders in children, CBT reduces the intensity of pain as well as improving the non-pain outcomes.

False: A systematic review of psychological treatment for chronic and recurrent pain in children and adolescents concluded that there was sufficient evidence that relaxation and CBT reduced the severity and frequency of chronic headaches but little evidence that they improved non-pain outcomes (Ecclestone et al 2003).

6. In cognitive therapy for depression, cognitive changes generally precede behavioural changes.

True: In cognitive therapy, the therapist and the patient initially work on modifying negative automatic thoughts that cause distress for the individual. Only after some change in these automatic thoughts has occurred will the patient be able to engage in behavioural tasks, which then in turn facilitate further challenging of automatic thoughts by providing evidence to the contrary (Hawton et al 1988, p. 200).

7. Collaborative empiricism is used in CBT.

True: Collaborative empiricism refers to the collaborative nature of the empirical enterprise central to cognitive therapy. In cognitive therapy, the therapist actively interacts with the patient, making it a collaborative venture, in contrast to some other forms of psychotherapy. The therapy is structured in order to engage the participation of the patient in the empirical investigation of their thoughts, inferences, conclusions and assumptions (Beck et al 1979; Johnstone et al 2004, p. 315; Sadock & Sadock 2005, p. 2599).

8. Contingency management includes consideration of internal motives.

False: Contingency management refers to a group of behavioural procedures based on the principle that behaviours persist as a result of reinforcement by some of their consequences. If these consequences are altered then the target behaviour will change. The reinforcement is withdrawn from the undesirable behaviours and is made contingent only on desirable behaviours. Contingency management is used to manage behavioural problems in people with learning disabilities and autism (Gelder et al 2006, p. 592).

9. An experienced psychotherapist can avoid countertransference.

False: Countertransference refers to the emotional response of the therapist towards the patient. In psychodynamic therapy this is considered to be an important source of information regarding the workings of the internal world of the patient. Experienced therapists are more able to recognize the counter-transference, but not able to avoid it (Brown & Pedder 1991, p. 61; Gelder et al 2006, pp. 584, 600).

10. Circular questioning is used in family therapy.

True: Circular questioning is an original feature of the Milan Associates Systemic model. It refers to a way of questioning in which responses are used to construct further questions that seek to bring out connections between behaviours, beliefs and relationships of individuals within the family. It allows the therapist and family to understand family processes from the perspectives of different family members and in doing so develop a complex picture of relationships, behaviours and beliefs (Gelder et al 2000, p. 1478; Stein et al 1999, p. 280).

11. Triangulation is a concept used in family therapy.

True: Triangulation refers to the process in which parents in conflict attempt to win the sympathy and support of their child, who is recruited by one parent as an ally in the struggle with the other. Triangulation may also refer to the process in which parents focus on a behavioural or health problem of the child as a strategy for diffusing relationship problems (Dallos & Draper 2000, p. 39; Sadock & Sadock 2005, p. 2244).

12. In structural family therapy, the therapist uses a directive approach.

True: The therapist in structural family therapy brings about change in family patterns to a healthier and more functional form based on a normative model of healthy family functioning using a more directive approach. In structural family therapy, the therapist negotiates a leadership role with the family, uses genograms, elaborates the structure of the family in terms of subsystems and relationships, makes use of reframing and uses directive and restructuring interventions (Stein et al 1999, p. 276).

13. Systems theory of family therapy assumes that the symptom in one member enables homeostasis.

True: Family systems, like other systems, have a tendency to maintain balance and equilibrium. Systems theory of family therapy suggests that a symptom in one or more members of the family is in fact an attempt to maintain equilibrium and attempts to change this will be met with resistance (Dallos & Draper 2000, p. 35; Sadock & Sadock 2005, p. 2587).

14. Foulkes is associated with the development of group analysis.

True: The work of Foulkes was fundamental in the development of group analysis. He also founded the Institute of Group Analysis in London.

15. Imparting of information by the therapist is a therapeutic factor in group psychotherapy.

True: Yalom described 11 therapeutic factors in group therapy: instillation of hope, universality, imparting information, altruism, corrective recapitulation of the primary family group, development of socializing techniques, imitating adaptive behaviours, interpersonal learning, group cohesiveness, catharsis and existential factors. Skills-based groups tend to focus more on imparting information to their members (Gelder et al 2006, p. 603; Johnstone et al 2004, p. 321; Sadock & Sadock 2005, p. 2570; Yalom 1995).

16. Advice is an important therapeutic factor in group therapy.

False: Direct advice from members invariably occurs in group psychotherapy. In dynamic groups this is usually in the early stages of the group or at a later stage when the group is confronted with some difficulty leading to temporary regression. In dynamic groups, group conductors generally do not offer direct instruction but in other forms of group therapy this may form an important part of the programme. See also answer to Q15 (Gelder et al 2006, p. 603; Johnstone et al 2004, p. 321; Sadock & Sadock 2005, p. 2570; Yalom 1995).

17. Resistance in group therapy may be expressed as scapegoating.

True: Resistance in a group hinders the ability of the group to continue with its task. This may manifest as scapegoating, i.e. subclassifying a group of people and attacking them and/or monopolizing the group (Barnes et al 1999, p. 111).

18. Contract marital therapy requires the cooperation of both partners.

True: Contract marital therapy involves an agreement between both partners to reward one another for behaviours and responses which each partner seeks from the other (Brown & Pedder 1991, p. 146).

19. In psychotherapy the term negative therapeutic reaction means that the patient idolizes the therapist.

False: Negative therapeutic reaction refers to the worsening or reappearance of symptoms following some progress in analysis. Initially it was thought of as an act of defiance but was later conceptualized as a paradoxical reaction to the accuracy of the interpretation. The negative therapeutic reaction is thought to be determined by aggressive and destructive instincts (Bateman & Holmes 1995, p. 165).

20. A diagnosis understandable in psychological terms is an indicator of likely response to psychotherapy.

False: A diagnosis understandable in psychological terms in its own right is not an indicator of likely response to psychotherapy. It does, however, help the assessment of suitability for psychotherapy, aid decisions regarding what type of therapy may be beneficial and guide ongoing therapy itself (Mace 1995, p. 169).

21. In supportive psychotherapy, it is not necessary to do a psychodynamic formulation.

True: Not all supportive psychotherapies are psychodynamic in orientation. A psychodynamic formulation is important in psychodynamic supportive therapy, but not necessarily in other forms of supportive therapy.

22. The ethos of therapeutic community includes normalization.

False: Normalization refers to the principle expressing the aims, attitudes and norms underpinning quality work with the mentally retarded. In essence it means making available to the mentally retarded the patterns and conditions in their everyday life as close to those of mainstream society as possible (Fraser & Kerr 2003, p. 2; Gelder et al 2000, p. 1503).

23. The therapist's account of the strength of a therapeutic relationship is related to the outcome.

True: Horvath & Symonds (1991) conducted a meta-analysis of studies looking at working alliance and outcomes in psychotherapy. They were able to demonstrate a moderate but reliable association between good working alliance and a positive outcome in psychotherapy. They also found that ratings of the working alliance by clients and therapists were both associated with positive outcome in psychotherapy, though the therapist's ratings were less predictive. They also concluded that the relation of the working alliance to outcome was independent of type of therapy and duration of treatment.

24. Underlying assumptions are processes that belong to the dynamic unconsciousness.

False: Assumptions or schemas in cognitive therapy refer to relatively stable cognitive structures developed as a means of organizing experiences and are part of normal cognitive development. Schemas influence automatic processes such as perception, affective responses and action responses. The dynamic unconscious is characterized by its use of primary process thinking. Primary process thinking displays the phenomena of displacement, condensation and symbolization and ignores categories of space and time. Secondary process thinking, on the other hand, obeys the laws of formal logic and grammar and is characteristic of conscious thinking (Beck et al 1979).

25. In psychoanalysis, working alliance is the same as transference relationship.

False: The working alliance is the agreement between patient and therapist that they will work together on the patient's emotional or psychological problems. The transference relationship refers to the patient's relationship to the analyst in which the individual transfers onto the analyst experiences, attitudes and feelings experienced in the past in relation to significant others (Butler & Pitt 1998, p. 54).

Research methodology – 1

Paul Wilkinson

	T	F

1. For a skewed distribution, the median is a more useful measure of central tendency than the mean. ☐ ☐

2. When comparing recovery rates between two samples, parametric statistics are best. ☐ ☐

3. For two studies with identical effect sizes, the p value will be smaller for the study with much larger numbers. ☐ ☐

4. If the confidence interval for the difference in Ham-D scores between treatment groups includes 0, we can conclude that it is likely that there is a real difference between treatments that is not due to chance. ☐ ☐

5. A type I error means that a result is falsely found to be statistically significant. ☐ ☐

6. A very low p value indicates that a result is clinically significant. ☐ ☐

7. An effectiveness study for a treatment for depression is more likely to include patients with co-morbid conditions than an efficacy study. ☐ ☐

8. The need for informed consent can limit the external validity of treatment studies. ☐ ☐

9. A scale must have good reliability for it to have good validity. ☐ ☐

10. We should assess the criterion validity of new scales that measure depressive symptoms. ☐ ☐

11. Log transformation is sometimes essential before parametric statistical tests are used. ☐ ☐

12. Non-parametric tests use the difference in medians and the inter-quartile range. ☐ ☐

13. Not taking into account dropouts from treatment may introduce bias. ☐ ☐

14. The use of intention to treat analysis may reduce accuracy of results. ☐ ☐

15. Subjects in cluster randomized controlled trials (RCTs) are analysed in exactly the same way as in standard RCTs. ☐ ☐

16. Crossover studies can have more power than using different patients in different treatment groups. ☐ ☐

17. Stratification can be used to control for confounding in a case-control study. ☐ ☐

T F

18. The *t*-test is commonly used to look at strength of association in case-control studies with a dichotomous exposure of interest. ☐ ☐

19. Multiple logistic regression is used to investigate the effects of variables on a continuous outcome measure. ☐ ☐

20. In multiple linear regression, if two covariates are highly correlated, there may be a type II error. ☐ ☐

21. Multiple linear regression cannot be used if there is a heavily skewed distribution of a proposed variable. ☐ ☐

22. For a screening test for schizophrenia, sensitivity will probably be lower for a random community sample than for a psychiatric inpatient sample. ☐ ☐

23. A meta-analysis will give more accurate and less biased results than one RCT. ☐ ☐

24. If the duration of illness is very long, incidence will be higher than prevalence. ☐ ☐

25. Administering the Beck Depression Inventory to a population is an accurate method of ascertaining population prevalence of depression. ☐ ☐

ANSWERS

1. For a skewed distribution, the median is a more useful measure of central tendency than the mean.

   True: The median gives the middle value, i.e. the 50th highest value if there are 99 values. In a skewed distribution, more values are a long way from the average, to one side of it. If positively skewed, values above the median are further from the median than values below the median. The mean will be over-affected by outliers if the distribution is skewed.

2. When comparing recovery rates between two samples, parametric statistics are best.

   False: When looking at recovery rates you are looking at numbers, or counts, of participants in different groups rather than comparing two outcome curves. Therefore, parametric statistics, which are used to compare two or more normal curves, cannot be used. Often the chi-squared test is used.

3. For two studies with identical effect sizes, the *p* value will be smaller for the study with much larger numbers.

   True: If there are larger samples we have more confidence that the difference is not due to chance. The statistics we calculate, for example *t* or *F* values, are often proportional to the square root of the number of participants.

4. If the confidence interval for the difference in Ham-D scores between treatment groups includes 0, we can conclude that it is likely that there is a real difference between treatments that is not due to chance.

False: If the confidence interval includes 0, this shows that the range of likely differences between populations includes 0, i.e. there is no actual difference.

5. A type I error means that a result is falsely found to be statistically significant.

True: In other words, the p value is below your threshold (often 5%) but there is not really a difference between two populations (such as all depressed people given a new antidepressant and all depressed people given a placebo). The difference is just a chance finding in a study. This can be important as we may conclude from a study that a new treatment is better than placebo when in fact there is no real difference. Bias, where poor methodology causes differences between groups, increases the risk of type I errors.

6. A very low p value indicates that a result is clinically significant.

False: A very low p value just means the difference between samples is very unlikely to be due to chance (statistical significance). It does not mean that the results are clinically meaningful. We must use our clinical judgement to decide that.

7. An effectiveness study for a treatment for depression is more likely to include patients with co-morbid conditions than an efficacy study.

True: Effectiveness studies are more likely to mirror real life clinical practice, such as including all possible patients with a condition, including those with co-morbid conditions. The results of these studies are therefore generally more relevant to clinical practice than efficacy studies, whose aim is to show whether a treatment can work in ideal circumstances.

8. The need for informed consent can limit the external validity of treatment studies.

True: External validity refers to how much the results of a study are generalizable to the population of interest. Unless there are exceptional circumstances, we can recruit only consenting subjects to research studies. If a lot of a population under study would not have the capacity to consent, such as patients suffering from psychosis, a study sample would not be fully representative of the population we want to treat. Research ethics committees have a difficult job in balancing the rights of the individual against the need for best information on treating a population when deciding whether there are 'exceptional circumstances' to allow inclusion of participants who do not have the capacity to give consent.

9. A scale must have good reliability for it to have good validity.

True: Validity (more strictly, internal validity) is how well a scale measures what it is supposed to measure. Reliability is whether the same scale gives the same results with the same subject when measured at different times by the same rater (intra-rater reliability) or different raters (inter-rater reliability). If a scale is not reliable, its measurements will not be valid. On the other hand, validity is *not* essential for reliability.

10. We should assess the criterion validity of new scales that measure depressive symptoms.

False: Criterion validity is how well a scale compares with an existing known quantity, such as height, or psychiatric diagnosis. It can be useful to compare a scale against DSM or ICD diagnosis, but it is not essential. Scales are more important in measuring the severity of symptoms and the changes in symptoms. It is more useful to test their reliability and concurrent validity, i.e. comparison against other valid rating scales.

11. Log transformation is sometimes essential before parametric statistical tests are used.

True: We need normally-distributed results to use parametric statistics. If results are skewed, we can log transform all values (in all groups!), and if the distributions are then normal, we can use parametric statistics.

12. Non-parametric tests use the difference in medians and the inter-quartile range.

False: Descriptive statistics like medians and inter-quartile ranges do not give us enough information to compare non-normally distributed groups. Instead, we must look at outcome scores of all participants in all groups and rank them from highest to lowest. We can then look at the total ranks of each group. Statistical tests, such as the Mann-Whitney test (for two independent samples) will tell us whether the difference in total ranks between the groups is statistically significant.

13. Not taking into account dropouts from treatment may introduce bias.

True: The reasons for dropout are likely to differ between groups. If one considers a study of psychotherapy for depression vs. waiting list control, it may be that the most unwell people in the treatment group are unable to travel to psychotherapy sessions. They may be more likely to drop out of the study than the equally unwell people on the waiting list. This would introduce systematic non-random error which would inflate the apparent efficacy of psychotherapy.

14. The use of intention to treat analysis may reduce accuracy of results.

True: You are not measuring outcome based on treatment given, so some accuracy may be lost. However, ITT reduces the effects of unknown bias caused by changes in treatment and is essential, as this bias cannot be measured. ITT may increase or decrease accuracy (we never know!) but it does minimize the chance of biased results.

15. Subjects in cluster randomized controlled trials (RCTs) are analysed in exactly the same way as in standard RCTs.

False: Cluster trials are RCTs where groups (for example GP practices or psychiatric units) rather then individual patients are randomly allocated to treatments. When analysing cluster RCTs we need to take into account intra-cluster correlation – participants in a cluster (such as GP practices) are likely to have certain things in common that they do not share with participants in other clusters. This may be because of shared environmental factors or different socio-economic status in different catchment areas. Because of these shared characteristics there may be large pre-treatment differences in outcome or risk variables in different groups. We can estimate the intraclass correlation and cluster size and use these to calculate a 'design effect'. We then increase the variance term in our calculations by this design effect.

16. Crossover studies can have more power than using different patients in different treatment groups.

True: In crossover studies, participants act as their own controls, alternating between different treatments at different time points. We therefore do not have to take into account possible error caused by between-subjects differences. Instead, more powerful repeat measures statistics can be used.

17. Stratification can be used to control for confounding in a case-control study.

True: Results are stratified into levels of a confounding factor, e.g. high levels, low levels or no levels of past cannabis use. We can look for an association between exposure of interest and outcome of interest at all strata, or use the Mantel–Haenszel procedure to calculate the association, controlling for this confounder. Stratification can also be used in cohort studies.

18. The *t*-test is commonly used to look at strength of association in case-control studies with a dichotomous exposure of interest.

False: We instead use the confidence interval of the odds ratio or the chi squared test. The *t*-test is used to compare groups with continuously distributed exposure of interest.

19. Multiple logistic regression is used to investigate the effects of variables on a continuous outcome measure.

False: Multiple logistic regression is used to investigate the effects of variables on a binary outcome measure, e.g. diagnosis/no diagnosis. Multiple linear regression is used to investigate the effects of variables on a continuous outcome measure.

20. In multiple linear regression, if two covariates are highly correlated, there may be a type II error.

True: In multiple regression, if two covariates correlate very highly (e.g. 0.9), the one with minutely better correlation with the outcome measure is selected first. The other variable will supposedly be a much less accurate predictor. This is called multicollinearity. This can lead to type II errors, as exposures of interest are wrongly deemed not to be associated with the outcome of interest.

21. Multiple linear regression cannot be used if there is a heavily skewed distribution of a proposed variable.

False: Normally-distributed data are needed. However, we can transform the distribution (e.g. log transformation) to make it normal.

22. For a screening test for schizophrenia, sensitivity will probably be lower for a random community sample than for a psychiatric inpatient sample.

True: Sensitivity is the proportion of those who truly have the diagnosis who are positive in a screening test. Sensitivity does not vary with prevalence. However, a lower severity of illness in a community group will increase the numbers who score below cut-off, thus reducing sensitivity.

23. A meta-analysis will give more accurate and less biased results than one RCT.

False: Not always. A good RCT is better than a meta-analysis of poor studies.

24. If the duration of illness is very long, incidence will be higher than prevalence.

False: Incidence is the proportion of a population with a new onset of illness over a time period. Prevalence is the proportion of a population who have an illness at any point during a time period. If there is long ongoing illness, relatively few get a new diagnosis and so incidence is lower than prevalence.

25. Administering the Beck Depression Inventory to a population is an accurate method of ascertaining population prevalence of depression.

False: The BDI is a self-rated measure of severity of depressive symptoms. It does not give a diagnosis. It may, however, be used in the first stage of a prevalence study.

All respondents with a BDI above a cut-off can receive a full diagnostic interview and a smaller proportion of those with lower BDIs are also seen, to ascertain the depression prevalence in this larger group.

Research methodology – 2

Paul Wilkinson

	T	F
1. Parametric statistics can be used if the distribution of results is Gaussian.	☐	☐
2. If standard deviations are larger, the effect size will be larger.	☐	☐
3. If $p < 0.05$, there is a real difference between populations under study.	☐	☐
4. The standard error of the mean (SEM) is used in calculating confidence intervals for differences between means of continuous measures.	☐	☐
5. If multiple tests are performed without adjusting significance thresholds, then a type II error is more likely.	☐	☐
6. If a hypothesized difference between populations is small, fewer subjects are needed to make a study adequately powered.	☐	☐
7. Development of the randomized controlled trial means that other types of treatment studies with less rigorous methodology are obsolete and of no use.	☐	☐
8. Randomization ensures that treatment groups are similar on known and unknown variables.	☐	☐
9. Convergent validity is often measured by correlating overall scores on a new outcome scale with overall scores on an established scale.	☐	☐
10. The Ham-D is a good scale to use to diagnose depression.	☐	☐
11. Parametric tests use the difference in means and the standard deviation.	☐	☐
12. The Kruskal–Wallis Test is a non-parametric test that can be used to compare more than two unrelated groups.	☐	☐
13. The use of per protocol analysis is a good way to take into account differential dropout rates between treatment groups.	☐	☐
14. The use of intention-to-treat analysis is a way to deal with attrition bias.	☐	☐
15. The use of a placebo run-in may overestimate treatment effects.	☐	☐
16. In a case-control study, if an exposure of interest increases rates of hospital admission, there may be a Berkson bias.	☐	☐
17. In a case-control study of the association between the diagnosis of alcohol dependence and the diagnosis of depression, the relative risk is the statistic that would give the most useful information on strength of association.	☐	☐

T   F

18. If the lower boundary of the confidence interval for the odds ratio for lifetime cannabis use and schizophrenia is greater than 1, we can conclude that it is likely that there is a real association between cannabis use and schizophrenia. ☐ ☐

19. In a case-control study, multiple linear regression can be used to prove that an exposure of interest causes an outcome of interest. ☐ ☐

20. Multiple linear regression is an appropriate statistical technique to use if there is a curvilinear relationship between variables. ☐ ☐

21. Before starting a screening programme, it is essential that there is a clear plan for what to do with cases screened as positive. ☐ ☐

22. For a screening test for schizophrenia, positive predictive value will be higher for a random community sample than for a psychiatric inpatient sample. ☐ ☐

23. In meta-analysis, publication bias may lead to a type I error. ☐ ☐

24. For prevalence, a time period must always be given. ☐ ☐

25. It is important to form an *a priori* hypothesis in qualitative research. ☐ ☐

ANSWERS

1. Parametric statistics can be used if the distribution of results is Gaussian.

   True: Parametric statistics, such as *t*-tests and ANOVAs, need normally distributed, or 'Gaussian', data.

2. If standard deviations are larger, the effect size will be larger.

   False: If there is a wider spread of results, the distributions of the two samples will overlap more, and therefore there will be less real difference between samples. The difference between samples is often given as the 'effect size', or 'Hedges' *g*', and is calculated by the difference in means divided by the weighted average standard deviation.

3. If *p* <0.05, there is a real difference between populations under study.

   False: This just means that there is a high probability (>95%) that they are truly different.

4. The standard error of the mean (SEM) is used in calculating confidence intervals for differences between means of continuous measures.

   True: The confidence interval is calculated with multiples of the difference in mean divided by the SEM for the difference. The SEM of a sample is the standard deviation divided by the square root of the sample size. It is therefore smaller as your sample gets bigger, and the confidence interval therefore becomes smaller as your sample sizes increase. When interpreting graphs with error lines, be sure to check whether standard deviation or SEM is used, as the SEM will appear much more impressive!

5. If multiple tests are performed without adjusting significance thresholds, then a type II error is more likely.

False: Type II errors occur when there is a real difference between populations, but a study finds no statistically significant difference. If a lot of statistical tests are performed on a dataset without adjusting significance thresholds, we are more likely to find a chance 'significant' result, when there is no real difference (i.e. a type I error). For example, if we perform 20 significance tests on samples where there is no real difference, the chances are that one of them (5%) will have a p value less than 5%. However, if multiple tests are performed without adjusting significance thresholds, there will be no effect on the chances of a type II error. If we reduce the significance thresholds, as we should to reduce type I errors, we do increase the rate of type II errors. Type II errors are generally less serious than type I errors. It is best to have a very small number of *a priori* hypotheses, to minimize chances of both types of errors.

6. If a hypothesized difference between populations is small, fewer subjects are needed to make a study adequately powered.

False: Before commencing a study, it is imperative to calculate the sample size needed to make a study adequately powered to find a statistically significant difference, if there is one. Power is increased (and a smaller sample size is needed) if: there is a larger hypothesized difference between groups; there is a smaller hypothesized standard deviation; parametric statistics can be used or if the necessary p value threshold is higher.

7. Development of the randomized controlled trial means that other types of treatment studies with less rigorous methodology are obsolete and of no use.

False: An RCT is the best study design, with the least bias; but other designs are useful if no RCTs have been performed. Other designs such as uncontrolled case series or open-label controlled trials are normally carried out to show there is a reasonable chance a treatment is effective before it is ethical to put patients in an RCT.

8. Randomization ensures that treatment groups are similar on known and unknown variables.

False: A major advantage of randomization is that it increases the chances that treatment groups are similar on known and unknown variables. If we non-randomly allocate to groups, we can ensure balance on known confounding variables, but there may still be an imbalance on important confounding variables we have not thought of. However, random allocation only increases the chance of balance. There may still be imbalance ('randomization error'), especially if groups are small.

9. Convergent validity is often measured by correlating overall scores on a new outcome scale with overall scores on an established scale.

False: That is concurrent validity. Convergent validity is whether measures which are expected to be correlated are indeed associated, e.g. correlation of emotional, cognitive and physical symptoms on a depression scale.

10. The Ham-D is a good scale to use to diagnose depression.

False: The Ham-D is a continuous scale that gives the level of symptoms, not the diagnosis. As with all continuous scales, some people with a diagnosis will get lower scores than some people without a diagnosis. Hence, beware of studies that state that all subjects have a diagnosis because they score above cut-off on a rating scale. Participants should only be interpreted as having a diagnosis if they meet certain diagnostic criteria, e.g. DSM, ICD, preferably rated using a standardized and valid interview, e.g. SCID, SADS.

11. Parametric tests use the difference in means and the standard deviation.

True: As we know the distribution is normal, the means and standard deviations (together with the numbers of participants) give us enough information about the data to compare different samples.

12. The Kruskal–Wallis Test is a non-parametric test that can be used to compare more than two unrelated groups.

True: It is rather like the ANOVA, a test to compare more than two groups, which can be used only if data is normally distributed.

13. The use of per protocol analysis is a good way to take into account differential dropout rates between treatment groups.

False: In most randomized controlled trials, some participants will drop out of treatment, or change treatment group. We then need to decide which group these people who have changed group should be analysed in: it could be as treated (what treatment they got); per protocol (only those who received the allocated treatment) or intention to treat (all participants analysed in the groups they were initially allocated to, ignoring the fact that they changed treatment). We should always use intention to treat (ITT) to take account of dropouts. Any other approach introduces bias. Also, ITT is more clinically useful: we need to know which treatment we should *offer* to our patients, when we do not know if they will drop out of treatment.

14. The use of intention-to-treat analysis is a way to deal with attrition bias.

True: Attrition bias is bias caused by differential dropout rates in different groups.

15. The use of a placebo run-in may overestimate treatment effects.

True: A placebo run-in is giving all participants a placebo and then including only those who do fail to respond to placebo in the main RCT. This increases any treatment effects. In real life, we are interested in the actual difference between a treatment and no treatment in the whole population; not the subpopulation of those who fail to respond quickly to placebo.

16. In a case-control study, if an exposure of interest increases rates of hospital admission, there may be a Berkson bias.

True: In the Berkson bias (admission rate bias or paradox), the exposure of interest leads to differential rates of hospital admission of cases and controls, rather than leading to different rates of the outcome of interest. For example, we may be more likely to admit a patient with depression if they have poor social support. A disproportionately high number of depressed inpatients would therefore have poor social support. A study where depressed cases are hospital inpatients may then make us think that there is an association between poor social support and depression. The solution is to try to use outpatient or community samples.

17. In a case-control study of the association between the diagnosis of alcohol dependence and the diagnosis of depression, the relative risk is the statistic that would give the most useful information on strength of association.

False: Unlike in cohort studies, we cannot calculate the relative risk from case-control studies, as we do not know the true numbers of people exposed to the exposure of interest. We must instead use the odds ratio, which approximates the relative risk if there is a very rare outcome.

18. If the lower boundary of the confidence interval for the odds ratio for lifetime cannabis use and schizophrenia is greater than 1, we can conclude that it is likely that there is a real association between cannabis use and schizophrenia.

True: An odds ratio (or relative risk) of 1 means there is no association at all between factors. If the CI includes 1, this shows that the range of likely associations includes 1, i.e. no real difference. If all points of the confidence interval are greater than 1, we can conclude that it is likely there is a real association.

19. In a case-control study, multiple linear regression can be used to prove that an exposure of interest causes an outcome of interest.

False: Observational studies show only a likely association between exposures and outcomes of interest. For example, the outcome measure may cause the exposure, or a third, confounding, factor, may cause both the exposure and outcome of interest. Randomized studies are needed to show 'causation'.

20. Multiple linear regression is an appropriate statistical technique to use if there is a curvilinear relationship between variables.

False: There must be linear relationship.

21. Before starting a screening programme, it is essential that there is a clear plan for what to do with cases screened as positive.

True: Screening is expensive and potentially harmful (especially by causing unnecessary anxiety in people with false-positive screens) and needs to be thought through. There must be a clear plan for what to do with people who screen positive, so that the benefits of early diagnosis outweigh the unnecessary anxiety.

22. For a screening test for schizophrenia, positive predictive value will be higher for a random community sample than for a psychiatric inpatient sample.

False: The positive predictive value of the test is the proportion of those screened positive that truly have the diagnosis. If there is lower prevalence, a higher proportion of the sample will not have the diagnosis and a higher proportion of those screened positive similarly will not have the diagnosis.

23. In meta-analysis, publication bias may lead to a type I error.

True: There is often a bias in favour of publishing positive findings. If only these studies are included, treatment effect is inflated. This may lead to the wrong conclusion that a treatment is better than a comparator.

24. For prevalence, a time period must always be given.

True: We need to say if it is point prevalence (at one point in time) or period prevalence (diagnosis at any time point during a time period).

25. It is important to form an *a priori* hypothesis in qualitative research.

False: In *quantitative* research we should form a hypothesis in advance (*a priori*). We then collect numerical data and use statistical tests to see how likely our hypothesis is to be correct. We can also test hypotheses in qualitative research though it is also often used to form hypotheses. Researchers try not to have pre-formed ideas and through methods such as focus groups and in-depth interviews, ideas and themes emerge. These can then be formulated as hypotheses to be tested in future research.

Schizophrenia

Fiona Hynes and Graham Murray

	T	F

1. Birth injury affects the age of onset of schizophrenia.

2. Schizophrenia is more common in those of Afro-Caribbean origin.

3. In expressed emotion, hostility is more detrimental than derogatory comments.

4. Both negative and positive symptoms lead to expressed emotion by carers.

5. The Camberwell Family Interview is a semi-structured interview to assess the level of expressed emotion.

6. Neuregulin 1 gene is implicated in the aetiology of schizophrenia.

7. Genes involved in myelination are implicated in the aetiology of schizophrenia.

8. The dysbindin gene is associated with schizophrenia.

9. In schizophrenia the gene for tau protein is abnormal.

10. 5% of elderly schizophrenics have a family history of schizophrenia in their first-degree relatives.

11. Having a relative with the disease is the largest single risk factor for schizophrenia.

12. In monozygotic twins discordant for schizophrenia, the risk of schizophrenia in their offspring is equal.

13. Oneiroid state was described by Mayer-Gross.

14. Somatization is an important factor in persistent delusional disorder.

15. Delusional disorder is associated with passivity phenomena.

16. Persistent delusional disorder is associated with persistent hallucinations.

17. There is no association between late onset schizophrenia and paranoid personality disorder.

18. The hippocampus is smaller in schizophrenia.

19. The information gating process is dysfunctional in schizophrenia.

20. The negative symptoms of schizophrenia are related to hypofunction of the pre-frontal cortex.

T F

21. Schizophreniform psychosis associated with temporal lobe epilepsy occurs most commonly shortly after seizures. ☐ ☐

22. In schizophrenia, intensive case management is more effective than standard care in preventing readmissions. ☐ ☐

23. Schneiderian first-rank symptoms predict outcome in schizophrenia. ☐ ☐

24. The mode of onset predicts prognosis in schizophrenia. ☐ ☐

25. Expressed emotion can affect the outcome of most psychiatric disorders. ☐ ☐

ANSWERS

1. Birth injury affects the age of onset of schizophrenia.

True: Perinatal complications have been associated with increased risk, earlier age of onset, negative symptoms and poorer prognosis of schizophrenia. The onset of schizophrenia tends to be earlier in males and in those with a positive family history, obstetric complications in gestation and delivery, especially, those that increase the risk of hypoxia, premorbid cognitive and behavioural deficits, low IQ, cannabis abuse, minor physical anomalies and deviances in brain structure (McKenna 2006, p. 128; Murray et al 1997, p. 295; Sadock & Sadock 2005, p. 1390).

2. Schizophrenia is more common in those of Afro-Caribbean origin.

True: Both Caribbean-born and UK-born Afro-Caribbeans have higher rates of schizophrenia compared to their white neighbours (Gelder et al 2000, p. 602; Stein & Wilkinson 1998, p. 326).

3. In expressed emotion, hostility is more detrimental than derogatory comments.

False: Expressed emotion includes critical comments, hostility, emotional overinvolvement, positive remarks and warmth. The levels of each component and their relative contributions vary across cultures. The first three are the most predictive of relapse. Further specification has not been possible (Gelder et al 2000, p. 626; Stein & Wilkinson 1998, p. 365).

4. Both negative and positive symptoms lead to expressed emotion by carers.

True: The carers of patients with schizophrenia are concerned about the negative symptoms, e.g. social withdrawal, lack of interaction, lack of interests, self-neglect, and the positive symptoms, e.g. disturbed or inappropriate behaviour and threats of violence. They can lead to expressed emotion and hence worsen the symptoms (Gelder et al 2006, p. 296).

5. The Camberwell Family Interview is a semi-structured interview to assess the level of expressed emotion.

True: The Camberwell Family Interview is a semi-structured, standardized interview to assess expressed emotion. The items are critical comments, hostility, emotional overinvolvment, warmth and positive comments. The interview is carried out with a relative and recorded on audiotape. Ratings are based on content and vocal tone (Stein & Wilkinson 1998, p. 364).

6. Neuregulin 1 gene is implicated in the aetiology of schizophrenia.

True: Abnormal glutamate neurotransmission is implicated in the aetiology of schizophrenia. An exon from the neuregulin 1 gene of chromosome 8p, called NRG1, is expressed in CNS synapses and plays a role in the expression and activation of neurotransmitter receptors, including glutamate receptors.

The Icelandic studies implicate NRG1 in the aetiology of schizophrenia. They found a core haplotype in 7.5% of the general population and in 15.4% of patients with schizophrenia. This would account for a 9% increase in risk for siblings of an affected individual. However, no single nucleotide polymorphism was associated with schizophrenia as significantly as the haplotype. This suggests that none of the identified variants were functional polymorphisms (Gelder et al 2006, p. 284; Sadock & Sadock 2005, p. 265).

7. Genes involved in myelination are implicated in the aetiology of schizophrenia.

True: Brains of patients with schizophrenia and bipolar disorders show downregulation of key oligodendrocytes and myelination genes, including transcription factors that regulate these genes, compared with control brains (Gelder et al 2006, p. 280; Wright et al 2005, p. 254).

8. The dysbindin gene is associated with schizophrenia.

True: There is an association between a single nucleotide polymorphism within the gene DTNBP1 encoding dysbindin (dystrobrevin binding protein) located on chromosome 6p22 and schizophrenia. Dysbindin is found both presynaptically and postsynaptically in a variety of neuron populations both cortically and subcortically. Dysbindin is involved in synaptic functioning and signalling. Reduced dysbindin expression has been seen in the dorsolateral prefrontal cortex, hippocampal formation and cingulate gyrus of patients with schizophrenia (Gelder et al 2006, p. 280; Wright et al 2005, p. 254).

9. In schizophrenia the gene for tau protein is abnormal.

False: Increased cerebrospinal fluid tau protein levels are considered a marker of neurodegenerative processes such as Alzheimer's disease. The more pronounced cognitive decline in older schizophrenic patients has been hypothesized to indicate a higher risk of developing Alzheimer's disease. However, no significant differences in cerebrospinal fluid total tau and phospho-tau levels between patients with schizophrenia and controls have been found (Schonknecht et al 2003).

10. 5% of elderly schizophrenics have a family history of schizophrenia in their first-degree relatives.

False: The genetic contribution to schizophrenia decreases with increasing age of onset. A positive family history of schizophrenia is commoner in those whose illness starts in early life or middle age. Recent studies have found no increased risk of schizophrenia in the first-degree relatives of patients with late onset schizophrenia-like psychosis. This suggests that schizophrenia-like psychoses with onset in late life are not genetically associated with schizophrenia (Butler & Pitt 1998, p. 156; Gelder et al 2006, p. 514; Johnstone et al 2004, p. 643).

11. Having a relative with the disease is the largest single risk factor for schizophrenia.

    True: The most powerful risk factor for schizophrenia is having a relative afflicted with the disorder. The prevalence of schizophrenia in the general population is approximately 0.85%. The lifetime risk of developing schizophrenia in relatives of patients with schizophrenia is: parents = 5%; siblings = 10%; children = 14%; children if both parents ill = 46% (Gelder et al 2000, p. 599; Gelder et al 2006, p. 281; Stein & Wilkinson 1998, p. 329).

12. In monozygotic twins discordant for schizophrenia, the risk of schizophrenia in their offspring is equal.

    True: This is because the unaffected twin has the same genetic susceptibility for developing schizophrenia as the affected twin, but for some reason the susceptibility was not expressed (Gelder et al 2006, p. 282).

13. Oneiroid state was described by Mayer-Gross.

    True: Mayer-Gross proposed an organic cause for schizophrenia and introduced the term oneiroid states (Oneiroide Erlebnisform) in 1924. He described it as consisting of acute psychotic symptoms with no organic features. The patient experiences narrowing of consciousness and scenic hallucinations. It can occur in schizophrenia and in intensive care patients who have to be totally passive and dependent on others. The atmosphere is perceived as strange and dream-like. The contents of oneiroid states are often remembered.

    However, Ladislas von Meduna described oneirophrenia in 1939 as a syndrome of endocrine origin characterized by acute confusion, dream-like quality of perceptions (hence the term oneirophrenia), anxiety, delusions, visual hallucinations and complete recovery (Gelder et al 2000, pp. 69, 645; McKenna 2006, p. 287; Sadock & Sadock 2005, p. 1514).

14. Somatization is an important factor in persistent delusional disorder.

    False: Delusional disorder is characterized by a single set of delusions or a set of related delusions, which are usually persistent and sometimes lifelong. The content of the delusions involves situations that occur in real life such as being followed, poisoned, infected, loved at a distance, deceived by spouse or lover, or having a disease (DSM-IV 1994, p. 296; ICD-10 1992, p. 97).

15. Delusional disorder is associated with passivity phenomena.

    False: Delusional disorder is characterized by a single set of delusions or a set of related delusions, which are usually persistent and sometimes lifelong. The content of the delusions involves situations that occur in real life such as being followed, poisoned, infected, loved at a distance, deceived by spouse or lover, or having a disease. Unlike in schizophrenia, the delusions are non-bizarre (DSM-IV 1994, p. 296; ICD-10 1992, p. 97).

16. Persistent delusional disorder is associated with persistent hallucinations.

False: Delusional disorder is characterized by a single set of delusions or a set of related delusions, which are non-bizarre, usually persistent and sometimes lifelong. Tactile or olfactory hallucinations may be present if they are related to the delusional theme. Clear, prominent and persistent auditory hallucinations and delusions of control are incompatible with the diagnosis (DSM-IV 1994, p. 296; ICD-10 1992, p. 97).

17. There is no association between late onset schizophrenia and paranoid personality disorder.

False: Lifelong paranoid or schizoid personality traits are found in 45% of patients with late onset schizophrenia (Gelder et al 2006, p. 514; Johnstone et al 2004, p. 644).

18. The hippocampus is smaller in schizophrenia.

True: Patients with schizophrenia have ventricular enlargement and small but significant reductions in brain weight and volume. There is volume loss in several areas including the hippocampus, prefrontal cortex and temporal cortex (Gelder et al 2006, p. 287; Stein & Wilkinson 1998, p. 344).

19. The information gating process is dysfunctional in schizophrenia.

True: When two sounds are delivered 0.5 seconds apart, normal individuals have a significantly decreased response to the second sound. A full response to the second sound occurs only if it is delayed 0.8 seconds. Thus, the two sounds of the pair are perceived quite differently, solely as a function of the time interval between them. This elementary form of habituation is called sensory gating.

The response to sound is measured using the P50 component of the auditory evoked potential. P50 is the positive wave that occurs 50 ms after the stimulus. Compared to the first sound, the amplitude of the P50 to the second sound is diminished by at least 50% in normals due to sensory gating. This inhibition of the P50 to the second sound, which is a measure of sensory gating, is impaired in most patients with schizophrenia. This may result in their inability to ignore irrelevant stimuli, resulting in feeling flooded with stimuli. They may cope by withdrawing and avoiding contact with others (Sadock & Sadock 2005, p. 1448).

20. The negative symptoms of schizophrenia are related to hypofunction of the pre-frontal cortex.

True: There is evidence from PET, SPECT and fMRI studies to suggest that the negative symptoms of schizophrenia are related to hypofunction of the dorsolateral prefrontal cortex. The hypofrontality may worsen with the duration of illness (Gelder et al 2000, p. 607; Gelder et al 2006, p. 287; Sadock & Sadock 2005, p. 1396).

21. Schizophreniform psychosis associated with temporal lobe epilepsy occurs most commonly shortly after seizures.

False: There are two types of psychoses associated with epilepsy:

1. The transient post-ictal psychosis usually starts 2–72 hours after the seizure and lasts 3–4 days. This is often associated with grandiosity, religious and mystical features.
2. Most epilepsy patients with a schizophreniform psychosis have a chronic interictal illness with no known direct relationship to ictal discharges or seizure events. The psychotic symptoms may worsen with increase in seizure frequency or anticonvulsant withdrawal. In a few, the psychosis may worsen on control of seizures. The terms alternating psychosis and forced paradoxical normalization refer to this antagonism between psychosis and seizures or EEG discharges (Johnstone et al 2004, p. 353; Mitchell 2004, p. 119; Sadock & Sadock 2005, p. 382; Yudofsky & Hales 2002, p. 683).

22. In schizophrenia, intensive case management is more effective than standard care in preventing readmissions.

False: No significant difference was found between intensive and standard case management in a 2-year follow-up study (Byford et al 2000).

23. Schneiderian first-rank symptoms predict outcome in schizophrenia.

False: First-rank symptoms are not predictors of outcome. Factors associated with good outcome include: acute onset, major precipitants, confusion or perplexity, prominent affective symptoms, female gender, good premorbid social adjustment, having no family history of schizophrenia and having a family history of affective disorder (Gelder et al 2006, p. 295; Johnstone et al 2004, p. 406; Stein & Wilkinson 1998, p. 305).

24. The mode of onset predicts prognosis in schizophrenia.

True: Acute onset, precipitating factors, older age of onset, and affective disturbance are associated with good prognosis (Gelder et al 2006, p. 295; Johnstone et al 2004, p. 406; Stein & Wilkinson 1998, p. 305).

25. Expressed emotion can affect the outcome of most psychiatric disorders.

True: Expressed emotion has been shown to predict outcome in schizophrenia, mood disorders, eating disorders and alcoholism (Johnstone et al 2004, p. 404).

Sex and reproduction

Konstantinos Stagias

56

	T	F
1. Penile erection occurs during slow wave sleep.	☐	☐
2. In erectile impotence due to medical causes nocturnal penile tumescence is reduced.	☐	☐
3. Homosexuals have higher rates of mental health problems than heterosexuals.	☐	☐
4. In premenstrual syndrome, the luteal oestrogen level is low.	☐	☐
5. Progesterone is the most effective treatment for premenstrual syndrome.	☐	☐
6. Thioridazine may cause ejaculatory failure.	☐	☐
7. SSRIs can cause erectile impotence.	☐	☐
8. Imipramine decreases libido in more than 25% of people.	☐	☐
9. Pseudocyesis is more common in those who have no children.	☐	☐
10. Psychological problems are more likely following an abortion due to malformation than if the baby was unwanted.	☐	☐
11. Approximately 50% of women experience the blues after pregnancy.	☐	☐
12. Feeling muddled is a common symptom of maternity blues.	☐	☐
13. The Edinburgh postnatal depression scale (EPDS) is a self-rating scale.	☐	☐
14. The Edinburgh postnatal questionnaire specifically asks about risks to the baby.	☐	☐
15. Postnatal depression hampers bonding.	☐	☐
16. Two-thirds of mothers with postnatal depression have bonding problems with their children.	☐	☐
17. Puerperal psychosis usually starts within 2 weeks of delivery.	☐	☐
18. Puerperal psychosis is usually a form of bipolar disorder.	☐	☐
19. The risk of postpartum psychosis is 20% in those who had a previous episode of postpartum psychosis.	☐	☐
20. Systematic desensitization is used in treating sexual dysfunction.	☐	☐
21. Masturbatory reconditioning is used as part of aversive therapy for fetishism.	☐	☐
22. Restriction of sexual contact is a feature of sensate focus therapy.	☐	☐

T F

23. In sex therapy, a male–female therapist pair is better than a single therapist. ☐ ☐

24. Sildenafil citrate acts by prolonging cGMP activity. ☐ ☐

25. Sildenafil is useful in antidepressant induced erectile failure. ☐ ☐

ANSWERS

1. Penile erection occurs during slow wave sleep.

False: Penile and clitoral erections occur during REM sleep or dream sleep. They are unrelated to the content of dreams (Gelder et al 2000, p. 996; Johnstone et al 2004, p. 773).

2. In erectile impotence due to medical causes nocturnal penile tumescence is reduced.

True: Organic causes for erectile dysfunction can be considered negligible if a man has good erections with masturbation or with partners other than his usual one, or has spontaneous erections at times when he does not plan to have intercourse, morning erections or erections during sleep. Erections during REM sleep or nocturnal penile tumescence can be measured using the 'stamp test' or strain gauge. In the stamp test postage stamps are stuck round the base of the penis at night. If in the morning they are broken it would indicate that he had an erection during sleep (Sadock & Sadock 2005, p. 1923).

3. Homosexuals have higher rates of mental health problems than heterosexuals.

True: Homosexuals have higher rates of anxiety, mood and substance use disorders, and suicidal ideation and suicide attempts compared with heterosexual populations. The risk of completed suicide is up to 13-fold greater than that of heterosexuals. This may be related to victimization and abuse during adolescence and stigmatization and discrimination during adulthood (Johnstone et al 2004, p. 769; Sadock & Sadock 2005, p. 1960).

4. In premenstrual syndrome, the luteal oestrogen level is low.

False: Premenstrual tension or premenstrual syndrome occurs cyclically during the luteal phase and resolves once menses start. Many, but not all, studies have found low progesterone, high oestrogen, or low progesterone to oestrogen ratio during the luteal phase (Sadock & Sadock 2005, p. 2317).

5. Progesterone is the most effective treatment for premenstrual syndrome.

False: More than 50 different treatments have been proposed, including progesterone, oral contraceptives, diuretics and psychotropics, indicating that there is no single effective cure. Moreover, placebo response has been as high as 65%. There have been encouraging reports of the effectiveness of SSRIs and CBT, especially for mood symptoms (Gelder et al 2006, p. 404; Sadock & Sadock 2005, p. 2319).

6. Thioridazine may cause ejaculatory failure.

True: Phenothiazines such as chlorpromazine and thioridazine impair erection and ejaculation in men and vaginal lubrication and orgasm in women due to their ability to block adrenergic and cholinergic receptors. Thioridazine may cause retrograde ejaculation in up to 50% of patients. Retrograde ejaculation is a startling but harmless condition in which the seminal fluid backs up into the bladder rather than being propelled through the penile urethra. Patients still have the orgasmic pleasure, but the orgasm is dry (Sadock & Sadock 2005, p. 1924).

7. SSRIs can cause erectile impotence.

True: SSRIs can cause erectile dysfunction. However, decreased libido, ejaculatory delay and anorgasmia are much more common than erectile dysfunction. Sexual side-effects including erectile dysfunction may be more common with paroxetine than with other SSRIs. Paroxetine may contribute to erectile dysfunction by inhibiting nitric oxide synthetase. Moreover, tricyclic antidepressants are more likely to cause erectile dysfunction than SSRIs. Overall, sexual side-effects most frequently occur with antihypertensives, antipsychotics, MAOIs and SSRIs (Cookson et al 2002, p. 253; Crenshaw & Goldberg 1996, p. 292; Gelder et al 2006, p. 477; King 2004, p. 588).

8. Imipramine decreases libido in more than 25% of people.

True: Imipramine causes sexual side-effects in more than 50% of patients. The commonest side-effects are decreased libido and delayed orgasm (Crenshaw & Goldberg 1996, p. 276).

9. Pseudocyesis is more common in those who have no children.

False: Pseudocyesis refers to the condition when a person who is not pregnant is convinced that she is pregnant and develops symptoms and signs of pregnancy. The differential diagnoses include:

1. Delusion of pregnancy which is not associated with the somatic symptoms of pregnancy
2. Simulated pregnancy and
3. Pseudopregnancy caused by endocrine tumours.

Pseudocyesis is usually associated with organic psychiatric disorders, schizophrenia and learning disability. Pseudocyesis has been associated with social deprivation, long-stay inpatients, being unmarried and widowhood.

10. Psychological problems are more likely following an abortion due to malformation than if the baby was unwanted.

True: Most of those who voluntarily abort suffer no adverse pychological effects, either in the short or the long term. The psychological consequences of termination are usually mild and transient, although they are greater for mothers who have cultural or religious beliefs against termination. Termination of a wanted pregnancy because of an abnormal karyotype or fetal abnormalities can be traumatic. The emotional consequences of miscarriage are comparable to those of perinatal death. They are likely to be less severe because there has been little time for attachment to the newly conceived, but such an event may still represent the loss of a greatly desired child. The incidence of depression is four times the rate in the general population (Gelder et al 2000, p. 1200; Gelder et al 2006, p. 401; Sadock & Sadock 2005, p. 1702).

11. Approximately 50% of women experience the blues after pregnancy.

True: About half of all mothers experience a brief period of lability of mood, irritability, crying, dysphoria and puzzlement at their condition. They frequently complain of feeling 'confused' and muddled. It occurs between the third and fifth days postpartum and usually lasts a few hours (Gelder et al 2000, p. 1202).

12. Feeling muddled is a common symptom of maternity blues.

True: Patients often complain of being confused but tests of cognitive function are normal (Gelder et al 2006, p. 401).

13. The Edinburgh postnatal depression scale (EPDS) is a self-rating scale.

True: The EPDS is a simple 10-item self-report scale. It can be completed in less than 5 minutes. The mother is asked to underline 1 of 4 possible responses that describes how she has been feeling over the previous 7 days. The EPDS reliably identifies women at high risk of developing depression. However, EPDS is not a diagnostic instrument and clinical judgement should always take precedence over any score obtained (Johnstone et al 2004, p. 751).

14. The Edinburgh postnatal questionnaire specifically asks about risks to the baby.

False: The 10 questions cover depressive symptoms including thoughts of self-harm. It does not ask about risk to the baby (Johnstone et al 2004, p. 751).

15. Postnatal depression hampers bonding.

True: Postnatal depression adversely affects the mother–infant relationship and the cognitive and emotional development of the infant. Evidence of negative consequences later in childhood is less clear (Gelder et al 2006, p. 403; Johnstone et al 2004, p. 749).

16. Two-thirds of mothers with postnatal depression have bonding problems with their children.

False: Mother–infant relationship or bonding disorders such as lack of emotional response, rejection of the infant and pathological anger occur in a quarter of cases of postnatal depression (Gelder et al 2000, p. 1204).

17. Puerperal psychosis usually starts within 2 weeks of delivery.

True: The onset of puerperal psychosis is usually within the first 1–2 weeks or the first month after delivery, but rarely may occur in the first 2 days (Gelder et al 2006, p. 402; Johnstone et al 2004, p. 747).

18. Puerperal psychosis is usually a form of bipolar disorder.

True: The majority of puerperal psychoses are affective in nature, with rapid fluctuations in mood and often a mixture of manic and depressive symptoms. The first episode of bipolar disorder is seven times more likely to occur in the postpartum period. The greatest risk factors are a past history of puerperal psychosis and past or a family history of bipolar disorder. There is also a specific familial risk for puerperal psychosis in bipolar disorder (Johnstone et al 2004, p. 747).

19. The risk of postpartum psychosis is 20% in those who had a previous episode of postpartum psychosis.

True: Women with a previous history of puerperal psychosis or bipolar disorder have a 20–30% risk of puerperal psychosis in subsequent pregnancies. The risk rises to above 50% in those who have a family history of bipolar disorder (Gelder et al 2000, p. 1203; Johnstone et al 2004, p. 747).

20. Systematic desensitization is used in treating sexual dysfunction.

True: Behaviour therapists view sexual dysfunction as a phobia of sexual interaction and use the traditional treatment for phobias, i.e. systematic desensitization (Sadock & Sadock 2005, p. 1931).

21. Masturbatory reconditioning is used as part of aversive therapy for fetishism.

False: In masturbatory reconditioning the subject picks a more appropriate and acceptable image to arouse himself and uses this while masturbating in order to recondition himself to a more appropriate stimulus. In aversive therapy the subject picks a non-acceptable deviant image and allows himself to become aroused before receiving an electric shock (www.soc.ucsb.edu/sexinfo).

22. Restriction of sexual contact is a feature of sensate focus therapy.

True: Sensate focus exercises are designed to allow the couple to develop an awareness of their arousal level by lessening the demand characteristics of the sexual experience and the associated anxiety. In a slow graduated fashion they take turns giving and receiving pleasure. Initially, the touching is restricted to non-genital/non-breast stimulation. They later progress to genital stimulation and intercourse (Gelder et al 2000, p. 892; Sadock & Sadock 2005, p. 1929).

23. In sex therapy, a male–female therapist pair is better than a single therapist.

False: There is no particular advantage of a co-therapy team over an individual therapist. A single female therapist may have advantages over a single male therapist. Similarly, there are no apparent advantages of daily over weekly or even monthly sessions.

24. Sildenafil citrate acts by prolonging cGMP activity.

True: The normal process of penile erection is as follows:

Sexual stimulation → nitric oxide activates enzyme guanylate cyclase → increased cyclic guanosine monophosphate (cGMP) → arteriole smooth muscle relaxation and vasodilatation in the corpus cavernosum → penile erection.

Sildenafil is a nitric oxide enhancer. It inhibits phosphodiesterase type 5 (PDE-5), the isoenzyme that degrades cavernosal cGMP. cGMP, the second messenger of nitric oxide, is the crucial mediator of penile erection. By inhibiting PDE-5, sildenafil protracts penile cGMP activity and prolongs erection. Sildenafil does not initiate erections, but solely augments erections that occur in response to a natural sexual stimulation (Gelder et al 2006, p. 481; Sadock & Sadock 2005, p. 1932).

25. Sildenafil is useful in antidepressant induced erectile failure.

True: Antidepressant drugs often cause decreased libido, impaired erection and delayed or absent ejaculation and orgasm. Erectile, ejaculatory and orgasmic side-effects respond to sildenafil, taladafil and vardenafil (Sadock & Sadock 2002, p. 980; Sadock & Sadock 2005, p. 1925).

Statistics – 1

Chittaranjan Andrade

	T	F

1. ANOVA is used to compare two groups.

2. Scales with multiple answers increase reliability in measuring attitude.

3. The chi-squared test of a 5 by 3 contingency table will have 15 degrees of freedom.

4. The chi-squared test could be used in a study of response to a new antidepressant in four different hospital populations.

5. Correlation is used to compare two groups.

6. Regarding correlation coefficient 'r', a value of +1 or –1, implies a cause–effect relationship.

7. Knowing the outcome status in a cohort study may lead to information bias.

8. A type II error occurs when a real difference is missed.

9. Observer-rated scales are prone to 'halo effect'.

10. The least squares method is used for dichotomous variables.

11. Logistic regression is done by the least squares method.

12. Means taken from large samples of a skewed distribution approximate to a normal distribution.

13. T^2 test is used for non-parametric variables.

14. Normal distribution is a requirement for parametric testing.

15. The power of a test varies with the size of the sample.

16. Volunteer bias would deter healthy people from responding to postal questionnaires.

17. R^2 usually increases if a further independent variable is added.

18. Operational definition of concepts used in rating scales increases reliability.

19. Newspaper advertising can be used for random sampling.

20. Psychiatric screening instruments used in a general hospital are usually used to detect uncommon syndromes.

21. In a trial of two antidepressants, failure to show a difference in outcome may be due to there being less than 5% of subjects with previous episodes of depression.

T F

22. A result statistically significant at a level of 5% implies that the correlation coefficient is 0.95. ☐ ☐

23. A sensitive test has a low number of false positives. ☐ ☐

24. Split-half reliability measures the validity of a test. ☐ ☐

25. In an experiment to determine whether drug therapy or hypnosis is better as a treatment to stop smoking, the results are measured by the number of cigarettes smoked after treatment. In this study, hypnosis is a dependent variable. ☐ ☐

ANSWERS

1. ANOVA is used to compare two groups.

True: ANOVA (analysis of variance) is a test used to compare means across two or more groups. Thus, we can use ANOVA to compare the mean IQ scores of men and women in a sample; or, we can use ANOVA to compare the mean baseline depression scores of patients randomized to experimental antidepressant drug (active control) and placebo (inactive control) groups. When there are only two groups, we often use the independent sample *t*-test because it is easier to compute.

2. Scales with multiple answers increase reliability in measuring attitude.

False: In general, the larger the number of categories in a variable, the more difficult it becomes for a test to yield significant results. Therefore, if a scale has multiple answers for each item, it becomes more difficult to achieve high reliability for a sample of given size.

3. The chi-squared test of a 5 by 3 contingency table will have 15 degrees of freedom.

False: The degrees of freedom for a chi-squared contingency table is computed by the formula (Rows–1) × (Columns–1). In this case, it will be (5–1)(3–1); that is, 4×2; that is, 8.

4. The chi-squared test could be used in a study of response to a new antidepressant in four different hospital populations.

True: True, if patients are classified as responders and non-responders. Then, we would compare the proportion of responders to non-responders in the four different hospital groups.

False, if response is assessed as a continuous variable, such as using the Hamilton Depression Rating Scale. One-way ANOVA would then be a more appropriate test.

Given that this question does not specify whether response is measured as a continuous variable or as a binary outcome the answer is true – chi-squared *could* be used.

5. Correlation is used to compare two groups.

False: Correlation is used to measure the strength of the relationship between two (usually continuous) variables. For example, we can use correlation to measure the strength of the association between IQ scores and marks obtained in an examination, or between serum antidepressant levels and percentage improvement in depression ratings. When the distribution of the variables is normal we use Pearson's product moment correlation. When the distribution is significantly non-normal the variables are ranked and a rank-order (Spearman's) correlation is performed.

6. Regarding correlation coefficient 'r', a value of +1 or −1 implies a cause–effect relationship.

False: Values of +1 or −1 indicate a perfect correlation, i.e. as the value of one variable changes by a certain degree, the value of the other variable changes by an exactly corresponding degree (though not necessarily the same in absolute value). Correlation measures only the strength of association between two variables; it never implies causality. Consider a hypothetical situation. We wish to determine the correlation between the number of eyeballs and the number of toes in different households in a residential area. We find that one household has 2 eyeballs and 10 toes altogether; in another household, there are 8 eyeballs and 40 toes, and so on. Assuming that nobody is handicapped or otherwise abnormal there will be a perfect correlation between the number of eyeballs and the number of toes. But, neither causes the other!

7. Knowing the outcome status in a cohort study may lead to information bias.

False: In cohort studies we try to measure the outcome status. Knowing the exposure status in a cohort study, or the outcome status in a case-control study, would lead to information bias.

8. A type II error occurs when a real difference is missed.

True: A type II (false negative) error is said to occur when the null hypothesis is mistakenly accepted, i.e. when a significant relationship between variables remains unrecognized. Type II errors occur when the sample size is small, when the sampling is biased, and when heterogeneity in the sample is large (and hence when the standard deviations are large).

The probability of a type II error is known as beta. The power of a test is a measure of how likely the test is to avoid a type II error.

9. Observer-rated scales are prone to 'halo effect'.

True: Halo effect is when the observer is biased by one positive aspect of the subject. For example, good looking candidates are more likely to pass viva examinations (Fear 2004, p. 32).

10. The least squares method is used for dichotomous variables.

False: The least squares method is used in regression to examine the relationship between continuous variables.

11. Logistic regression is done by the least squares method.

False: It is linear regression which employs the least squares method. The least squares method refers to the technique by which linear regression lines are fitted to a scatter plot of individual data points. The vertical distances between the individual data points and the line are calculated, squared and added together. The line of best fit is that line which has the smallest 'sum of squares' (Puri & Tyrer 1998, p. 278).

12. Means taken from large samples of a skewed distribution approximate to a normal distribution.

False: If the population distribution is skewed, this will be reflected in its standard deviation. A random sample drawn from such a sample will also be skewed, and this will also be reflected in the standard deviation of the sample. As the standard error of the mean (which describes the distribution of means of samples drawn from the population) is computed by dividing the standard deviation by the square root of the sample size, it follows that the standard error will also reflect the skewness. Hence, the means will NOT approximate to a normal distribution.

13. T^2 test is used for non-parametric variables.

False: The Hotelling's T^2 test is used in multivariate analysis of variance (MANOVA), and is applied to continuous variables. NB: This is different from the student *t*-test.

14. Normal distribution is a requirement for parametric testing.

True: Tests such as the *t*-test, ANOVA, ANCOVA, RMANOVA, MANOVA and Pearson's correlation are parametric procedures. They test dependent variables which are continuous in nature, i.e. operationalized along interval or ratio scales. For parametric testing, the dependent variable should be normally distributed. Incidentally, this requirement notwithstanding, parametric tests are generally robust to violations of normality, unless the skewness or kurtosis is marked.

If distributions are significantly non-normal, non-parametric alternatives, e.g. Wilcoxon test, Mann–Whitney test, Kruskall–Wallis test and Spearman's correlation procedure are used. These tests are conducted on ranked data.

15. The power of a test varies with the size of the sample.

True: A larger sample is associated with greater statistical power.

16. Volunteer bias would deter healthy people from responding to postal questionnaires.

True: Persons who suffer from the problem addressed in the questionnaire would be more interested in the subject than healthy persons, and would therefore be more likely to take the trouble to respond to a postal questionnaire.

17. R^2 usually increases if a further independent variable is added.

True: The extent of increase in R^2 depends on the extent to which the new independent variable correlates with the dependent variable and explains an additional proportion of the variance in the dependent variable.

Here is the explanatory note. In multiple regression, R is the correlation between the actual value of the dependent variable in an index case and the value of the dependent variable predicted by the regression equation for that case. Expressed otherwise, R is the multiple correlation coefficient, much as r is the correlation coefficient between two continuous variables. Just as r^2 (the square of the correlation coefficient) is the proportion of the dependent variable explained by the independent variable, so too is R^2 the proportion of the dependent variable explained by the different independent variables in the multiple regression equation.

18. Operational definition of concepts used in rating scales increases reliability.

True: Operationalization of a variable is the procedure whereby a variable is defined in a way that permits its accurate (or at least standardized) measurement.

For example, the question 'How did you sleep last night?' may have three choices as answers: Very poorly, Poorly, and Well. Different patients may make different choices despite having slept for the same period. This can be more reliably assessed if the choices are operationalized as follows:

- Well: Had the necessary quota of sleep, felt refreshed on awaking
- Poorly: Experienced disturbed sleep, lost up to 2 hours of sleep
- Very poorly: Lost more than 2 hours of sleep.

19. Newspaper advertising can be used for random sampling.

False: Subjects recruited through newspaper advertisements are those who have direct or indirect access to a newspaper, those who are interested in the subject of the study, those who have the personality characteristics which make them more likely to respond or volunteer, those who may be impoverished and thereby more interested in the inconvenience reimbursements offered for completing the study, etc. Such subjects, by virtue of these biases, are not representative of the population. Newspaper advertisements for sampling are useful when recruitment for the study is slow or difficult.

20. Psychiatric screening instruments used in a general hospital are usually used to detect uncommon syndromes.

False: Screening instruments are used to quickly and conveniently identify patients who may have a disorder. Thus, screening instruments can be applied in group settings, or to large samples of patients. Thereby, screening is a time-cost-energy effective substitute for more accurate but more expensive or time-consuming procedures, and can be used to detect any syndrome, common or uncommon.

21. In a trial of two antidepressants, failure to show a difference in outcome may be due to there being less than 5% of subjects with previous episodes of depression.

False: Insufficient statistical power or a genuine lack of any difference between the two drugs would be the only reasons. Insufficient statistical power could be due to:

1. Insufficient sample size
2. The use of a categorical outcome variable (which would require a larger sample size) instead of a continuous outcome variable
3. Sample heterogeneity (which would increase the standard deviation and hence necessitate a large sample size)
4. High similarity of antidepressant effect of the two drugs (which would require a larger sample size to detect the small difference).

22. A result statistically significant at a level of 5% implies that the correlation coefficient is 0.95.

False: Statistical significance may relate to means, proportions, or other matters, and not necessarily to the correlation coefficient. In the case of the correlation coefficient, a very large correlation coefficient may not be significant if the sample size is small. And, a very small correlation coefficient may well be significant if the sample size is very large.

23. A sensitive test has a low number of false positives.

False: It has few false negatives.

Sensitivity is the ability of the test to identify the presence of disease.

Sensitivity = true positives/total cases.

Specificity is the ability of the test to identify the absence of disease.

Specificity = true negatives/total non-cases.

Positive predictive value is the proportion of cases that actually have the disease out of the total number of cases predicted by the test to have the disease.

Negative predictive value is the proportion of cases that actually are disease free out of the total number of cases predicted by the test to be disease free.

Efficiency is the ability of the test to correctly identify presence and absence of disease, i.e. the proportion of cases correctly classified.

Note that sensitivity and specificity are often inversely related. A sensitive test often has low specificity, and vice versa.

24. Split-half reliability measures the validity of a test.

False: Split-half reliability is one way to measure the internal consistency of a test which purports to measure a single construct. It is a test of reliability. In split-half reliability, the items in the test are split into two equal halves and the scores for the two halves are correlated. If the correlation is high, the test is internally consistent, i.e. the halves of the test are likely measuring the same thing. Cronbach's alpha is a special way of measuring split-half reliability. It is the average correlation of all the possible ways in which the test items can be divided into two halves.

25. In an experiment to determine whether drug therapy or hypnosis is better as a treatment to stop smoking, the results are measured by the number of cigarettes smoked after treatment. In this study, hypnosis is a dependent variable.

False: Treatment (drug therapy vs. hypnosis) is the independent variable, and number of cigarettes smoked is the dependent variable.

Statistics – 2

Chittaranjan Andrade

	T	F

1. Analysis of variance enables a test of significance of multiple repeated mean scores on a measure of a normally distributed variable. ☐ ☐

2. The Barnum effect explains in part people's belief in astrology. ☐ ☐

3. The chi-squared test can be used to compare the Ham-D scores between patients treated with an experimental antidepressant drug and placebo. ☐ ☐

4. The chi-squared test could be used in a study of response to a new antidepressant at four 3-monthly intervals in one hospital population. ☐ ☐

5. Correlation coefficient refers to how one variable alters with change in another paired variable. ☐ ☐

6. Correlation coefficient 'r' may be used when studying non-linear relationships. ☐ ☐

7. In a normal distribution, 68% of the population lie within one standard deviation of the mean. ☐ ☐

8. Standard error of a proportion will depend on the proportion in the wider population. ☐ ☐

9. The Hawthorne effect can be a source of error. ☐ ☐

10. The least squares method is used for normally distributed continuous data. ☐ ☐

11. Logistic regression is used for categorical variables. ☐ ☐

12. The arithmetic mean is equal to the median when the distribution of scores is unimodal and symmetrical. ☐ ☐

13. The null hypothesis is that the two populations being compared are different. ☐ ☐

14. Parametric statistics are generally more powerful than non-parametric tests. ☐ ☐

15. If, in a 60-year-old man, the probability of having A is 0.2, and B is 0.1, and both are independent, then the probability of having neither is 0.7. ☐ ☐

16. Logistic regression is done by the least squares method. ☐ ☐

17. In the design of an experimental study, prospective methods are relatively inexpensive. ☐ ☐

18. In psychological assessment, the response set is the responses the subject believes the interviewer wants. ☐ ☐

T   F

19. Snowballing can be used for random sampling. ☐ ☐

20. In a study of the ego-strength of 16-year-old females working in a clothes factory, as an indicator of the ego-strength of all 16-year-old girls in the same city, the sample is biased. ☐ ☐

21. A treatment trial shows no significant difference in efficacy between two antidepressants. This may be because the sample size considerations were based on active drug versus placebo comparison. ☐ ☐

22. A result statistically significant at a level of 5% implies that the result could not be accepted as valid. ☐ ☐

23. A specific test has a low number of false negatives. ☐ ☐

24. Instruments need to result in a normal distribution of results to have validity. ☐ ☐

25. A researcher investigates the effect of smoking marijuana on motivation. He finds motivation levels lower in smokers than in a control population. In this study, marijuana smoking is the independent variable. ☐ ☐

ANSWERS

1. Analysis of variance enables a test of significance of multiple repeated mean scores on a measure of a normally distributed variable.

True: For example, if we obtain Ham-D scores in one or more groups of patients at several different points in time, we may want to know whether there has been a significant change in the scores across time. If there is more than one group, we may also want to know if the rate of change across time differs between groups. We use repeated measures analysis of variance (RMANOVA) for this design. To examine changes in only one group across time, we use a one-way RMANOVA; the 'one way' refers to differences across time. To examine changes in two or more groups across time, we use a two-way RMANOVA; one of the 'two ways' refers to differences across time, and the other to differences between groups.

2. The Barnum effect explains in part people's belief in astrology.

True: The Barnum effect is named after the American circus proprietor P. T. Barnum, some of whose exhibits were frauds which preyed upon the gullibility of the audience. Astrological columns present generalizations which apply to most people; people who read these columns are struck by the seeming relevance of the column to their own life and experiences, and therefore credit astrology with the status of a science.

The Barnum effect is also known as the Forer effect, after psychologist B. R. Forer who found that people tend to accept vague and general personality descriptions as uniquely applicable to themselves without realizing that the same description could be applied to almost anyone.

This effect is also known as the subjective validation effect, or the personal validation effect, because the validation of the construct under consideration is based on subjectivity, personal experience, and credulity.

3. The chi-squared test can be used to compare the Ham-D scores between patients treated with an experimental antidepressant drug and placebo.

False: The chi-squared test is used to compare proportions between two or more groups. For example, it could be used to compare the proportion of responders to non-responders in antidepressant- and placebo-treated groups.

The chi-squared test cannot be used to compare a quantitative variable, such as Ham-D scores, between groups.

For example, suppose 10 men and 15 women were randomized to receive a new antidepressant drug and 12 men and 12 women were randomized to receive placebo. We wish to find out whether the two treatment groups were similar in sex distribution at baseline. We use the chi-squared test to determine whether the sex distribution differed significantly between antidepressant- and placebo-treated groups.

4. The chi-squared test could be used in a study of response to a new antidepressant at four 3-monthly intervals in one hospital population.

False: Antidepressant response is commonly assessed as a continuous variable using measures such as the Ham-D. Repeated assessments of the same variable across time are tested using RMANOVA. As there is only one group being tested, the test would be one-way RMANOVA.

5. Correlation coefficient refers to how one variable alters with change in another paired variable.

False: Linear regression tests how one variable alters with changes in another paired variable. Correlation examines only the strength of association between two paired variables. Linear regression and correlation are related procedures.

6. Correlation coefficient 'r' may be used when studying non-linear relationships.

False: The Pearson's product-moment correlation coefficient is used only when the relationship between the variables is linear (hence the concept of linear regression). It cannot be used when the relationship between the variables is nonlinear (hence the concept of curvilinear regression). Curvilinear relationships may be U-shaped, sigmoid, or of other shapes.

7. In a normal distribution, 68% of the population lies within one standard deviation of the mean.

True: In general, continuous variables in nature are normally distributed. This means that 68.3% of the population lies within one standard deviation of the mean; 95.5% lies within two standard deviations of the mean; and 99.7% lies within three standard deviations of the mean. A characteristic of the normal distribution is that the curve of variable value (X-axis) and frequency (Y-axis) is bilaterally symmetrical and shaped like a bell. Hence, the normal distribution is also known as the bell-shaped curve. It is also called the Gaussian distribution, after the mathematician Gauss. In the normal distribution, the mean, median, and mode coincide.

8. Standard error of a proportion will depend on the proportion in the wider population.

True: The standard error of a proportion is given by the square root of:

$P(1-P)/n$ where P is the value of the proportion and n is the sample size.

9. The Hawthorne effect can be a source of error.

True: The Hawthorne effect can be a source of error in any type of research. The Hawthorne effect is said to occur when the act of measurement influences that which is being measured. For example, when the behaviour of subjects is measured by observation, the subjects know that they are being observed, they become self-conscious and behave less naturally. Another example is when the pupil of the eye is measured. When light is thrown into the eye so that the pupil can be visualized, the pupil constricts. When measuring the length of the penis, touching can alter the variable being measured.

10. The least squares method is used for normally distributed continuous data.

True: The least squares method is used in regression to examine the relationship between continuous variables. One of the assumptions of the procedure is that the variables are normally distributed. If this assumption is not met, the procedure is carried out after log-transforming one or both variables. Alternatively, the procedure can be applied on the ranked data.

11. Logistic regression is used for categorical variables.

True: Logistic regression is used to predict or explain the value of a categorical variable which is dichotomous. It cannot be used when the variable is classified into three or more categories.

12. The arithmetic mean is equal to the median when the distribution of scores is unimodal and symmetrical.

True: A unimodal distribution has only one mode, and a symmetrical distribution is a normal distribution. In a normal distribution, the mean, median, and mode coincide.

13. The null hypothesis is that the two populations being compared are different.

False: The null hypothesis states that the populations under comparison do not differ significantly, or that the relationship between two variables is not significant. It is the alternative hypothesis which states that the populations are different, or that there is a significant relationship between variables.

14. Parametric statistics are generally more powerful than non-parametric tests.

True: This is why, wherever possible, variables should be operationalized along interval or ratio scales. Data so collected should never be split into categories unless there is a very definite reason to do so (e.g. a non-normal distribution, or a non-linear relationship between variables to be compared, or the existence of natural categories within the data).

Note that 'powerful' tests are those which are less vulnerable to a type II (false negative) error.

15. If, in a 60-year-old man, the probability of having A is 0.2, and B is 0.1, and both are independent, then the probability of having neither is 0.7.

False: The probability of NOT having A is $1.0 - 0.2 = 0.8$. The probability of NOT having B is $1.0 - 0.1 = 0.9$. The probability of occurrence of BOTH of two independent events is given by the product of their individual probabilities. Therefore, the probability of occurrence of both 'A absent' and 'B absent' is $0.8 \times 0.9 = 0.72$. Note that the value of probability can range from 0 to 1. A probability of 1 means that the event will certainly occur, whereas a probability of 0 means that the event will certainly not occur.

16. Logistic regression is done by the least squares method.

False: Linear and multiple regression, which are applied to continuous variables, employ the least squares method. Logistic regression makes use of the binomial distribution in making its parameter estimates.

17. In the design of an experimental study, prospective methods are relatively inexpensive.

False: In retrospective designs, data are drawn from the charts of subjects already treated in the past. Prospective methods require a fresh sample to be drawn from the population. This may take much time, especially if the study selection criteria are rigorous. Longitudinal prospective studies are even more lengthy than cross-sectional studies. As a result, expenses mount. The advantages of retrospective designs are lower time and financial costs. Furthermore, more data may be available with retrospective designs. Retrospective research has many disadvantages. Subjects would not have been randomized. Data might not have been obtained in a standardized fashion. Data might not have been reliably recorded. All the relevant variables might not have been addressed. Appropriate assessment tools might not have been used. Situations might have changed. Cohort effects might be present due to changes in patterns of patient attendance, changes in assessment and treatment styles down the years, etc. Overall, therefore, retrospective studies are good when we want a large body of data, or data to formulate hypotheses. Prospective studies are preferable when we want to confirm hypotheses.

18. In psychological assessment, the response set is the responses the subject believes the interviewer wants.

False: Response set is a source of error in self-rated and certain other instruments. The simplest example of response set is when a subject answers 'yes' to a borderline question after answering 'yes' to a series of preceding questions; or, in the Wisconsin Card Sorting Test, when the subject sticks to the same rule of card sorting even after the rules have changed. Thus, a series of questions puts the subject into a frame of mind, and this frame of mind influences his responses to subsequent questions. Rating scales in which closely similar items are placed together are prone to 'response sets'.

19. Snowballing can be used for random sampling.

False: Snowball sampling is the procedure whereby one subject recruits those of his contacts who are willing to participate in the study, and each of these contacts recruits further contacts. Snowballing is biased because only persons known to or through the initial contact are eligible for recruitment and they may not be representative of the population.

Snowballing is useful when it is hard to locate the population, e.g. to locate homosexuals in a society which does not allow the open expression of gay behaviour.

20. In a study of the ego-strength of 16-year-old females working in a clothes factory, as an indicator of the ego-strength of all 16-year-old girls in the same city, the sample is biased.

True: The ego-strength is likely to vary between, for example, girls who study in college and those who work in a factory. Therefore, girls who work in a factory cannot be considered representative of all girls of that age in the city.

21. A treatment trial shows no significant difference in efficacy between two antidepressants. This may be because the sample size considerations were based on active drug versus placebo comparison.

True: The difference between an antidepressant drug and placebo is likely to be large and, hence, a smaller sample size will be sufficient to adequately power the study to identify the difference to a statistically significant extent. In contrast, the difference between two antidepressant drugs is likely to be small and, therefore, larger sample sizes will be required to demonstrate the statistical significance of the difference. If power calculations are based on antidepressant vs. placebo, the sample size will not be adequate to identify true differences between two antidepressants.

22. A result statistically significant at a level of 5% implies that the result could not be accepted as valid.

False: It means that the null hypothesis is rejected and the alternative hypothesis is accepted.

23. A specific test has a low number of false negatives.

True: Specificity is the ability of the test to identify the absence of disease.

Specificity = true negatives/total non-cases. See Q23 in Statistics – 1.

24. Instruments need to result in a normal distribution of results to have validity.

False: If the Ham-D is administered to persons in the general population, most will obtain very low scores, but those who are depressed will obtain high scores.

Thus, the distribution will be non-normal. However, Ham-D is still a valid measure of the severity of depression.

25. A researcher investigates the effect of smoking marijuana on motivation. He finds motivation levels lower in smokers than in a control population. In this study, marijuana smoking is the independent variable.

True: And motivation is the dependent variable.

Statistics – 3

Chittaranjan Andrade

	T	F
1. ANOVA is appropriate in a study with a repeated measures design.	☐	☐
2. In a double-blind controlled study on the effect a new drug has on anxiety levels, patients are not told whether they are receiving drug or placebo.	☐	☐
3. The chi-squared test could be used in a study of comparison of pay vs. job satisfaction in two groups of workers, one male and the other female.	☐	☐
4. Chi-squared could be used to analyse the results of a questionnaire measuring level of anxiety in a random sample of the population.	☐	☐
5. The variation in a variable can be explained by the square of its correlation coefficient with another variable.	☐	☐
6. The closer the correlation coefficient 'r' is to zero, the fewer errors made in prediction.	☐	☐
7. In an IQ test showing normal distribution with a mean of 100 and a standard deviation of 15, approximately 15% of the population have an IQ less than 70.	☐	☐
8. The Fisher exact probability test should not be used for small numbers.	☐	☐
9. Incidence includes cases that are no longer current.	☐	☐
10. Non-parametric statistics can be measured by least squares.	☐	☐
11. The Mann–Whitney test could be used to analyse the results of a questionnaire measuring level of anxiety in a random sample of the population.	☐	☐
12. The mode is a measure of central tendency.	☐	☐
13. In an experiment to determine whether drug therapy or hypnosis is better in treatment to stop smoking, the results are measured by the number of cigarettes smoked after treatment. In this study the null hypothesis postulates there will be a significant difference between drug therapy and hypnosis in reduction of cigarette smoking.	☐	☐
14. A population pyramid can be used to describe the sex and age structure of a population.	☐	☐
15. The primacy effect includes deciding about a person by their physical appearance.	☐	☐
16. In categorical independent variables, regression is usually by the method of least squares.	☐	☐

T F

17. Scores obtained on two successive administrations correlated 0.90 indicate reliability and not validity of a personality questionnaire.

18. A new 'treatment' is tried on gifted children, all of whom have an IQ greater than 140. If the mean IQ of the sample is 150, and if the treatment has no effect on IQ, the mean IQ that one would expect on re-testing 1 year later is slightly greater than 150.

19. The telephone directory can be used for random sampling.

20. Standard deviation is a measure of precision of an estimate.

21. A statement that an association between two variables is statistically significant means that, if the study is repeated, chances are that the significance of the association would be the same.

22. A result statistically significant at a level of 5% implies that there is a 5% chance that the results suggest a wrong conclusion.

23. Stratification increases the power of a study.

24. The T^2 test is used for non-parametric variables.

25. In an experiment designed to investigate the effect of home background on intelligence, the family size is a dependent variable.

ANSWERS

1. ANOVA is appropriate in a study with a repeated measures design.

True: A repeated measures design is one in which subjects are assessed at two or more time points. If there is only one group and only two time points, and if the dependent variable is a continuous variable, the paired t-test is the simplest procedure. However, a model of ANOVA known as repeated measures ANOVA can also be performed. It is the only test possible when there is more than one group or more than two time points.

If there are only two assessment points, the mixed-model procedure is used. If there are more than two assessment points, the assumptions of the mixed-model (sphericity, homogeneity of variances, etc.) are often violated, and repeated measures multivariate ANOVA is the more appropriate procedure. It can be executed using the Hotelling's T-square, Pillai's, Wilk's, or Roy's procedures.

2. In a double-blind controlled study on the effect a new drug has on anxiety levels, patients are not told whether they are receiving drug or placebo.

True: Single-blind studies are those in which the investigator does not know the experimental condition to which the subject belongs, but the subject is aware of the assignment. Double-blind studies are those in which neither subject nor investigator is aware of the treatment assignment. Subject blindness is necessary to ensure that subject expectations about the treatment do not bias their response, or their report of response. Investigator blindness is necessary to ensure that investigator expectations from treatment or pressures on the investigator do not contaminate their assessments.

3. The chi-squared test could be used in a study of comparison of pay vs. job satisfaction in two groups of workers, one male and the other female.

False: Pay and job satisfaction are usually both measured as continuous (quantitative) variables along a ratio scale. The relationship between pay and job satisfaction would be tested using a method of correlation. However, if we wished to determine whether the relationship between pay and job satisfaction differs between males and females, we would need to use logistic regression with gender as the dependent (grouping) variable, and with pay and job satisfaction as the independent variables. We would need to specify an interaction term between pay and job satisfaction.

4. Chi-squared could be used to analyse the results of a questionnaire measuring level of anxiety in a random sample of the population.

False: There is no hypothesis stated here. All that can be done is to compute descriptive statistics, such as range, mean and standard deviation, median, mode, etc.

5. The variation in a variable can be explained by the square of its correlation coefficient with another variable.

True: If the correlation between age and speed of performance on a test is 0.6, the variance is 0.36, i.e. 36%. This means that 36% of the variance (variation) in speed of performance is explained by variations in age. This variance should not be confused with variance which is the square of the standard deviation, which is used in computing statistics such as the t-value or the F value.

6. The closer the correlation coefficient 'r' is to zero, the fewer errors made in prediction.

False: The closer the correlation coefficient is to zero, the weaker is the relationship between the variables, and hence the less accurately does the independent variable predict the dependent variable.

7. In an IQ test showing normal distribution with a mean of 100 and a standard deviation of 15, approximately 15% of the population have an IQ less than 70.

False: In a normal distribution, 68.3% of the population lie within 1 standard deviation of the mean, i.e. between 85 and 115; 95.5% lie within 2 standard deviations of the mean, i.e. between 70 and 130. Therefore, 4.5% lie below 70 and above 130, or, 2.25% lie below 70 and 2.25% lie above 130. Moreover, if 68.3% lie between 85 and 115, and if 95.5% lie between 70 and 130, 27.2% (95.5–68.3) lie between 70 and 85, and between 115 and 130. Or, 13.6% lie between 70 and 85, and 13.6% lie between 115 and 130.

In this example, if the mean is 100, the median and mode are also 100 because the distribution is normal.

8. The Fisher exact probability test should not be used for small numbers.

False: The chi-squared test has certain assumptions. One of these is that the expected frequency in at least 80% of cells should be 5 or above, and no expected frequency should be <1. In this context, expected frequency for a cell is given by the product of the row and column totals (for that cell) divided by the grand total (that is, the sample size).

In 2×2 and 2×3 chi-squared contingency tables, if the expected frequency assumption is not met, the Fisher's exact test can be used. Some researchers routinely use the Fisher's exact test if the sample size is <20.

The Fisher's exact test is far more computationally intensive than the chi-squared test.

9. Incidence includes cases that are no longer current.

False: Incidence refers to the occurrence of new cases in a population during a specified period of time. Incidence is usually described as the number of new cases per 100 (or 1000, or 100 000, as appropriate) population.

10. Non-parametric statistics can be measured by least squares.

True: Here, Spearman's procedure is the non-parametric equivalent of Pearson's procedure. Spearman's procedure is conducted on data that have been ranked rather than on the raw data. Spearman's procedure is applied when the distribution of the raw data is non-normal, or when the primary data were collected as ranked data.

11. The Mann–Whitney test could be used to analyse the results of a questionnaire measuring level of anxiety in a random sample of the population.

False: The Mann–Whitney test is a non-parametric procedure which compares a continuous variable between two groups when the assumptions for the *t*-test are not met.

In the question above, no groups are specified. Had two groups been specified (e.g. males vs. females), and had the distributions of anxiety scores been non-normal, the Mann–Whitney test could have been used.

12. The mode is a measure of central tendency.

True: The mean, median and mode are measures of central tendency.

There are different kinds of mean, i.e. arithmetic, geometric, and harmonic. In statistics, we almost always consider the arithmetic mean, or average, which is the sum of the terms divided by the number of the terms.

The median is the middle term when the terms are arranged in ascending or descending order of magnitude. If the number of terms in the sample is even, the median is the average of the middle two terms.

The mode is the most commonly occurring term in the sample.

The mean is used for most statistical descriptions and procedures. Tests of the mean are more powerful, i.e. less vulnerable to a type II error.

The median is used when the distribution is non-normal. The mode is used when we are most interested in the frequently occurring values.

13. In an experiment to determine whether drug therapy or hypnosis is better in treatment to stop smoking, the results are measured by the number of cigarettes smoked after treatment. In this study the null hypothesis postulates there will be a significant difference between drug therapy and hypnosis in reduction of cigarette smoking.

False: The null hypothesis states that there will be no difference in the reduction in cigarette smoking between the two treatments. It is the alternative hypothesis which states that the two treatments will differ significantly in their effect on smoking.

14. A population pyramid can be used to describe the sex and age structure of a population.

True: The X-axis describes the population and the Y-axis describes age groups. A separate graph is formed for males and for females, and a mirror image of one is placed adjacent to the original graph of the other to produce the shape of a pyramid.

15. The primacy effect includes deciding about a person by their physical appearance.

False: The primacy effect is when an initial situation influences the interpretation or effect of a later one. For example, we often make persistent judgements about people based upon first impressions. This is a classic example of the primacy effect.

In contrast, the recency effect is when a recent situation is associated with a greater influence than an earlier situation. For example, if we are asked to remember a word list, we most easily remember the words which were read out last.

16. In categorical independent variables, regression is usually by the method of least squares.

True: In a multiple regression procedure a dichotomous categorical independent variable will be coded as 0 or 1. If the variable is divided into more than two categories, dummy variables are created, and the presence or absence of each of the categories is coded as 0 or 1. Incidentally, ANOVA can be thought of as linear regression with coded categorical independent variables. Like simple linear regression, multivariate regression makes use of the least squares technique.

17. Scores obtained on two successive administrations correlated 0.90 indicate reliability and not validity of a personality questionnaire.

True: Reliability means replicability. A reliable instrument is one which yields the same or very similar results no matter how many times it is administered to the same individual (test–retest reliability) or no matter how many different persons administer it to the same individual (inter-rater reliability).

There are different methods to assess reliability, and correlation is not one of the recommended ones!

18. A new 'treatment' is tried on gifted children, all of whom have an IQ greater than 140. If the mean IQ of the sample is 150, and if the treatment has no effect on IQ, the mean IQ that one would expect on re-testing 1 year later is slightly greater than 150.

False: If the treatment has no effect, the mean IQ should remain the same, i.e. 150. However, as it is unrealistic to expect that the children will perform in exactly the same manner as they did the previous year, the mean IQ at re-testing could be either above 150 or below 150 but not significantly different from 150. Note that as the variation in performance on re-testing is random, we cannot expect that the mean on re-testing will be greater than the baseline mean.

19. The telephone directory can be used for random sampling.

False: Persons who own a telephone and who are listed in the directory comprise a socio-economic subset of the population and do not represent the population. Therefore, a sample drawn from the telephone directory will be a biased sample.

The telephone directory can be used for random sampling only if the population is defined as all those who own telephones. This, for example, is meaningful if the subject of the study is telephone behaviour or usage.

If the telephone directory is used for recruitment, it must be recognized that this is a convenience sample. In a way, almost all studies are conducted on convenience samples. For example, every sample drawn in a hospital setting is a convenience sample because patients who come to the hospital are likely to systematically differ from those in the general population. The only way to obtain a truly random sample is to use population-based methods of sampling, as in epidemiological studies.

20. Standard deviation is a measure of precision of an estimate.

False: The standard deviation is a measure of dispersion. That is, it is a measure of the extent of scatter of the individual terms (in the sample) around the mean. The mean of a sample is only an estimate of the population mean. The standard error of the mean, and the confidence intervals for the mean, are measures of the accuracy of the mean.

21. A statement that an association between two variables is statistically significant means that, if the study is repeated, chances are that the significance of the association would be the same.

True: If two variables are significantly associated and we repeat our study, we should find a significant association 95 times out of 100.

22. A result statistically significant at a level of 5% implies that there is a 5% chance that the results suggest a wrong conclusion.

True: It means that there is a 5% probability that the result is due to chance factors, and a 95% probability that the result is due to genuine reasons.

23. Stratification increases the power of a study.

True: This is because stratification seeks to balance the groups on important, potentially confounding (independent) variables. As a result, variability resulting from heterogeneity across groups is diminished. As power is inversely related to variability, reducing the variability through stratification will increase the power of the study.

24. The T^2 test is used for non-parametric variables.

False: The Hotelling's T^2 test is one of the ways of executing a multivariate analysis of variance (MANOVA). In this test, several means are simultaneously compared between groups to reduce the risk of a false positive (type 1) error which may arise if each mean is compared separately between the groups.

25. In an experiment designed to investigate the effect of home background on intelligence, the family size is a dependent variable.

False: Family size is an independent variable and intelligence is the dependent variable. Other home background characteristics which may be examined as independent variables include parental intelligence, parental aspirations for the child, parental socio-economic status, etc. Dependent variables could be the child's IQ score, the child's examination results, etc.

60 Statistics – 4

Chittaranjan Andrade

		T	F

1. Semantic differential scales are used in attitude measurement.

2. A cut-off point on the scores of the Present State Examination can be used to define caseness for screening purposes in epidemiological research.

3. The chi-squared test could be used in a study of comparison of pay vs. job satisfaction in two groups of workers aged 20 and aged 30.

4. Path analysis is used to develop classification systems.

5. Correlation between IQ and reading ability in a school-wide sample of children is found to be +0.55. Among a group of learning disabled children of similar age group, one might expect the correlation to be much greater.

6. In the design of an experimental study, 'crossover' means patients are paired and then swapped.

7. For a normally distributed variable the mean and standard deviation provide a sufficient statistical description.

8. The halo effect can be a source of error in experimental psychology.

9. Incidence is usually higher than prevalence for schizophrenia.

10. A Likert scale allows for a 5-point response.

11. Two samples significantly different on the Mann–Whitney test can have the same median.

12. Multivariate statistics can be measured by least squares.

13. In a study of the ego-strength of 16-year-old females working in a clothes factory, as an indicator of the ego-strength of all 16-year-old girls in the same city, the parameter is the mean ego-strength of 16-year-old females in the factory.

14. The power of a study is 1 minus type 2 error.

15. The Beck Depression Inventory is a self-rated questionnaire.

16. Regression is used to compare two groups.

17. In the construction of a psychometric rating scale, high test-retest reliability may impair the detection of individual change.

18. Every 10th name on a hospital admission register can be used for random sampling.

T F

19. Psychiatric screening instruments used in a general hospital should have normative data.

20. In the construction of a psychometric rating scale, the type of population chosen for standardization must be different from the population for which the scale is intended.

21. A treatment trial shows no significant difference in efficacy between two antidepressants. This may be because the outcome measurement was based on a scale measuring traits rather than state.

22. If an association between two variables is statistically significant, it means that a causal association has been established.

23. The t-test is used to compare two groups.

24. In an experiment to determine whether drug therapy or hypnosis is better as a treatment to stop smoking, the results are measured by the number of cigarettes smoked after treatment. In this study, the number of cigarettes smoked before treatment is a dependent variable.

25. In a placebo-controlled trial of a new antidepressant where the subjects are matched in pairs and a suitable rating scale is used, a Wilcoxon test would be more sensitive than a t-test.

ANSWERS

1. Semantic differential scales are used in attitude measurement.

True: The semantic differential scale asks a person to express an attitude along a 7-point scale which has a bipolar adjective at the ends. For example, a person may be asked:

Do you believe that women in managerial positions are

1. Competent
2.
3.
4.
5.
6.
7. Incompetent.

Ratings may also be aligned horizontally as:

Good   Bad

3   2   1   0   1   2   3

The subject is required to make a choice between the adjectives and along the continuum.

2. A cut-off point on the scores of the Present State Examination can be used to define caseness for screening purposes in epidemiological research.

False: The Present State Examination is a 140-item tool which evaluates different categories of psychopathology towards establishing a clinical diagnosis.

In psychiatry, the most common instrument used to define caseness is presently the DSM-IV. Sometimes, caseness may be defined in terms of a cut-off on a rating scale. For example, a cut-off may be specified on the Goldberg General Health Questionnaire to define caseness when screening for psychiatric disorders in a large sample. A cut-off of 7 on the Mood Disorders Questionnaire may be used to define caseness when screening for bipolar disorders. A cut-off of 18 on the Ham-D may be used to define caseness when recruiting for a clinical trial in which patients who are only mildly depressed are to be screened out.

3. The chi-squared test could be used in a study of comparison of pay vs. job satisfaction in two groups of workers aged 20 and aged 30.

False: Pay and job satisfaction are usually both measured as continuous (quantitative) variables along a ratio scale. The relationship between pay and job satisfaction would be tested using a method of correlation. However, if we wish to determine whether the relationship between pay and job satisfaction differs between two age groups, we would need to use logistic regression with age group as the dependent (grouping) variable, and with pay and job satisfaction as the independent variables. We would need to specify an interaction term between pay and job satisfaction to answer the question asked.

4. Path analysis is used to develop classification systems.

False: Path analysis is used to test a model with several independent and several dependent variables set out in the form of a path.

For example, we know that stress causes depression, that depressed patients are often anxious, and that mood disturbance impairs quality of life. We may hypothesize (a) that stress raises anxiety scores, which in turn raise depression scores, which in turn lower quality of life scores, and (b) that anxiety also directly lowers quality of life scores. In other words, we indicate paths of how different variables directly or indirectly result in downstream effects. Paths can converge, diverge, or intersect. Such models can be tested through correlation coefficients derived through path analysis.

5. Correlation between IQ and reading ability in a school-wide sample of children is found to be +0.55. Among a group of learning disabled children of similar age group, one might expect the correlation to be much greater.

False: Among children with learning disabilities, reading ability is compromised no matter what the IQ is. In consequence, the relationship between IQ and reading ability is much weakened. The result is a lower correlation coefficient.

6. In the design of an experimental study, 'crossover' means patients are paired and then swapped.

False: Crossover means that patients are exposed first to one experimental condition, e.g. active drug, and then to the other, e.g. placebo. Patients are usually randomized to one or the other condition and subsequently crossed over to the condition to which they have not been exposed. There is usually a washout interval between exposures to the two conditions. Crossover designs may also involve more than two conditions, e.g. experimental condition, active control and inactive control.

7. For a normally distributed variable the mean and standard deviation provide a sufficient statistical description.

True: The range may be added to provide additional information.

8. The halo effect can be a source of error in experimental psychology.

True: The halo effect is said to occur when the response to one variable influences the response to other variables. For example, when a patient is depressed, he may rate his activities of daily living as being worse than they actually are. This is because depression makes him see everything in a negative light. Another example is when an individual is judged based on a single attribute, e.g. if he tells a single lie, he is judged to be dishonest by nature.

The practice effect is another source of error. If the same ISQ, or a similar ISQ, is administered repeatedly, the subject's performance improves not because he knows better but because he has 'learnt' how to perform in that test. However, knowledge improves if the candidate studies the explanations also.

Subject variables are also a source of error. For example, more intelligent subjects may show certain responses, males may show certain responses, younger persons may show certain responses, etc. These can be controlled for by proper randomization or group matching, or can be reduced through analysis of co-variance if the assumptions of ANCOVA are met.

9. Incidence is usually higher than prevalence for schizophrenia.

False: Incidence describes the occurrence of new cases in a population over a specified time period, while prevalence describes the total number of cases in a population over a specified time period. The chronic nature of schizophrenia is therefore reflected in the prevalence being greater than incidence. Point prevalence is the proportion of cases at a specific point in time. One-year prevalence is the proportion of persons who were already cases or who became cases during that year. Lifetime prevalence is the proportion of persons who become cases during their lifetime.

10. A Likert scale allows for a 5-point response.

True: A Likert scale measures the extent to which a person agrees or disagrees with a statement. The most common scale is 1 to 5. Often the scale will be 1=strongly disagree, 2=disagree, 3=not sure, 4=agree, and 5=strongly agree.

11. Two samples significantly different on the Mann–Whitney test can have the same median.

True: Although the Mann–Whitney test is sometimes described as a test which compares medians between two groups (much as the *t*-test compares means between two groups), what the Mann–Whitney test actually compares are the mean ranks. The mean ranks can vary even if the medians are the same. This is because the median is a single term; the values of the numbers on either side can differ widely between groups, resulting in differences in mean ranks. If the difference in mean ranks is sizeable, the Mann–Whitney test will emerge significant.

12. Multivariate statistics can be measured by least squares.

True: More specifically, multiple regression analysis uses the least squares method.

13. In a study of the ego-strength of 16-year-old females working in a clothes factory, as an indicator of the ego-strength of all 16-year-old girls in the same city, the parameter is the mean ego-strength of 16-year-old females in the factory.

False: The population of 16-year-old females working in a clothes factory is a biased subset of 16-year-old females in the city. This is because factory workers are likely to belong to a specific socio-economic status, and would therefore differ from girls who work elsewhere in education, income, quality of residence, and other variables.

'Parameter' is the term used to describe values such as mean, median, mode, standard deviation, etc. for the population. The equivalent for a sample is 'statistic'.

14. The power of a study is 1 minus type 2 error.

True: The power of a test is the probability that a type 2 error will not occur, i.e. 1 minus the probability of the type 2 error.

15. The Beck Depression Inventory is a self-rated questionnaire.

True: Other self-rated instruments include personality inventories, e.g. Eysenck Personality Questionnaire, Cattell's 16-PF self-report questionnaire; quality of life scales, e.g. WHO-QOL; the General Health Questionnaire and the Michigan Alcohol Screening Test.

Clinician-rated instruments include the Ham-D, Ham-A, Montgomery–Asberg Depression Rating Scale, the Young Mania Rating Scale, the Bech–Rafaelson Mania Rating Scale, the Brief Psychiatric Rating Scale, the PANSS, the Clinical Global Impression of severity and the Clinical Global Impression of change.

Neuropsychological measures are almost all clinician-administered, e.g. WAIS, Wechsler Memory Scale, Halstead-Reitan battery, the Luria-Nebraska battery, etc.

The Raven's Standard and Advanced Progressive Matrices and the Coloured Progressive Matrices are self-administered.

The Zung depression scale has both self-rated and observer-rated versions.

16. Regression is used to compare two groups.

False: Regression is used to explain or predict the value of a dependent variable given the value of an independent variable. For example, we can use regression to derive an equation which explains or predicts the seizure threshold given the patient's age. Linear regression is used when there is one independent variable and one dependent variable. Multiple regression is used when there are several independent and one dependent variables.

17. In the construction of a psychometric rating scale, high test–retest reliability may impair the detection of individual change.

False: If the test–retest reliability is high, it means that repeated administration of the test to the same individual yields the same or very similar results. The assumption is that the individual has himself not changed, and therefore the test correctly reports the same results.

If the individual does change, a tool with high test–retest reliability must necessarily identify the change. The better the test–retest reliability, the better the tool will be at identifying the change.

18. Every 10th name on a hospital admission register can be used for random sampling.

False: This is systematic sampling, a form of non-random sampling. Systematic sampling is acceptable when it is believed that the distribution of subjects in the sample is reasonably free of bias. For example, in this situation, taking every 10th name is an acceptable form of sampling if it can be reasonably assumed that there is no bias in the manner in which the names are entered in the hospital admission register.

Random sampling assumes that every subject in the population has an equal opportunity of being selected no matter what the previous selections have been. In contrast, in systematic sampling (to use this example), once the initial subject has been chosen, the next 9 subjects have no chance of being chosen, the 10th subject will definitely be chosen, the next 9 will not, etc.

19. Psychiatric screening instruments used in a general hospital should have normative data.

True: Psychiatric screening instruments used in a general hospital should have normative data based on which a cut-off score (with appropriate sensitivity and specificity) can be selected. This cut-off score can be used to separate cases who are likely to have a psychiatric disorder from those who are unlikely to have a psychiatric disorder.

20. In the construction of a psychometric rating scale, the type of population chosen for standardization must be different from the population for which the scale is intended.

False: Psychometric instruments are standardized for the populations for which they are intended. This is because the reliability and validity of a particular version of an instrument can vary across populations.

21. A treatment trial shows no significant difference in efficacy between two antidepressants. This may be because the outcome measurement was based on a scale measuring traits rather than state.

True: Antidepressant drugs treat symptoms such as depression and anxiety. These are states. States are things which alter over time whereas traits are more stable. Antidepressant drugs do not usually influence personality characteristics, i.e. personality traits, and these are therefore unlikely to differ between groups treated with different antidepressant drugs.

22. If an association between two variables is statistically significant, it means that a causal association has been established.

False: There are several possible indicators of causality, and statistical significance is one of them. However, none of the indicators decisively establishes causality.

For example, in children aged 0–2 years, a significant correlation is identified between the number of words the child knows and the number of teeth the child has. This does not establish that vocabulary improves dentition, or that dentition improves vocabulary. Rather, both are explained by a third variable, age.

23. The *t*-test is used to compare two groups.

True: The independent sample *t*-test is used to compare means between two groups. The paired *t*-test, in contrast, is used to compare the means of the same variable obtained from the same group at two different points in time.

The *t*-test can be used to compare levels of depression measured using Ham-D in a random sample of high school boys and girls. Here, gender is the grouping variable and depression score is the variable being compared between the two groups.

24. In an experiment to determine whether drug therapy or hypnosis is better as a treatment to stop smoking, the results are measured by the number of cigarettes smoked after treatment. In this study, the number of cigarettes smoked before treatment is a dependent variable.

False: The number of cigarettes smoked before treatment is an independent variable. Treatment, i.e. drug therapy vs. hypnosis, is also an independent variable. Whereas treatment is the primary independent variable, pretreatment smoking is a potentially biasing independent variable, and can be treated as a co-variate in the analysis. In this example, the number of cigarettes smoked after treatment is the dependent variable.

25. In a placebo-controlled trial of a new antidepressant where the subjects are matched in pairs and a suitable rating scale is used, a Wilcoxon test would be more sensitive than a *t*-test.

False: Parametric tests are more powerful than nonparametric tests in the identification of a true difference in means. Therefore, the paired *t*-test would be superior to the Wilcoxon test.

The Wilcoxon test would be desirable only if the paired t-test cannot be performed, e.g. when the sample size is small or when the distribution of the differences between pairs of values is non-normal.

Incidentally, the paired t-test or the Wilcoxon test are usually performed on pre- vs. post-data, i.e. on repeated measures. A situation in which subjects are matched and compared using a paired test (paired t-test or Wilcoxon test) is unusual in research.

61 Suicide

Chris O'Loughlin

	T	F
1. The term 'Deliberate self-harm' was coined by Morgan.	☐	☐
2. 'Anomie' explains suicide bombing.	☐	☐
3. A British household survey found 1% of adults had suicidal ideation in the preceding week.	☐	☐
4. Living with spouse is a risk factor for repeated deliberate self-harm (DSH).	☐	☐
5. Risk of repeated DSH is high in the first 3 months after an episode of DSH.	☐	☐
6. Repetition of self-harm is more likely in antisocial personality disorder.	☐	☐
7. A history of criminal conviction is a risk factor for repeated deliberate self-harm.	☐	☐
8. The rate of repetition of DSH is 50% within the first year.	☐	☐
9. Attempted suicide in the elderly is more common in men than in women.	☐	☐
10. Deliberate self-harm in the elderly is less common in comparison with teenagers.	☐	☐
11. In old age self-harm is rarely a failed suicide attempt.	☐	☐
12. The suicide rate in pathological gambling is around 15%.	☐	☐
13. Depressed women are more likely to commit suicide than depressed men.	☐	☐
14. Identical twins are more prone to committing suicide.	☐	☐
15. Having a child aged below 2 years reduces the risk of suicide in women.	☐	☐
16. Suicide in the elderly is commonly associated with alcoholism.	☐	☐
17. 25% of suicides are committed by those aged above 65 years.	☐	☐
18. Suicide is less common in the elderly when compared to the general population.	☐	☐
19. In the elderly, suicide is not usually due to mental health disorders.	☐	☐
20. Suicide is commonly associated with physical illness in old age.	☐	☐
21. Suicide in the elderly is more common in women than in men.	☐	☐
22. A 65-year-old depressed man is more likely to kill himself than a 30-year-old depressed man.	☐	☐
23. Adolescent girls with intentional self-harm have usually experienced parental criticism immediately preceding the episode.	☐	☐

T F

24. When considering a suicide attempt in a 15-year-old, parental criticism is usually the cause. ☐ ☐

25. Reducing the availability of means of suicide does not reduce suicides in the long term. ☐ ☐

ANSWERS

1. The term 'Deliberate self-harm' was coined by Morgan.

True: Before the 1950s little distinction was made between those who killed themselves and those who survived after an apparent suicidal act. In 1952 Stengel differentiated between suicide and attempted suicide. The terms evolved further:

- Stengel (1952) Attempted suicide
- Kessel (1965) Deliberate self-poisoning and Deliberate self-injury
- Morgan (1975) Deliberate self-harm
- Kreitman (1977) Parasuicide.

More recently, patient groups have advocated dropping the word 'deliberate' as it is felt by some to be pejorative and stigmatizing (Gelder et al 2006, p. 418; Johnstone et al 2004, p. 670).

2. 'Anomie' explains suicide bombing.

False: Emile Durkheim in 1897 described four basic types of suicide:

1. Anomic: The individual is out of step with society because of changes in life circumstances and the weakness of the society, e.g. an alcoholic who has lost his job, is rejected by his family and falls between services.
2. Altruistic: The individual dies for a cause where society exerts a strong influence on him to take his own life, e.g. suicide bombing.
3. Egoistic: Lonely, withdrawn individuals, who are not integrated into or dependent on society, e.g. arranging an assisted suicide.
4. Fatalistic: Result of strict rules in society which are decisive for the individual, e.g. suicide of a slave, or a widow in certain cultures (Gelder et al 2000, p. 1035; Sadock & Sadock 2005, p. 2442).

3. A British household survey found 1% of adults had suicidal ideation in the preceding week.

True: The British psychiatric morbidity survey found that 10% had depressive symptoms and amongst them 1 in 10 had suicidal ideation (Jenkins et al 1998).

4. Living with spouse is a risk factor for repeated deliberate self-harm.

False: Living alone and being single, divorced, separated or widowed are associated with increased risk (Gelder et al 2000, p. 1043; Gelder et al 2006, p. 420; Johnstone et al 2004, p. 661).

5. Risk of repeated DSH is high in the first 3 months after an episode of DSH.

True: The risk of repetition of DSH is highest in the 3 months after an episode of DSH. Amongst those admitted to hospitals for DSH, one-half are first-timers and the others are repeaters. The rates of repetition after DSH are:

- Within 3 months = 10%
- Within 1 year = 15% (12–26%)
- Within 4 years = 21% (12–30%)
- Long-term = 23% (12–32%).

Bancroft & Marsack in 1997 proposed three patterns of repetition: chronic repetition due to recurrent crisis, bursts of repetition during periods of stress and one-off repetition during severe crisis. Repeaters with >20 admissions account for 4% of DSH patients (Gelder et al 2000, p. 1043; Johnstone et al 2004, p. 677).

6. Repetition of self-harm is more likely in antisocial personality disorder.

True: DSH and repetition of DSH are associated with personality disorders, especially antisocial personality disorder. DSH is also associated with impulsivity, criminal record, history of violence, history of traumatic events (including a 'broken home'), family violence, physical and mental maltreatment by partners and unstable living conditions (Gelder et al 2000, p. 1043; Gelder et al 2006, p. 421; Sadock & Sadock 2005, p. 2448).

7. A history of criminal conviction is a risk factor for repeated deliberate self-harm.

True: Features that predict repetition of DSH include unemployment, lower social class, criminal record, history of violence, high suicidal intent, hopelessness, past psychiatric history, history of traumatic events including broken homes, family violence, physical and mental maltreatment by partners, unstable living conditions, substance misuse and non-compliance.

There is a high incidence of self-harm amongst prisoners, particularly female prisoners. The lifetime prevalence of deliberate self-harm among sentenced prisoners is 32% in women and 17% in men (Gelder et al 2000, p. 1043; Gelder et al 2006, p. 420; Johnstone et al 2004, p. 675).

8. The rate of repetition of DSH is 50% within the first year.

False: Among those who present with their first episode of DSH, 12–26% (mean = 15%) repeat within a year. Approximately half of those presenting to the hospital with DSH are first-timers, the other half are repeaters, 30% having self-harmed at least twice (Gelder et al 2000, p. 1043; Johnstone et al 2004, p. 677).

9. Attempted suicide in the elderly is more common in men than in women.

False: Deliberate self-harm is more common in women than men at all ages but the ratio decreases in the elderly. The absolute number of DSH episodes in women is higher with a 3:2 ratio. However, the rates are more similar because there are fewer elderly men than elderly women. DSH in the elderly accounts for 5% of all cases of DSH. Among elderly DSH patients, 90% have depression, 60% have physical illness, 50% are admitted to a psychiatric facility and 8% commit suicide within the next 3 years. DSH in the elderly is often precipitated by bereavement, up to 44% in one series (Jacoby & Oppenheimer 2002, p. 677; Johnstone et al 2004, p. 648).

10. Deliberate self-harm in the elderly is less common in comparison with teenagers.

True: DSH declines with age (Gelder et al 2000, p. 1041).

11. In old age self-harm is rarely a failed suicide attempt.

False: DSH in older people is more likely to represent suicide attempts failed due to confusion from physical illnesses, polypharmacy and alcohol misuse. DSH is relatively uncommon in older age groups, contributing only 5–15% of the total number of episodes of DSH. Compared with younger subjects, repetition of DSH is less common, but completed suicides are more common in the elderly (Gelder et al 2000, p. 1659; Johnstone et al 2004, p. 648).

12. The suicide rate in pathological gambling is around 15%.

False: The rates of suicidal ideation, suicide attempts and suicide are higher in pathological gamblers. This may be related to their high impulsivity, high rates of co-morbid psychiatric conditions as well as social disruptions. The incidence of attempted suicide among pathological gamblers is approximately 8 times that of the general population. Even though there is little specific information on suicide rates in pathological gambling, the rates are unlikely to be as high as 15% (Gelder et al 2000, p. 992).

13. Depressed women are more likely to commit suicide than depressed men.

False: Suicide is 3 times more common in men than in women (Gelder et al 2006, p. 410; Johnstone et al 2004, p. 662).

14. Identical twins are more prone to committing suicide.

False: Twins have a reduced risk of suicide (Tomassini et al 2003).

15. Having a child aged below 2 years reduces the risk of suicide in women.

True: Having a child aged below 2 years is significantly protective for women (Johnstone et al 2004, p. 662).

16. Suicide in the elderly is commonly associated with alcoholism.

False: Substance misuse is a risk factor for suicide in the elderly. However, primary substance use disorders account for a smaller proportion of suicides than in younger age groups (Gelder et al 2006, p. 410; Jacoby & Oppenheimer 2002, p. 679).

17. 25% of suicides are committed by those aged above 65 years.

False: Around 20% of all suicides are committed by those aged above 65 years. They form only 15% of the population. The rates declined in the 1960s following detoxification of the gas supply. The rates are three times higher in men than in women. The rates in men increase with advancing age, while the female rates gradually fall. The main predictive factors in old age are age, male gender, physical illness (in 35–85% of cases), social isolation, widowed or separated status, alcohol abuse and current depression or a history of depression (80%). Up to 15% have no psychiatric illnesses (Johnstone et al 2004, p. 648; www.Samaritans.org).

18. Suicide is less common in the elderly when compared to the general population.

False: Around 20% of all suicides are committed by those aged above 65 years, who form only 15% of the population. In most countries, the highest suicide rates are in those aged over 75 years (Gelder et al 2000, p. 1658; Gelder et al 2006, p. 412; Johnstone et al 2004, p. 648).

19. In the elderly, suicide is not usually due to mental health disorders.

False: Current or past history of depression, social isolation and physical health problems are the most important risk factors for suicide in the elderly. 70–80% of elderly suicides are associated with mental illness, most commonly depression. Up to 15% may have no psychiatric illness (Gelder et al 2000, p. 1660; Gelder et al 2006, p. 412; Johnstone et al 2004, p. 648).

20. Suicide is commonly associated with physical illness in old age.

True: Suicide in the elderly is associated with physical illness (20–85%), mental illness (70–80%), especially depression and/or substance abuse, separated or widowed status, and social isolation, increasing age and male gender (3 times). Terminal illness is under-represented in suicide victims (Jacoby & Oppenheimer 2002, p. 679; Johnstone et al 2004, p. 648).

21. Suicide in the elderly is more common in women than in men.

False: Suicide is more common in men than women at all ages, showing a ratio of approximately 3:1 (Jacoby & Oppenheimer 2002, p. 678; Johnstone et al 2004, p. 648).

22. A 65-year-old depressed man is more likely to kill himself than a 30-year-old depressed man.

False: Suicide rates used to be higher in older people and depression used to be more frequently associated with suicide in the elderly than in the young. However, in the past decade there has been a marked shift in suicide epidemiology. The suicide rates in young men have increased dramatically, though in the past couple of years the rates have been falling. The rates in the elderly have come down. Currently, in the UK, the rate of suicide for young men is higher than for older adults.

23. Adolescent girls with intentional self-harm have usually experienced parental criticism immediately preceding the episode.

True: Deliberate self-harm behaviour in adolescent girls is usually impulsive and occurs in the context of a dispute within the family or a significant relationship (Gelder et al 2000, p. 1805).

24. When considering a suicide attempt in a 15-year-old, parental criticism is usually the cause.

False: The large Oxford study of under 16s who had attempted suicide showed that arguments with parents were usually the most common problem for the young people. This may include parental criticism. However, it cannot be concluded that the cause for the suicide attempt is usually parental criticism.

25. Reducing the availability of means of suicide does not reduce suicides in the long term.

False: A proportion of people who attempt to kill themselves are ambivalent about their plan. Hence, restricting the availability of methods is likely to decrease the likelihood of suicides. One-third of individuals who fail to commit suicide with one method will not switch to an alternative. Population-based measures basically aim at decreasing the availability of the means to kill oneself. In Britain, during 1948–50, domestic coal gas accounted for 40% of suicides in men and 60% in women. The introduction of non-toxic North Sea gas reduced suicides by a third. Erecting a physical barrier on the Clifton suspension bridge in Bristol reduced suicides by jumping from the bridge. The results of reducing the toxicity of car exhausts (7% reduction in male suicides expected) and substituting tricyclics with SSRIs are awaited. Adding methionine to paracetamol has been predicted to reduce female suicides by 5% (Gelder et al 2006, p. 418; Johnstone et al 2004, p. 670).

References and further reading

Most of the references are common to more than one topic. Others refer only to specific topics. Therefore, the common references are listed first, followed by topic specific references. Some topics have no specific references other than those listed under 'Common references'.

Common references

ABPI 2005 Medicines compendium. Datapharm Communications, Surrey

American Psychiatric Association 1994 Diagnostic and statistical manual of mental disorders, 4th edn. APA, Washington, DC (DSM-IV)

American Psychiatric Association 2000 Diagnostic and statistical manual of mental disorders, 4th edn, text revision. APA, Washington, DC (DSM-IV-TR)

Anderson IM, Reid IC 2002 Fundamentals of clinical pharmacology, 2nd edn. British Association for Psychopharmacology/Martin Dunitz, London

Atkinson RL, Atkinson RC, Smith EE et al 2000 Hilgard's Introduction to psychology, 13th edn. Harcourt College Publishers, Fort Worth

Bateman A, Holmes J 1995 Introduction to psychoanalysis: Contemporary theory and practice. Routledge, London

Bateman A, Tyrer P 2004 Psychological treatment of personality disorders. Advances in Psychiatric Treatment 10: 378-388

Bazire S 2005 Psychotropic drug directory. Fivepin, Salisbury

Beck AT, Rush AJ, Emery G et al 1979 Cognitive therapy of depression. The Guilford Press, New York

Bennett PN, Brown MJ 2003 Clinical pharmacology, 9th edn. Churchill Livingstone, Edinburgh

Bluglass R, Bowden P 1990 Principles and practice of forensic psychiatry. Churchill Livingstone, Edinburgh

BMA and RPSGB 2005 British national formulary 50 (BNF)

Bouras N 1999 Psychiatric and behavioural disorders in developmental disabilities and mental retardation. Cambridge University Press, Cambridge

Butler R, Pitt B 1998 Seminars in old age psychiatry. Gaskell, London

Chick J, Cantwell R 1994 Seminars in alcohol and drug misuse. Gaskell, London

Cookson J, Taylor D, Katona C 2002 Use of drugs in psychiatry, 5th edn. Gaskell, London

Copeland JRM, Abou-Saleh MT, Blazer DG 2002 Principles and practice of geriatric psychiatry, 2nd edn. Wiley, Chichester

Crenshaw TL, Goldberg JP 1996 Sexual pharmacology. Norton, New York

Fear C 2004 Essential revision notes in psychiatry for MRCPsych. PasTest, Cheshire

Fraser W, Kerr M 2003 Seminars in the psychiatry of learning disabilities, 2nd edn. Gaskell, London

Gelder MG, Andreasen NC, Lopez-Ibor JJ 2000 New Oxford textbook of psychiatry. Oxford University Press, Oxford

Gelder M, Harrison P, Cowen P 2006 Shorter Oxford textbook of psychiatry, 5th edn. Oxford University Press, Oxford

Ghodse H 2002 Drugs and addictive behaviour: A guide to treatment, 3rd edn. Cambridge University Press, Cambridge

Goodyer IM, Herbert J, Tamplin A 2003 Psychoendocrine antecedents of persistent first-episode major depression in adolescents: a community-based longitudinal enquiry. Psychological Medicine 33: 601-610

Gross R 2001 Psychology. The science of mind and behaviour, 4th edn. Hodder & Stoughton, London

Hodges JR 1994 Cognitive assessment for clinicians. Oxford University Press, Oxford

Jacoby R, Oppenheimer C 2002 Psychiatry in the elderly, 3rd edn. Oxford University Press, Oxford

Johnstone EC, Cunningham Owens DG, Lawrie SM et al 2004 Companion to psychiatric studies, 7th edn. Churchill Livingstone, Edinburgh

Kandel ER, Schwartz JH, Jessell TM 2000 Principles of neural science, 4th edn. McGraw-Hill, New York

Kaplan HI, Sadock BJ, Sadock VA 2000 Pocket handbook of psychiatric drug treatment, 3rd edn. Lippincott Williams & Wilkins, Philadelphia

King DJ (ed.) 2004 Seminars in clinical psychopharmacology, 2nd edn. Gaskell, London

Lawlor B 2001 Revision psychiatry. MedMedia, Dublin

Lawrie SM, McIntosh A, Rao S 2000 Critical appraisal for psychiatry. Churchill Livingstone, Edinburgh

Lishman WA 1997 Organic psychiatry, 3rd edn. Blackwell Science, Oxford

McKenna PJ 2006 Schizophrenia and related syndromes, 2nd edn. Psychology Press, Hove

Mitchell AJ 2004 Neuropsychiatry and behavioural neurology explained. Saunders, Edinburgh

Munafo M 2002 Psychology for the MRCPsych, 2nd edn. Hodder Arnold, Oxford

Murray R, Hill P, McGuffin P 1997 Essentials of postgraduate psychiatry, 3rd edn. Cambridge University Press, Cambridge

National Institute for Health and Clinical Excellence. Online. Available: http://www.nice.org.uk (NICE)

Neal MJ 1992 Medical Pharmacology at a glance, 2nd edn. Blackwell Science, Oxford

Norman IJ, Redfern SJ 1996 Mental health care for elderly people. Churchill Livingstone, Edinburgh

Parsons T 1951 The social system. Free Press, Glencoe

Pilowsky I 1969 Abnormal illness behaviour. Psychological Medicine 42: 347-351

Puri BK, Tyrer PJ 1998 Sciences basic to psychiatry, 2nd edn. Churchill Livingstone, Edinburgh

Puri BK, Hall AD 2004 Revision notes in psychiatry, 2nd edn. Hodder Arnold, London

Rutter M, Taylor E 2002 Child and adolescent psychiatry, 4th edn. Blackwell Science, Oxford

Sadock BJ, Sadock VA 2002 Kaplan & Sadock's synopsis of psychiatry, 9th edn. Lippincott Williams & Wilkins, Philadelphia

Sadock BJ, Sadock VA 2005 Kaplan & Sadock's comprehensive textbook of psychiatry, 8th edn. Williams & Wilkins, Philadelphia

Sato T et al 2002 Syndromes and phenomenological subtypes underlying acute mania: a factor analytic study of 576 manic patients. American Journal of Psychiatry 59: 968-974

Sims A 2004 Symptoms in the mind, 3rd edn. Saunders, London

Stahl SM 2000 Essential psychopharmacology: Neuroscientific basis and practical applications, 2nd edn. Cambridge University Press, Cambridge

Stein G, Wilkinson G 1998 Seminars in general adult psychiatry. Gaskell, London

Stone JH, Roberts M, O'Grady J et al 2000 Faulk's basic forensic psychiatry. Blackwell Science, Oxford

Taylor D, Paton C, Kerwin R 2005 The Maudsley prescribing guidelines, 8th edn. Taylor & Francis, London

World Health Organization 1992 The ICD-10 classification of mental and behavioural disorders. WHO, Geneva (ICD-10)

World Health Organization 2001 International classification of functioning, disability and health. WHO, Geneva

Wright P, Stern J, Phelan M 2005 Core psychiatry, 2nd edn. Saunders, London

Yudofsky SC, Hales RE 2002 Textbook of neuropsychiatry and clinical neurosciences. American Psychiatric Publishing, Arlington, VA

Alcohol

Barcelous DG et al 2002 American academy of clinical toxicology practice guidelines on the treatment of methanol poisoning. Journal of Toxicology: Clinical Toxicology 40: 415-446

Antidepressants

Scott A 2005 College guidelines on electroconvulsive therapy: an update for prescribers. Advances in Psychiatric Treatment 11: 150-156

Child and adolescent psychiatry

Baron-Cohen S et al 1997 Another advanced test of theory of mind: evidence from very high functioning adults with autism or Asperger syndrome. Journal of Child Psychology and Psychiatry 38: 813-822

Bernstein GA et al 2000 Imipramine plus cognitive-behavioral therapy in the treatment of school refusal. Journal of the American Academy of Child and Adolescent Psychiatry 39: 276-283

Black D, Cottrell D 1993 Seminars in child and adolescent psychiatry. Gaskell, London

Dodge KA et al 2003 Peer rejection and social information-processing factors in the development of aggressive behaviour problems in children. Child Development 74: 374-393

Goodman R, Scott S 1997 Child psychiatry. Blackwell Science, Oxford

Goodyer IM, Herbert J, Altham PM 1998 Adrenal steroid secretion and major depression in 8- to 16-year-olds, III. Influence of cortisol/DHEA ratio at presentation on subsequent rates of disappointing life events and persistent major depression. Psychological Medicine 28: 265-273

Hazell P et al 2002 Tricyclic drugs for depression in children and adolescents. Online. Available: www.cochrane.org

Kaufman J et al 2001 Are child-, adolescent-, and adult-onset depression one and the same disorder? Biological Psychiatry 49: 980-1001

March J et al 2004 Fluoxetine, cognitive-behavioural therapy, and their combination for adolescents with depression: Treatment for Adolescents With Depression Study (TADS) randomized controlled trial. Journal of the American Medical Association 292: 807-820

Tourette's Syndrome Study Group 2002 Treatment of ADHD in children with tics: a randomized controlled trial. Neurology 58: 527-536

Drug abuse

Baciewicz GJ 2005 Injecting drug use. Online. Available: http://www.emedicine.com/med/topic586.htm

Bierut LJ et al 1998 Familial transmission of substance dependence: alcohol, marijuana, cocaine, and habitual smoking: a report from the Collaborative Study on the Genetics of Alcoholism. Archives of General Psychiatry 55: 982-988

Coleman T 2004 ABC of smoking cessation: Use of simple advice and behavioural support. BMJ 328: 397

http://www.drugabuse.gov (NIDA)

Kendler KS, Prescott CA 1998 Cannabis use, abuse and dependence in a population-based sample of female twins. American Journal of Psychiatry 155: 1016-1022

Lancaster T, Stead LF 2004 Physician advice for smoking cessation. Online. Available: www.cochrane.org

Solowij N 1998 Cannabis and cognitive functioning. Cambridge University Press, Cambridge

Eating disorders

Forman-Hoffman V 2004 High prevalence of abnormal eating and weight control practice amongst US high school students. Eating Behavior 5: 325-336

Hay PJ, Bacaltchuk J 2004 Psychotherapy for bulimia nervosa and bingeing. Online. Available: www.cochrane.org

Pratt BM, Woolfenden SR 2002 Interventions for preventing eating disorders in children and adolescents. Online. Available: www.cochrane.org

Szmukler G, Dare C, Treasure J (eds) 1995 Handbook of eating disorders. Theory, treatment and research. John Wiley, Chichester

Treasure J, Schmidt U 2005 Anovexia nervosa. Online. Available: www.clinicalevidence.com

Virkkunen M, Narvanen S 1987 Plasma insulin, tryptophan and serotonin levels during glucose tolerance test among habitually violent and impulsive offenders. Neuropsychobiology 17: 19-23

Forensic

Barron P et al 2002 Offenders with intellectual disability: The size of the problem and therapeutic outcomes. Journal of Intellectual Disability Research 46: 454-463

Chiswick D, Cope R 1995 Practical forensic psychiatry. Gaskell, London

Coid J et al 2002 Ethnic differences in prisoners. The British Journal of Psychiatry 181: 481-487

d'Orban PT 1979 Women who kill their children. The British Journal of Psychiatry 134: 560-571

Fazel S et al 2002 Prevalence of epilepsy in prisoners: systematic review. BMJ 324(7352): 1495

Gunn J, Taylor PJ 1993 Forensic psychiatry. Clinical, legal and ethical issues. Butterworth-Heinemann, Oxford

Hanson RK, Bussiere MT 1998 Predicting relapse: a meta-analysis of sexual offender recidivism studies. Journal of Consulting and Clinical Psychology 66: 348-362

Shaw J et al 2006 Rates of mental disorder in people convicted of homicide. National clinical survey. The British Journal of Psychiatry 188: 143-147

Taylor PJ, Gunn J 1999 Homicides by people with mental illness; myth and reality. British Journal of Psychiatry 174: 9-14

Learning disabilities

Craft M, Bicknell J, Hollins S 1985 A multi-disciplinary approach to mental handicap. Balliere Tindall, London

Harris JC 2000 Developmental neuropsychiatry, Vol. 2. Assessment, diagnosis and treatment of developmental disorders. Oxford University Press, Oxford

McGuffin, P et al 1994 Seminars in psychiatric genetics. Gaskell, London

Mood disorders

Bain M et al 2000 Obstetric complications and affective psychoses. British Journal of Psychiatry 176: 523-526

Bradley B, Matthews A 1983 Negative self-schema in clinical depression. British Journal of Psychology 22: 173-181

Cardno AG et al 2002 A twin study of genetic relationships between psychotic symptoms. American Journal of Psychiatry 159: 539-545

Cook N et al 1986 Clinical utility of the dexamethasone suppression test assessed by plasma and salivary cortisol determinations. Psychiatry Research 18: 143-150

Lee MA et al 1988 Chronic caffeine consumption and the dexamethasone suppression test in depression. Psychiatry Research 24: 61-65

Murali V, Oyebode F 2004 Poverty, social inequality and mental health. Advances in Psychiatric Treatment 10: 216-224

Murphy E 1982 Social origins of depression in old age. British Journal of Psychiatry 142: 111-119

Paykel ES 1992 Handbook of affective disorders, 2nd edn. Churchill Livingstone, Edinburgh

Paykel ES 2003 Life events and affective disorders. Acta Psychiatrica Scandinavica (suppl 418): 61-66

Spataro J et al 2004 Impact of child sexual abuse on mental health: Prospective study in males and females. British Journal of Psychiatry 184: 416-421

Vinokur AD et al 1995 Impact of the JOBS intervention on unemployed workers varying in risk for depression. American Journal of Community Psychology 23: 39-74

Zeanah CH et al 1993 Do women grieve after terminating pregnancies because of fetal anomalies? A controlled investigation. Obstetrics and Gynaecology 82: 270-275

Neuropsychiatry

Alberts B, Johnson A, Lewis J et al 2000 The molecular biology of the cell, 4th edn. Garland Science, New York

Blichert-Toft M 1992 Breast conserving therapy for mammary carcinoma: psychosocial aspects, indications and limitations. Annals of Medicine 24: 445-451

Feinstein A 1999 The clinical neuropsychiatry of multiple sclerosis. Cambridge University Press, Cambridge

Fitzgerald MJT 1996 Neuroanatomy basic and clinical, 3rd edn. Saunders, London

Lindsay KW, Bone I 2004 Neurology and neurosurgery illustrated, 4th edn. Churchill Livingstone, Edinburgh

Pennington K et al 2005 The role of proteomics in investigating psychiatric disorders. British Journal of Psychiatry 187: 4-6

Schneerson J 2000 Handbook of sleep medicine. Blackwell Science, Oxford

Stern JM, Engel J 2004 Atlas of EEG patterns. Lippincott Williams & Wilkins, Philadelphia

Trimble M, Schmitz B (eds) 2002 The neuropsychiatry of epilepsy. Cambridge University Press, Cambridge

Neurotic disorders

Bosma H et al 1997 Low job control and risk of coronary heart disease in Whitehall II (prospective cohort) study. BMJ 314: 558

Dolan M 2004 Psychopathic personality in young people. Advances in Psychiatric Treatment 10: 466-473

Kivimaki M et al 2003 Sickness absence as a global measure of health: Evidence from mortality in Whitehall II (prospective cohort) study. BMJ 327(7411): 364

Klein DF 1993 False suffocation alarms, spontaneous panics, and related conditions. An integrative hypothesis. Archives of General Psychiatry 50: 306-317

Mechanic D 1962 The concept of illness behaviour. Journal of Chronic Diseases 15: 189-194

Old age psychiatry

Bluming AZ 2004 Hormone replacement therapy: the debate should continue. Geriatrics 59: 30-31, 35-37

Briley DP et al 2000 Does leukoaraiosis predict morbidity and mortality? Neurology 54: 90-94

Brodaty H et al 2003 Meta-analysis of psychosocial interventions for care-givers of people with dementia. Journal of American Geriatrics Society 51: 657-664

Esiri MM et al 2004 Neuropathology of dementia, 2nd rev. edn. Cambridge University Press, Cambridge

Payne B, Cikovic R 1995 Empirical examination of the characteristics, consequences and causes of elder abuse in nursing homes. Journal of Elder Abuse and Neglect 74: 61-74

Roose SP, Sackeim HA 2004 Late-life depression. Oxford University Press, Oxford

Schweitzer I et al 2002 Is late onset depression a prodrome to dementia? International Journal of Geriatric Psychiatry 17: 997-1005

Pharmacology

Cooper JR, Bloom FE, Roth RH 2003 The biochemical basis of neuropharmacology, 8th edn. Oxford University Press, Oxford

Rang HP, Dale MM, Ritter JM et al 2003 Pharmacology, 5th edn. Churchill Livingstone, Edinburgh

Psychology

Cohen S 1992 Folk devils and moral panics, 30th anniversary edn. Routledge, New York

Egusa G et al 2002 Influence of the extent of westernisation of lifestyle on the progression of preclinical atherosclerosis in Japanese subjects. Journal of Atherosclerosis and Thrombosis 9: 299-304

Farrington DP 1995 The development of offending and antisocial behaviour from childhood: key findings from the Cambridge Study in delinquent development. Journal of Child Psychology and Psychiatry 36: 929-964

Giddens A 1997 Sociology, 3rd edn. Polity Press, Cambridge

Gleitman H 1996 Basic psychology, 4th edn. WW Norton, New York

Hayes N 1994 Foundations of psychology. Routledge, London

Holmes TH, Rahe RH 1967 The social readjustment rating scale. Journal of Psychosomatic Research 11: 213-218

Illich I 2001 Limits to medicine. Medical nemesis: The expropriation of health, new edn. Marion Boyars, New York

Osgood CE, Tannenbaum PH 1955 The principle of congruity in the prediction of attitude change. Psychological Review 62: 42-55

www.publications.parliament.uk/pa/cm200304/cmselect/cmodpm/45/45.pdf (The Home Office)

Psychometry

Aiken LR 2000 Psychological testing and assessment, 10th edn. Allyn and Bacon, Massachusetts

Halligan P, Kischka U, Marshall JC 2003 Handbook of clinical neuropsychology. Oxford University Press, Oxford

Lezak MD 1995 Neuropsychological assessment, 3rd edn. Oxford University Press, Oxford

Psychotherapy

Aveline M, Dryden W (eds) 1988 Group therapy in Britain. Open University Press, Milton Keynes

Barnes B, Ernst S, Hyde K 1999 An introduction to group work. A group-analytic perspective. Palgrave Macmillan, Basingstoke, Hampshire

Brown D, Pedder J 1991 Introduction to psychotherapy: An outline of psychodynamic principles and practice, 2nd edn. Routledge, London

Dallos R, Draper R 2000 Introduction to family therapy. Open University Press, Milton Keynes

Eccleston C et al 2003 Psychological therapies for the management of chronic and recurrent pain in children and adolescents. Online. Available: www.cochrane.org

Hawton K, Salkovskis P, Kirk J, Clark D (eds) 1988 Cognitive behavioural therapy for psychiatric problems. A practical guide. Oxford University Press, Oxford

Horvath AO, Symonds BD 1991 Relation between working alliance and outcome in psychotherapy: A meta-analysis. Journal of Counselling Psychology 38: 139-149

Kreeger L (ed.) 1975 The large group. Dynamics and therapy. Karnac Books, London

Mace C (ed.) 1995 The art and science of assessment in psychotherapy. Routledge, London

Minuchin S 1974 Families and family therapy. Routledge, London

Stein SM, Haigh R, Stein J (eds) 1999 Essentials of psychotherapy. Butterworth-Heinemann, Oxford

Turner JA, Clancy S 1988 Comparison of operant behavioural and cognitive-behavioural group treatment for chronic low back pain. Journal of Consulting & Clinical Psychology 56: 261-266

Yalom I 1995 The theory and practice of group psychotherapy, 4th edn. Basic Books, New York

Research methodology

Altman D 1991 Practical statistics for medical research. Chapman and Hall, London

Gilbody S, Whitty P 2002 Improving the delivery and organization of mental health services: beyond the conventional randomized controlled trial. British Journal of Psychiatry 180: 13-18

Haynes RB, Richardson WS, Rosenberg W et al 2005 Evidence based medicine, 3rd rev. edn. Churchill Livingstone, Edinburgh

Howitt D, Cramer D 1997 An introduction to statistics in psychology. Prentice Hall, Harlow

Schizophrenia

Byford S et al 2000 Cost-effectiveness of intensive vs. standard case management for severe psychotic illness: UK700 case management trial. British Journal of Psychiatry 176: 537-543

Schonknecht P et al 2003 Cerebrospinal fluid tau protein levels in schizophrenia. European Archives of Psychiatry and Clinical Neurosciences 253: 100-102

Statistics

Ajetunmobi O 2002 Making sense of critical appraisal. Hodder Arnold, London

Streiner DL, Norman GR 2003 PDQ Statistics. 3rd rev. edn. Decker, Ontario

Zar JH 1999 Biostatistical analysis, 4th edn. Prentice Hall, New Jersey

Suicide

Jenkins R et al 1998 British psychiatric morbidity survey. British Journal of Psychiatry 173: 4

Tomassini C et al 2003 Risk of suicide in twins: 51 year follow up study. BMJ 327: 373-374

Useful websites

http://www.cambridgecourse.com
http://www.cochrane.org
http://www.prepdublin.com
http://www.rcpsych.ac.uk
http://www.superego-cafe.com
http://www.trickcyclists.co.uk

Index

B

C

E

I

M

N

O

P

U

V

Commissioning Editor: Michael Parkinson
Development Editor: Ailsa Laing
Project Manager: Frances Affleck
Designer: Erik Bigland

WM 18·2 MIC

1500 Questions in Psychiatry
for the MRCPsych

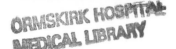